Studies in American Sociology
under the
General Editorship
of
Stanford M. Lyman

Volume VI

ROADS TO DYSTOPIA

Sociological Essays on the Postmodern Condition

Stanford M. Lyman

Manufactured in the United States of America

05 04 03 02 01 5 4 3 2 1

Designed by Ellen Beeler

♾ The paper used in this publication meets the minimum requirements of the American National Standard for Permanence of Paper for Printed Library Materials Z39.48–1984.

Library of Congress Cataloging-in-Publication Data

Lyman, Stanford M.
Roads to dystopia : sociological essays on the postmodern condition / Stanford M. Lyman.
p. cm. — (Studies in american sociology ; v. 6)
Includes bibliographical references and index.
ISBN 1-55728-711-2 (cloth : alk. paper)
1. Postmodernism—Social aspects. 2. Sociology. 3. Social problems. I. Title. II. Series.
HM449 .L94 2001
301—dc21

2001001999

To Arthur J. Vidich,
colleague, critic, friend

Let me recall: the overwhelming preponderance of collectivity with its scientific, technological and economic machinery, the increasing incapacity of individual consciousness to cope with the abstract anarchy of its environment, and its surrender to the collective consciousness that operates anonymously and dispersedly in our social and intellectual institutions—all this has shifted the center of gravity of our world from existential to functional, instrumental, and mechanical ways of life. At the same time, the hypertrophy of rationalization has produced an overcompensating irrationality, reversing to the bodily concrete or spiraling to the absurd.

—ERICH KAHLER, *Out of the Labyrinth: Essays in Clarification*

Acknowledgments

Most of the essays in this book were presented at various round tables, academic conventions, lectures, colloquia, and meetings of professional associations and have been published in assorted journals and publications:

"Gunnar Myrdal's *An American Dilemma* after a Half Century: Critics and Anticritics," presented in Montreal, July 26–July 28, 1998, at the World Congress of Sociology that included a session on Gunnar Myrdal and the Chicago School, published in the *International Journal of Politics, Culture and Society* 12:2 (winter 1998): 327–89. Reprinted by permission of Kluwer Academic/Human Sciences Press.

"The 'Yellow Peril' Mystique: Origins and Vicissitudes of a Racist Discourse," presented at a session of the American Sociological Association's annual meeting in Washington, D.C., August 12–August 16, 2000, published in the *International Journal of Politics, Culture and Society* 13:4 (summer 2000): 683–747. Reprinted by permission of Kluwer Academic/Human Sciences Press.

"The Chinese Question and America's Labor Historians: A Wrong Turn in a Quest for a Usable Past," presented at a session of the Ethnic Studies Program (Florida Atlantic University-Boca Raton campus), February 28, 2000, and at a "Workplace Topics Forum" cosponsored by the Center for Labor Research and Studies, the Department of History, and the Asian Studies Program at Florida International University, on March 3, 2000, published as "The Chinese Question and America's Labor Historians" in *New Politics* 7:4 (new series) Whole #28 (winter 2000): 113–48, plus the reference notes that appeared in the *New Politics* web site: *www.Wilpaterson.edu/~newpol/issue28/lyman28.htm* Reprinted by permission of New Politics.

"The Lost Tribes of Israel as a Problem in History and Sociology," presented at the annual meeting of the International Committee on Social Structures and Institutions at the Inter-University Centre, Dubrovnik, Croatia, May 4–May 9, 1998, published in the *International Journal of Politics, Culture and Society* 12:1 (fall 1998): 7–42. Reprinted by permission of Kluwer Academic/Human Sciences Press.

"Postmodernism and the Construction of Ethnocultural Identity: The Jewish-Indian Theory and the Lost Tribes of Israel," presented at the twenty-second annual meeting of the Mid-South Sociological Association, Little Rock, Arkansas, October 30–November 2, 1996, and delivered as the Symposium Keynote Address to the Department of Sociology, Anthropology and Social Work at Middle Tennessee State University on the occasion of its fifth annual Tennessee Undergraduate Social Science Symposium, November 13–November 17, 1996, published in *Sociological Spectrum* 17:3 (July–September 1997): 259–82. Reprinted by permission of Taylor and Francis, publishers.

"Dramas, Narratives, and the Postmodern Challenge," presented at the conference on "Sociological Aspects of Literature," New York City, April 28–April 29, 1995, published in *Alfred Schutz's "Sociological Aspect of Literature": Construction and Complementary Essays,* ed. Lester Embree (Dordrecht/Boston/London: Kluwer Academic Publishers, 1998), pp. 197–218. Reprinted by permission of Kluwer Academic Publishers.

"Cinematic Ideologies and Societal Dystopias: Filmmaking in the United States, Japan, Germany, and the Soviet Union, 1900–1996," published in the *International Journal of Politics, Culture and Society* 10:3 (spring 1997): 497–542. Reprinted by permission of Kluwer Academic/Human Sciences Press.

"Community: A Theoretical Perspective on Its Dilemmas, Contradictions, and Possible Future," presented at the Reubin O'D. Askew Institute on Politics and Society, first annual conference of the Florida Institute of Government, Gainesville, Florida, November 9–November 11, 1995, published in *Amid Political, Cultural and Civic Diversity: Building a Statewide Community in Florida,* ed. Lance deHaven-Smith and David Colburn (Dubuque, Iowa: Kendall/Hunt Publishing Company, 1998), pp. 247–84. Reprinted by permission of Kendall/Hunt Publishing Company.

Over the course of years of study and reflection I have benefited from the lectures, writings, and personal communication of teachers, colleagues, students, and friends. I am especially indebted for how much I have learned from Gary Abraham, Patti Adler, Peter Adler, David Altheide, the late Herbert Blumer, Alan Berger, Richard Harvey Brown, Tony Carnes, the late Horace Cayton, Randall Collins, Ying-jen Chang, Donna Darden, Yen LeEspiritu, Arthur Evans Jr., Franco Ferrarotti, Gary Alan Fine, the late Erving Goffman, Cecil Greek, Rom Harré, Herbert Hill, Roscoe Hinkle, Gisela Hinkle, the late Nat Huggins, Michael Hughey, Monica Humer, Robert Jackall, Gary Jaworski,

John M. Johnson, Tetsuden Kashima, Joseph Kotarba, Peter Kwong, Him Mark Lai, Paul Leslie, James Liu, Mary Lydon, David Maines, Peter K. Manning, E. Doyle McCarthy, Pyong Gap Min, Guy Oakes, Gary Okihiro, Virginia Olesen, Michael Omi, Tudor Parfitt, Robert Prus, Marvin B. Scott, Emanuela Trevisan Semi, Dmitri Shalin, Alvin Y. So, the late Hans Speier, John Kuo Wei Tchen, Stephen Park Turner, Arthur J. Vidich, Jacqueline Wiseman, and Morrison Wong. Special words of thanks are owed to Harvard Lyman for supplying me with articles about and an understanding of DNA, to Princeton Lyman for catching and correcting an error in one of my endnotes, and to Sylvia Lyman for her support and encouragement of this project.

Funded in part by the work-study program at Florida Atlantic University, my student research assistants Stanley Tang, Connie Tang, Ceecee Tang, Eiji Murai, and James McCluskie have rendered yeoman service as hunters and gatherers of materials. The word-processing of this manuscript has been carried out by Charlotte Steinberg to whom I owe much not only for deciphering the scribblings made by my premodern word processor, a pencil, but also for retyping disks that had eroded, and contributing several stylistic improvements. The index has been prepared by John Huckle. Larry Malley and his staff of editors have once again served this series with acuity in proofreading, excellence in manuscript styling, and the quality in artistic design that a scholarly work deserves. For all errors, I take full responsibility.

Stanford M. Lyman
Boca Raton, Florida
October 2000

Contents

PART I

Introduction

Introduction

> The innermost structure of the mentality of a group can never be as clearly grasped as when we attempt to understand its conceptions of time in the light of its hopes, yearnings, and purposes.
>
> —KARL MANNHEIM, *Ideology and Utopia*

> What we are witnessing . . . is a sort of interregnum, a moment between myths when the old versions of the past are either redundant or unacceptable, and new ones have yet to surface.
>
> —TONY JUDT, "The Past Is Another Country: Myth and Memory in Postwar Europe"

The Postmodern Turn

As the twentieth century closes and the still clouded vistas of the twenty-first century begin to appear before our eyes, we, the inhabitants of something far less consolidated than the much-vaunted "global village," are reminded of William Graham Sumner's mordant view of the *fin de siècle* of the previous century: "We are like spectators at a great national convulsion . . . The mores which once were are a memory. Those which any one thinks ought to be are a dream."[1] In the United States there were numerous reactions to this and any other less than sanguine outlook on America's and the Occident's future: An "age of reform,"[2] accompanied by the preaching of a "social gospel,"[3] a variety of ideologically driven social movements,[4] and programs and politics of governmental intervention, offering a "new deal," a "fair deal," a rebirth of "Camelot," a "war on poverty," a "thousand points of light," an end to the "Cold War," and a provision for a "peace dividend," delivered promissory notes for a brighter future.[5] If the social problems toward which these notes had been written proved recalcitrant, Americans could fall back on what Richard Hofstadter calls the country's vulnerability to a "paranoid style"[6] of believing, explaining, and acting—that is, insisting that the actions taken by members of hostile conspiracies directed against the nation, its culture, morals, and ways of life, and carried out by immigrants (Asiatics, Jews, southern and eastern Europeans), or bearers of alien ideologies (anarchists, syndicalists, communists, fascists, illuminati) are subverting progress and undermining the nation's future.

Wracked by what are now called "culture wars," Americans of the current *fin de siècle* are, to use Todd Gitlin's words, living in the twilight time of their once common but now shattered dreams.[7] Caught between rebellion and repentance,[8] the central structures of the long dominant ethos of pragmatism[9] seem to be coming apart. The nostrums of mainstream sociology—the optimism of George Lundberg's affirmative answer to his own question, "Can science save us?";[10] the stability in the midst of change that Parsonsian structural-functionalism had offered[11]—had shown themselves to be less than effective two decades before the century ended. Thus chastened, the historian of the age of reform, gloomily concluded on a Yeatsian note: "The nation seems to slouch onward into its uncertain future like some inarticulate beast, too much attainted by wounds and ailments to be robust, but too strong and resourceful to succumb."[12] All that was once solid, as Marshall Berman—echoing Marx—put it, had "melt[ed] into air."[13]

The end of the Second World War in 1945, was, as Modris Eksteins points out, the "center of our century and [of] our meaning." He continues:

> Our historical sense is derived . . . from two directions: from the buildup that were the events of the pre-1945 past, with its inherent notions of agency and cause, and from the confusions of our own end-of-century, end-of-millennium present, with its immediacy and contradiction.

And then he concludes, "We arrive, on the one hand, from a prior imperial age whose gist was coherence, and on the other hand, from a postcolonial present whose logic is fragment."[14] It is no wonder, then, that the present millennial moment is conceptualized as one "in between" another, as one whose condition can only be designated as *post*-modernity, with no name for the age and situation that will follow.[15] It is a moment in a time-out-of-time, whose appropriate mode of self-expression can only be, as Eksteins tells us, "a pastiche of styles, an assemblage of fragments, . . . a mélange of memory, reflection, and narrative."[16] It is one, so it is alleged, wherein the traditional humanistic and social disciplines do not apply. Nevertheless, it is also a moment that combines enlightenment (but not necessarily *The Enlightenment*)[17] with despair,[18] critique with hope.[19]

Perhaps no discipline has been more affected by the alleged failures of social science to deliver on its original promise than sociology. Recognizing that a condition of postmodernity has come to pass—that is, a condition wherein old social issues have not only not been resolved but also taken on new definitions and concomitants, while a rising set of technological innovations, cybernetic advancements, and globalizing processes has catalyzed the emergence of new forms of social and political power[20]—sociologists have begun to reexamine and critically appraise their own discipline. Their commentaries and conclusions, however, diverge so much from one another that they serve more to illustrate the epistemological crisis introduced by postmodernity[21] than to formulate a new social science of and for society. Thus, Alan Wolfe has asserted that practitioners of the discipline that once considered itself to be "the queen of the sciences" have been so chastened that "sociologists are no longer certain they have anything to offer the world."[22] Less pessimistic but still skeptical, Barry Smart, while admiring Zygmunt Bauman's proposal for a sociology that would "try to promote forms of autonomy and solidarity through a postmodern strategy that 'refers to values rather than laws; to assumptions instead of foundations; to purposes and not to groundings,'"[23] nevertheless points out that "the implications . . . of a post-modern shift from an 'onto-epistemological' . . . to a 'value-theoretical'[24] tradition have as yet to be fully explored."[25] Charles Lemert, who holds that *Postmodernism Is Not What You Think,*[26] argues that "social theories of the postmodern are interpretations of that world, the reality (or hyperreality) of which is much more in the experience of living than thinking";[27] hence, he calls for living "a sociological life," one that would entail "the courage to accept what we cannot change in order to do what can de done about the rest."[28] But, how, in light of postmodernism's disprivileging of all discourses,[29] sociologists would be able to distinguish the immobile from the dynamic phenomena of the postmodern world worries Alan Sica, who, after looking over the ideas of several contemporary social theorists, notices that "missing from all this [epistemological discussion] is the self-confidence of theory 50 years ago, the certainty then entertained about the salutary relations among theorizing, social research, and the creation of an improved social sphere . . . The slippery slope on which theorists now must pitch their tents have very little in common with the 'strong empirical foundations' that *seemed* reasonably attainable to earlier generations. It is, alas, a good time to theorize—for those who are warmed by the uncertain and entropic."[30] And, to go one step further toward the abyss of unknowing, it is worth noticing that at one point in his many writings lamenting the postmodern condition and expressing doubt about the very possibility of knowledge under its epistemological regime,[31] Jean-Francois Lyotard (1924–1998) offered what seems to be a counsel of utter despair: "In a world in which success means saving time, thinking has only one disadvantage, but it is an irredeemable disadvantage: it makes you waste time."[32] Thus does postmodernist thought, as Chris Jenks, one of its more astute critics, charges, subvert not only the cognitive underpinnings of the social sciences, but also foreclose on the very possibility of knowledge itself: "Postmodernism does not proffer alternative ways of knowing from whence we might appropriately confront and appreciate the 'new,' but instead it insinuates into all discourse, through a continuous scything at the knees of existing epistemologies, a sustained reduction and depotentiation of explanations that is premised upon the wholly unprivileged quality of all discourses."[33] With all this, one is virtually compelled to acknowledge the point made by Jeffrey C. Alexander, who, after examining how in the past one hundred years both Occidental thought and Western institutions have become trapped "between progress and apocalypse," concludes that "a taut dialogue between pessimism and optimism, reason and unreason, defines social theory in the twentieth century."[34]

In what follows, I shall discuss what I regard as the elementary dynamics of certain social processes that, in the century just ended, moved from dreams of eudaemonic fulfillment to nightmares of *anomie*-laden dystopia.

Burdens of the Past, Promises of the Future: An American Dilemma

In 1988, Leslie Berlowitz observed that "since the nineteenth century the struggle over identity and origins has distinguished the political and cultural life of all major nations," but went on to point out that this "potentially dangerous struggle has been especially problematic for Americans, who . . . often responded to [a] 'fear' of pastlessness by making rigid assertions about the founding myths and symbols and by insisting upon the constancy of certain values which, they have argued, constitute the moral core of America."[35] Among these myths, and likely at their core, is the belief that the American people are and will continue to be a *nation.* However, how to make a single peoplehood—if, indeed, that is what a nation is supposed to be[36]—out of the many races, subnations, ethnic groups, religious believers, and freethinkers who have and continue to populate the United States has been a challenge from the time of America's first years of postcolonial independence.[37]

In the first chapter of this book, I explore the fate of ideas and proposals contained in Gunnar Myrdal's *An American Dilemma,*[38] perhaps the single most important study of the race problem in the United States. A pithy commentary on what has resulted from that then so promising investigation is Charles Lemert's gloomy observation, "Race is no less an 'obsession' today than it was in the 1940s when Myrdal wrote *An American Dilemma,* or at the turn of the century when Du Bois declared the color line the problem of the 20th century, or in 1835 when Tocqueville declared race 'America's most formidable evil threatening its future.'"[39] For most postmodernists, however, it is the Enlightenment that is held responsible for the persistence of America's and the Occident's race problem. However, that is not the position I hold—

for justice, the rule of reason, and modernist ideas of equality, all elements of the Enlightenment's legacy,[40] ought not be jettisoned so quickly from the epistemological, juridical, and praxiological approaches still being or yet to be applied in order to solve that problem. As Todd Gitlin points out—and, on this point, my position is the same as his—"[T]he Enlightenment is best understood as an aspiration, an invitation, a commitment to a process that seriously aims to bring about understandings that do not yet exist."[41]

American Orientalism

Like most investigations of the race problem in America, Myrdal focused his study on the relations between blacks and whites. However, as one of the members of President Clinton's Advisory Board on his Initiative on Race would explain to her colleagues in July 1997, it would be necessary for both social research and public policy to move beyond the "dualistic approach that American society has become comfortable with" if the tripling of the Asian Pacific American population in the next several decades is properly recognized as likely to "re-shape human relations and race relations in dramatic ways."[42]

In chapters 2 and 3, I address one aspect of this issue—the belief that the peoples of Asia constitute a threat to the national, economic, cultural, and moral security of the Occident in general and the United States in particular. Despite the changing situations and the more varied ethnic composition of the peoplehood now classified as "Asian and Pacific Americans,"[43] there remains a deeply embedded prejudice—summed up in the term *yellow peril*[44]—against those so designated. The existence and expressions of such primordial ties as culture, territory, and language are conceived all too often by non-Asians as signs of a failure to assimilate,[45] or, more insidiously, as warnings of a subversive intention on the part of Chinese, Japanese,[46] or—more recently, but with less intensity than that which responded to the original Asian migrants—of Korean, Vietnamese, Hmong, and other Asian Pacific peoples.[47]

While advocates of multiculturalism call for revisions in the histories and cultures of Asian Pacific Americans,[48] challenge the assertion that assimilation must be the only acceptable outcome of immigration,[49] and support the "blended race" offspring of interracial and interethnic marriages in their claim to choose their own ethnoracial identity,[50] certain labor historians—to one of whom's work chapter 3 of the present book is devoted[51]—are seeking, on the one hand, to absolve members of the nineteenth-century white working class of much of the culpability for the shabby treatment inflicted on Asian immigrants (e.g., exclusion from emigrating to the United States, denial of the opportunity to apply for American citizenship, and debarment from labor union membership), and, on the other, suggesting that interracial class solidarity in fact did triumph over racism.[52] Unfortunately, for those who believe that an about-to-be-revived color blind orientation will soon relieve Americans of their multifaceted race problems, the facts of America's past labor history and the privileges still associated with what David Roediger calls the "wages of whiteness,"[53] suggest otherwise. Furthermore, a solidarity arising out of technological breakthroughs in this computer age is not likely to culminate in a class-based global village. As Jerry Kang observes in his path-breaking essay on the possibilities opened up by the current cybernetic revolution: "Race continues to be a fundamental axis of social, economic, cultural, and political organization . . . affect[ing] both the symbolic and material realms of our lives, shaping our self-conceptions and altering our life-chances . . . We should not presume that by logging into cyberspace, we enter some digital promised land that deletes centuries of racial conflict or downloads into our brains an antiracist patch that encodes us all to 'get along.'"[54]

The special character of America's "yellow peril" imagery of Asians is that it has engrafted a species of "Orientalism"[55] on to the American dilemma, a species that cannot be eradicated by the ordinary mechanisms of policy-making. For, as Neil Gotanda has pointed out, "Critique and criticism of stereotypes in popular culture are an insufficient basis for [the instauration] of an anti-Orientalist politics."[56] The threat of an insidious yellow peril is deeply embedded in American political, cultural, and social institutions. "We need," Robert G. Lee observes, "to understand the [ideas attached to the American picture of the] Oriental as a complex field of racial representation . . . , [one that] contains multiple, contradictory images and stereotypes."[57] In chapters 2 and 3 I offer a history and critical analysis of this imagery showing it to be a singular aspect of a complex racial ideology. Grasping the character of this ideology provides a deeper understanding of race as a social practice and, perhaps, gives us a tool for dismantling it. As the millennium dawns, however, the prospects for the forging of this tool are not bright.

A Jewish Question

Postmodernity is a retreat into the present, Keith Tester has noted. But as such it "is a milieu which is not so much without history, . . . [as it is one] which deliberately refuses to accept the perceived requirements of linear time."[58] One development that has challenged the modernist ideologies of progress and their attendant epistemologies[59] directly and empirically is the revival of the quest for—and the claim of the discovery of—remnants of the "lost tribes of Israel." Chapters 4 and 5 investigate this matter; for if, as Dorothy Ross has argued, "the global theories of progress and the analytical theories of structure and process . . . have been employed to stabilize the uncertainties of modern history,"[60] the designation of certain contemporary peoples as descendants of the ten tribes expelled from the Northern Kingdom of Israel in 722 B.C.E. punctures a deep fissure in the equilibrium that conventional history and accepted modes of historiography provide. A premodern event could be understood in postmodern terms.

The problematic introduced by the recent resurfacing of the ten lost tribes—when, between the last week of November 1984 and the first week of January 1985, a joint but secret plan, called "Operation Moses," put together by special operatives from the United States, Sudan, and the State of Israel, flew five thousand of the so-called Falasha Jews from Ethiopia to Israel (their right to enter and be awarded instant citizenship under the latter country's "Law of Return" having been secured when the Sephardi Chief Rabbi of Israel, Ovadia Yosef, declared that the Falasha are descendants of the lost tribe of Dan and hence are "Jews who must be saved from absorption and assimilation")[61] —is that of a disruptive "intrusion"[62] on both sacred and secular thought. While secular scholars, Jewish and gentile, had dismissed the likelihood that there could still exist findable descendants of the tribes expelled from Israel twenty-seven hundred years earlier, religious Jews as well as evangelical Christians would not abandon a prophetic tradition that entailed an eschatological apocalypse: The biblical prophets, "unwilling to accept the finality of exile and assimilation, [had] kept alive the hope that the Ten Tribes continued to exist . . . [Thus, the] prophetic promises of return . . . inspired a messianic quest which persisted for centuries: . . . [so that] the final redemption might be expedited."[63] The pious of both orthodox Judaism and evangelical Christianity insisted that there would some day in the future come a rediscovery and an ingathering of the lost tribes, who would thereby be reunited with the Judean brethren from whom they had so long been separated. And, with that penultimate event, a Christian chiliastic and a Jewish messianic age would be imminent.

Without warning, claims of a discovery of the lost tribes of Israel have not only intruded upon annalists but also added unexpected issues for policy-makers. It all began when, in 883 C.E., Eldad the Danite, a traveler to north and east Africa and its environs, informed his coreligionists in Spain that he had obtained definite knowledge of the locations of all ten of the erstwhile Israelite tribes: Issachar, Zebulon, Reuben, Ephraim, both halves of the tribe of Menasseh, Simeon, Dan, Naphtali, Gad, and Asher.[64] Said to be living somewhere beyond the mystical Sambatyon River, the lost tribes would figure in occasional reports of sightings or intelligence during the next eight centuries,[65] their most significant role occurring in the age of European expansion and the confrontations of both Judaism and Western Christendom with Islam.

The puzzle introduced into the Occident's ethnological ideas about human origins by Columbus's encounter with dark-skinned peoples inhabiting what soon proved to be a double-continent separated from both Europe and Asia by two oceans, led more than one cosmologist to designate the newly named "Indians" as descendants of ancient Israel's lost tribes.[66] Not only might such a conjectural imputation resolve their presence in the Americas with what was the then accepted Bible-based Noachian flood ethnology,[67] but also it could be used in support of secular political and cultural aims. Thus, what is now called the "Jewish-Indian theory" was employed from 1649 to 1659 by Amsterdam's Rabbi Menasseh ben Israel in an only partially successful attempt to persuade Oliver Cromwell to revoke a royal edict that had prohibited Jewish settlement in the British Isles since 1290;[68] by England's James Adair, in 1775, to propose an Anglo-Indian alliance that would not only rescue these newly found Jews from the terrors of the Spanish inquisition, but also wrest Florida from Spain;[69] by one of early America's most energetic evangelists, Elias Boudinot, in 1816, to urge the speedy conversion of the Cherokees, Creeks, and neighboring tribes as a prelude to returning them to their ancestral home, Palestine;[70] and by the Tammany Hall leader, Mordecai Noah, in 1825, who, in order to counter the missionary endeavors being carried out by Boudinot's followers, invited the American Indians, whose ancient Israelite ancestry he would proclaim until his dying day, to settle in "Ararat," the Jewish "homeland" that he founded in that year on Grand Island, New York.[71]

In 1945, in the immediate aftermath of the horrors of the Holocaust, Erich Kahler took note of what seemed to be a peculiar feature characterizing the whole of Jewish history, namely, "the magnitude of the demands which their God, or their destiny, or their aspiration, whatever we may call it, has made upon them."[72] To these imperatives one must now include the euphoric and utopic promises and the not infrequent dysdaemonic and perhaps dystopic outcomes that have occurred and continue to occur as Occidental Jewry confronts and is confronted by the claims of, or for the descendants of, their once-lost-and-now-allegedly-found tribal brethren.[73] Thus, to give one less than sanguine reaction, although, or perhaps, precisely because he had come to believe "that all the inhabitants of the Indies are the descendants of the Jews," the mid-sixteenth-century bishop Diego de Landa ordered the Spanish soldiers under his command to burn as many of the seemingly Hebraic Mayan bark-cloth books as they could find, thus destroying what might have been evidence of an ancient Israelite presence in the Americas.[74] Among the seventeenth-, eighteenth-, and early nineteenth-century missionaries and explorers, those who disliked the greed and covetousness that they thought they perceived in the American aborigines attributed such insalubrious traits to the latter's Jewish origins; while others thought the Indians too noble in their magnificent savagery to be avaricious and mendacious Israelites; and still others supposed that the "redmen" might be the accursed spawn of Ham's son Canaan, and thus unredeemable.[75] Nor did any of the liberationist usages of the "Jewish-Indian" theory prove efficacious: England's anti-Jewish immigration policy was only partially undone by Menasseh ben Israel's mission to Cromwell, and not solely in response to the Amsterdam Rabbi's adroit usage of lost tribe eschatology; Adair's proposal that England ally with and arm Florida's "Jewish" Indians and undertake an imperial war against Spain was not accepted; Boudinot's followers' evangelization missions among the southeastern America's tribalized "Israelites" did not bring a halt to the "trail of tears" along which the Cherokee exiles from Georgia were driven to their dismal reservation existence in Oklahoma; Mordecai Noah's refuge for both the American Indian "lost tribes" and the rest of the Jews in diaspora had to be abandoned for lack of funds. Native Americans of the present era do not believe they have an Israelite heritage, and they do not seek a redemptive *aliyah* to the State of Israel.

Nor have the recent claims to lost tribe ancestry by several dark-skinned postcolonial peoples been met with widespread joyous acceptance from all elements of Occidental Jewry or with ready incorporation into the State of Israel. The erstwhile "Falasha," now called "Beta Israel," some twenty thousand of whom have been admitted to Israel under its Law of Return and declared to be descendants of the lost tribe of Dan, were housed in trailer camps and, later, ghettos, and required to go through a symbolic conversion ceremony. Employed primarily as menials, their children were compelled to go to religious or away-from-home boarding schools, but perhaps most disheartening, their freely donated blood was discarded as a cautionary preventive against AIDS.[76] To the present day, their brethren still in Ethiopia are classified as "Falas Mora" and denied admission to Israel,[77] while the land that was once the biblical Kingdom of Israel from which they are allegedly descended, is scheduled to become part of a yet-to-be-established Palestinian state.[78] Not presently a "land of milk and honey," Israel has yet to ensure its promise of ingathering dispersed Jewry. The condition and future of the Ethiopian Jews[79] add a postmodern dimension to the age-old question, what does it mean to be a Jew? "As Jewish identity is refracted through the prism of Beta Israel's experience," Hagar Salamon has observed, "Judaism will continue to reveal itself in a dynamic and not always coherent fashion, joining competing voices and engaged in multiple and changing dialogues."[80]

One less than coherent factor of this new aspect of the "Jewish Question" finds a situs in the recent introduction of genetic science into the unresolved ethnoreligious identity of the Lemba, a people living in Zimbabwe, Mozambique, and other parts of southern Africa, whose claims of ancient Judean or Israelite ancestry have been contested by the authorities in Israel. That people's situation has become an unintended feature of the identity politics that characterize what might be called the current postzionist as well as postmodernist phase of Jewish history.[81] On the one hand, bringing finis to the status of "otherhoodedness," the condition par excellence from which postmodernist perspective seeks liberation, requires an unstinting critique of the dolorous effects that biologic theories of group identity have wrought;[82] on the other hand, the new possibilities for uncovering both personal and collective ancestry provided by recent advances in DNA research threaten to turn the construction of ethnocultural origins into a global natural science.[83] In the case of the Lemba, many of whom profess Christianity but insist on proclaiming their genetic and ethnocultural Jewishness, DNA studies have shown that a statistically significant number of men in one of its lineage segments carry the Y chromosome with the "*cohen*" signature, evidence of ancient Hebraic ancestry.[84] Adherents to the two eschatologies—one Christian-evangelical, the other Jewish-messianic—are now confronted by the imperatives of a genetic determinant that, if accepted by those empowered to answer the question, *who is a Jew?,* could seriously affect individual choice, faith-based religiosity, and conversion-oriented endeavors. Those more secular persons who look forward to an inner-worldly utopia wherein Jewish identity has become "banalized"[85] —that is, when Jews are neither pilloried for being "killers of Christ," "ugly and smelly," "uncivilized and wicked," "degenerate," "feminine, hysterical and mad," nor praised for being "witty," "emotional," "clever and modern," nor provoked by dint of being "alienated," "capitalistic," or "socialist revolutionaries" —what Juliet Steyn calls the "all-too-familiar catalogue that passes from the ideological to the museological—the detritus of the death camps"[86]—are, even if the "museological fate" is not repeated, not likely to realize their dream in the DNA-determined world that is now emerging. A genetic component bids fair to become a significant aspect of the "map of meaning"[87] that is given to the peoples scattered over the globe, a new biocultural feature of the postmodern "geography of identity."[88]

Dramas and Cinemas of Dystopia

In "Social Reality as Theater: Dramas, Narratives, and the Postmodern Challenge," I array features of the *condition* of postmodernity against the *epistemologies* of postmodernist thought. Whereas the former describes a *Lebenswelt* that meets many of the requirements of a dismal dystopia desperately in need of deliverance, the latter all too often denies the dispossessed subalterns the agency that is needed to deliver them.[89] Thus, to give one example that here will stand in for many others, Charlene Spretnak points out that what she calls "deconstructive-postmodern aesthetics regards the world . . . [as] a repressive labyrinth of 'social production,' a construction of pseudoselves who are pushed and pulled by cultural dynamics and subtly diffused 'regimes of power' . . . [a world wherein values] and ethics are deemed arbitrary, . . . [and] 'history' . . . viewed as one group or another's self-serving selection of facts."[90] It is not that such a description of the real world is necessarily wrong, rather that it mistakes the topic for investigation for the resource needed to conduct that investigation.[91] Just as the structural-functional followers of Talcott Parsons assume the existence of a societal social system motored by an equilibrium-seeking entelechy, so the postmodernists believe that the once-proud and powerful system that he described has crumbled under the weight of events and processes that it could not absorb. But these are matters that need to be proved, not presumed. As a remedy, I propose borrowing concepts and insights from Kenneth Burke, Erving Goffman, and Alfred Schutz to formulate both an epistemology and a method of research so that one might enter the world armed with open-ended conceptualizations of agents and agency, space and territory, scenes and scenarios, time and duree, character and personification.[92] What is "out there" is to be discovered in and through the individual and collective actions and sentiments of people.[93] Whether spectators at a great abyss, as Sumner believed, or participant observers in revolts or revolutions,[94] theatrical or mundane scenes of everyday life,[95] or dramas of the routine,[96] our epistemology is and ought to be dramaturgy. Theirs, that is, the people, each of whom is a *socius,* is to perform, to act and be acted upon, to be a subject and a subaltern, to be empowered and subordinated as *virtu* and authority provide shifting scenarios of a sometimes free but usually constrained existence.[97]

Popular culture, but more especially cinematic drama, occupies a "thirdspace" (to borrow Edward W. Soja's wonderfully sensitizing concept)[98] in the representational geography of modern and postmodern human affairs. The shapes and scenes on the movie screen depict real or imagined persons and ways of life, perhaps, as Herbert Blumer noticed so many years ago, also undermining localized mores while they reaffirm deeply embedded values.[99] Among cinema's value-laden themes are political ideologies that one cineaste defines as "integrated assertions, theories and aims that constitute a governmental policy,"[100] but that are in fact broader in scope and reach to the sometimes unarticulated hopes and dreams of peoples in quest of a more promising future, often enough of a utopia.

In chapter 7, I trace out ideological trajectories in the films of four modern societies—the United States, Japan, Germany, and the Soviet Union. I argue that, however the utopic dream was cinematically imagined—as a problem-solving, world-saving American Protestant endeavor, as a fascist dream of establishing a globally expanding land of *Übermenschen,* as a domestic response to Japan's defeated hope for a "Great Eastern Cooperative commonwealth of Asian nations," or as a communist wonderland of abundant, productive, and liberated proletarian joyousness—it ended in denial, escapism, or economic disillusion.

Although the year 2001 opens the way to a new millennium, America's cinema is continuing down the fateful path already established. The family, a Hollywood casualty of dysfunction for two decades—that is, since *Kramer vs. Kramer* (1979) and *Ordinary People* (1980) laid out its utter failure as a nurturing institution,[101] is sunk in a slough of despond—for example, *American Beauty* (1999), which, as Steve Vineberg observes, "regurgitates a long line of hollowly cynical portraits of our suburban life that present moral decrepitude as the natural inhabitant of well-off, WASP households, a poison that apparently creeps off the manicured lawns and hangs ominously in the moneyed air";[102] or *Virgin Suicides* (2000), that treats its five teen-age sisters' self-destroying depression as the basis for a melancholy black comedy, no other emotion being suitable for the utter hopelessness of adolescence. Nor are the nations of the world any more secure from ever-threatening assaults by their domestic, foreign, or extraterrestrial enemies than they were at the end of *Independence Day* (1997), the "date" on which a motley band of misfits managed to save what was left of the earth's human population from destruction by monstrous marauders from outer space. Films of the twenty-first century thus far seem more interested in looking back to those wars in which there were clearly defined enemies and an equally clearly defined band of nondeviant and heroic men to be America's defenders. Thus, the box office smash hit of April and May 2000 is *U-571,* a filmic recreation of a World War II mission in which an American submarine crew must board a German U-boat and capture a secret coding device. Such nostalgia for unblemished heroes speaks to the longing for an older heroic America and boldly contrasts with Hollywood's current crop of deviance-drenched dramas—for example, *28 Days,* in which a party girl (Sandra Bullock), who is also a successful New York City writer, achieves moral and medical redemption by spending a month at a court-ordered rehabilitation center; *Where the Heart Is,* in which a pregnant seventeen-year-old woman (Natalie Portman), abandoned by her boyfriend, gives birth in a chain store, achieves fulfillment with new friends, and finds that she has a useful talent that will support her; *High Fidelity,* in which a man (John Cusack), in a failing business who is also unable to build a relationship with a woman, revisits his former girlfriends in a quest to discover what went wrong in his many attempts at family life; *Keeping the Faith,* in which two longtime friends, one a sworn-to-celibacy Catholic priest (Edward Norton), the other an unmarried Jewish rabbi (Ben Stiller), become romantically involved with a gentile woman (Jenna Elfman) who is forbidden fruit for each; *American Psycho,* in which a high-fashion, self-obsessed Wall Street broker (Christian Bale) goes on a brutal, misogynistic killing spree while his colleagues, utterly soulless representatives of the new high-tech capitalism, remain studiously indifferent. Unable to find soulful solace or satisfying security among his living contemporaries, and longing for the loving parents he knew as a child, one cinematic hero of the year 2000 (Jim Caviezel) employs the wonderful accident of a freak sunspot phenomenon to reach back in time, rescue his firefighter father from both a raging inferno and the deadly cancer that cigarette-smoking can cause, and to save his mother from death at the hands of a serial killer (*Frequency*), and thus to restore through the magic realism of the movies what the philosopher-sociologist Alfred Schutz had seen as death's barrier separating predecessors from their successors.[103]

And what hope does Hollywood hold out for us because of the advances in science and the triumphs of rational thought over superstition? Where once, as Sigmund Freud (1856–1939) put it, "We believe that it is possible, for scientific work to discover something about the reality of the world through which we can increase our power and according to which we can regulate our life,"[104] now, with the aid of what science has wrought and Hollywood's take on the matter, we are more likely to regard science as a thing gone mad, as a fateful illusion of modernist culture, and to hear—in place of the cool voice of a scientist's rational thought—the horrifying screams of his (un)reason. As David J. Skal points out, "In the twentieth century science has amply demonstrated its power to grind *Homo sapiens* into material insignificance while simultaneously offering transcendent fantasies of power and dominion."[105]

Continuing the Eclipse of Community

It has been more than forty years since Maurice R. Stein published *The Eclipse of Community,* documenting and critically appraising not only a half-century's social scientific work on the history, structures, and processes attendant on intimate human association, but also pointing out how those ties, so often celebrated as the *summum bonum* of human existence, are eroding.[106] Noting that "substantive values and traditional patterns are continually being discarded or elevated to fictional status whenever they threaten the pursuit of commodities or careers"; that community ties are becoming "increasingly dispensable"; and that those feelings and imperatives that once bound members of nuclear families to one another seem far less efficacious as "we are forced to watch children dispens[e] with their parents at an ever earlier age in suburbia," Stein pointed to two doleful effects: "On the one hand, individuals become increasingly dependent upon centralized authorities and agencies in all areas of life . . . , [and, on] the other, personal loyalties decrease their range with the successive weakening of national ties, family ties, and finally, ties to a coherent image of one's self."[107] Not much has happened to halt this erosion since Professor Stein gave it particular notice in 1960.

In chapter 8, I explore further dimensions of this sociocultural dynamic, tracing its intellectual origins through a close examination of the writing of Rousseau, Montesquieu, Ferdinand Toennies, John Dewey, and the Chicago School sociologists, the effects of postmodern thought, and my own critique of the new "communitarian" movement. Once closely associated with the adaptive strategies of new immigrant groups in America, the idea of community has not yet disappeared altogether. Indeed, its recent resurgence among many of America's ethnic groups speaks not only to a disillusion with the promises of a "melting pot" America—from which, according to utopian writers from J. Hector de Crevecoeur[108] to Israel Zangwill,[109] would emerge a wholly new set of persons—but also to the uninspiring new pluralist and multiculturalist movements—whose spokespersons sometimes fail to credit their ideational origin to Horace Kallen[110] and Randolph Bourne[111]—that are neither territorially based nor necessarily intimate in character. As Michael W. Hughey and Arthur J. Vidich observe, "Faced with the inability to give cultural content to Americanism and with the rootlessness and personal isolation that seems to be fostered by the very fabric of American life, the most primitive biological form of identification—that of descent—has been reasserted as a major basis for organizing the lives of all immigrant groups, regardless of how many generations they have resided in the United States."[112] Thus does disillusion find a semblance of sublimation in reaching into the primordial past as allusion—"a poetic dimension . . . created by the simultaneous presence of two different realities whose competition with one another produces a single more complex reality"[113]—a reality whose communitarian promise, like that of the once beckoning greensward of suburbia, is uncertain.

Beyond Dystopia: To Struggle Is All

The essays in this book speak to a burgeoning period of human existence that some believe is best described as "*post-histoire,*" defined by Henrik de Man as a moment in time when humankind gains unwanted "entry into a phase of world events that does not fit into history at all, because the otherwise historically verifiable connections between causes and effects are not forthcoming."[114] The great metanarratives heralded the coming of a utopia in which the problems that plague humankind would lose their intransigence before the ultimate will of God, the forces of history, or the capabilities of inspired human agency.[115] With Lyotard's "incredulity toward metanarratives"[116] bidding for the paramount place in social and political thought, the hope for these solutions dissolves into nothingness.

But we do not need to accept such a doleful conclusion. This book is offered to those who choose to resist the pessimistic fatalism of postmodernism, those who—chastened by Simmel's recognition that there can never be an utterly free-floating *life* without its attendant constraining *forms*[117]—nevertheless struggle on in its quest.

PART II

Legacies of the American Dilemma

CHAPTER ONE

Gunnar Myrdal's *An American Dilemma* after a Half Century

Critics and Anticritics

> [T]he United States is distinguished by an emphasis on adversarial relations among groups, and by intense, morally based conflicts about public policy, precisely because its people quarrel sharply about how to apply the basic principles of Americanism they purport to agree about.
>
> —SEYMOUR MARTIN LIPSET,
> *American Exceptionalism: A Double-Edged Sword*

Introduction

In 1944 Harper and Brothers published the most monumental sociological study of the black American to date—*An American Dilemma,* the fruits of a mammoth interdisciplinary research project carried out under the sponsorship of the Carnegie Corporation and the general guidance of the Swedish social scientist Gunnar Myrdal. Not since the comprehensive work by the distinguished (though largely forgotten) black historian George Washington Williams—*The History of the Negro in the United States,* published in 1883—had such a compendium of data been made available.[1]

In its 1,024 pages of text *An American Dilemma* includes sections on the nature of the black problem, population and migration, economics, politics, and justice; social inequality and social stratification; leadership and concerted action; and the black community. Moreover, the appendices contain theoretical discussions of the place of values in social science, general aspects of sociological methodology, and a brief discussion of the place of women in American society, which Myrdal saw as a parallel to the race problem. In no other single work will the student of race relations find so much information carefully compiled, clearly presented, and cogently organized.

Myrdal's great work not only offers a thoroughgoing critique of what approaches then existed in the minds of those U.S. sociologists concerned to understand and contribute to a solution to America's race problem, but also proposes a unique normative socio-psychological resolution of that problem. Myrdal's basic orientation is rooted in his thesis that the "American Creed," an ideal allegedly internalized by all Americans, is antithetical to, and will eventually triumph over, the race prejudices that so debilitate the nation:

> The "American Dilemma" . . . is the ever-raging conflict between on the one hand, the valuations preserved on the general plane which we call the "American Creed," where the American thinks, talks and acts under the influence of high national and Christian precepts, and, on the other hand, the valuations on specific planes of individual and group living, where personal and local interests; economic, social, and sexual jealousies; considerations of community prestige and conformity; group prejudice against particular persons or types of people; and all sorts of miscellaneous wants, impulses, and habits dominate his outlook.[2]

And Myrdal insisted on his main argument, namely, that "the American Negro problem is a problem in the heart of the American . . . The moral struggle goes on within people and not only between them . . . There are no homogeneous 'attitudes' behind human behavior but a mesh of struggling inclinations, interests, and ideals, some held conscious and some suppressed for long intervals but all active in bending behavior in their direction."[3] Despite his original distinction between the nonprejudicial valuation of the American Creed on the one hand, and the negrophobic valuations of individual and group living that take place in accordance with "personal and local interests" on the other, Myrdal held that "the Negro problem is an integral part of, or a special phase of, the whole complex of problems in the larger American civilization . . . There is no single side of the Negro problem—whether it be the Negro's political status, the education he gets, his place in the labor market, his cultural and personality traits, or anything else—which is not predominantly determined by its total American setting."[4]

The Swedish scholar admitted the difficulties under which he, an outsider, labored to comprehend and present to the American people an understandable vision of their perhaps most distressing problem. Speaking of himself in the third person, Myrdal observed, "He is under the pressure to state to himself what he thinks about this somewhat strange culture."[5] Moreover, he conceded that while his study was one carried out in terms of reason-based social science, "at least in the present stage of social research, it is next to impossible to judge rationally our most general assumptions concerning a civilization."[6] What he offered as the American dilemma, he concluded, is a "picture . . . that . . . faithfully represents what the author, upon careful consideration, believes to be true."[7] Nevertheless, near the end of his long (1898–1986) and productive life (he had been awarded the Nobel Prize in economics in 1974, the Swedish Academy believing his best efforts were to be found in *An American Dilemma, Asian Drama,* and *The Political Element in the Development of Economic Theory*),[8] Myrdal had begun work on a revision of *An American Dilemma.*[9] However, blindness and his final illness made supervising page proofs impossible.[10] At his request, the unpublished manuscript was to be placed with his other papers at the Arbetarrörelsens Arkiv in Stockholm. Our debt—and those of the critiques and anti-critiques—is to the first edition.

Even before his project had begun, and continuously since its publication, Myrdal's investigation of America's race problem has been fraught with controversy. His invitation to direct the study had come from Frederick Keppel, president of the Carnegie Corporation, a corporate foundation that had been established in 1911 as the institutional embodiment of its millionaire industrialist namesake's philanthropy.[11] That sponsorship aroused the scorn of Marxists,[12] especially after it became known that corporation president Keppel believed that in the United States "the race question was so 'charged with emotion' that no American scholar could be entrusted to provide the principal intellectual focus for such an inquiry."[13] Moreover, despite its supposedly close association with the early actions of the leaders of the civil rights movement, Myrdal and, even more, Ralph Bunche, his perhaps most valuable research associate on the project, were decidedly lukewarm about the efforts then being put forth by such organizations as the National Association for the Advancement of Colored People.[14] As for American contributions to scholarship on the race question, there is, in addition to Keppel's implied denigration of nearly a half century of studies on the issues entailed therein, Myrdal's own observations, especially as they are presented in "Appendix 2: A Methodological Note on Facts and Values,"[15] including his devastating critique of the perspectives of such luminaries of American social science as William Graham Sumner,[16] Robert E. Park,[17] W. I. Thomas,[18] William Fielding Ogburn,[19] Franklin H. Giddings,[20] and W. Lloyd Warner[21]—sociologists, that is, known in America not only for their prodigious scholarship but also for wide disagreements with one another on both substantive matters and methodological issues. But, while excepting Lester Ward, Simon Patten, Louis Wirth, John Dollard, and Robert MacIver[22] from his withering assault on what he characterized as "a do-nothing (*laissez-faire*) valuation of . . . [social] situations" (a perspective that he alleged was ubiquitous in the mainstream of American social science),[23] Myrdal went even further, virtually indicting the whole of Occidental scholarship for the same offense: "The tendencies criticized" [in

American social science], he wrote, "are, however, common in all social sciences in the entire Western world."[24] Opposed to the calls for a value-free social science, Myrdal asserted its opposite: "A 'disinterested social science' is . . . pure nonsense. It never existed. It never will exist. We can make our thinking strictly rational in spite of this, but only by facing the valuations, not by evading them."[25] However, Myrdal did more than face these valuations; his critics responded, sometimes negatively, to his own characterizations of American values and to the primacy he placed on them.

Critics Then and Now

In 1989, Gerald Jayne and Robin M. Williams Jr., writing as coeditors of the report by the National Research Council's Committee on the Status of Black Americans, observed, "We write 45 years after Gunnar Myrdal in *An American Dilemma* challenged Americans to bring their racial practices into line with their ideals. Despite clear evidence of progress against each problem, Americans face an unfinished agenda: many black Americans remain separated from the mainstream of national life under conditions of great inequality. The American dilemma has not been resolved."[26] Seven years later, in 1996, Reynolds Farley, recalling that in 1944 Myrdal had "described the deleterious consequences of racial residential segregation for blacks,"[27] went on to note, in support of the thesis advanced in a 1993 study conducted by Douglas Massey and Nancy Denton,[28] as well as on the basis of data from the United States Bureau of the Census, that "continuing apartheid is the strong backbone of the system of black-white stratification . . . , truncat[ing] educational and employment opportunities . . . , generat[ing] a ghetto culture that is dysfunctional in our achievement-oriented society . . . , [and] producing that tangle of pathology now known as the urban underclass."[29] One year later, John Hope Franklin, newly appointed chairman of the advisory board for President William J. Clinton's Initiative on Race and Reconciliation—perhaps echoing the cautious optimism of 1944, when Myrdal had closed *An American Dilemma* by enunciating his belief that "in the long run . . . the conservative white Southerner . . . can be won over to equalitarian reforms in line with the American Creed,"[30] and announcing that "America can demonstrate that justice, equality and cooperation are possible between white and colored people"[31]—observed about the work to be accomplished by his six-person panel, "I hope it will turn the corner for this nation once and for all with respect to the question of race . . . I don't mean it will all be solved by that time. But I hope it will have the significance of turning the corner so we can look back and say this was the decisive moment, this was the watershed."[32] However, turning that corner would involve bringing to resolution the divisive issues of affirmative action and multiculturalism—issues that have so divided the nation, its leaders, and its peoples that one can no longer speak of either a liberal or a conservative consensus on America's race problem.[33] These are issues that entail not only the eradication of unjust inequalities affecting persons of varying colors, cultures, and faiths, but, more significantly, the crafting of equality in a democratic state with an increasing and increasingly group-conscious sense of its multiracial and multiethnic composition.[34]

Researched and written before the modern court-and-legislation-oriented civil rights movement proved effective—and toward which Myrdal's study would contribute, most notably in the school desegregation cases[35]—Myrdal and his colleagues had had to face challenges quite different from those that would confront later advocates. The latter, unlike Myrdal and his co-workers, would be seeking to establish equality in the years after the worst features of America's government-supported racist practices had been nullified by the Supreme Court or obliterated by congressionally enacted civil rights guarantees.[36] It would prove hard enough for Myrdal and his supporters to confront the prevailing Jim Crow features of the South as well as the more subtle forms of racism in the North and West. At virtually every turn, Myrdal and his coworkers had had to contend with the "racial etiquette" that prevailed in the states of the former Confederacy.[37] Ralph Bunche (1904–1971), the future Nobel laureate who served as one of Myrdal's principal researchers,[38] and who in one instance as the only black American accompanying Myrdal and Arthur Raper through the South, had had to help the group depart "hurriedly from several explosive situations in Alabama and Georgia after whites took offense at their pointed questions about race issues . . . [T]he thought of a lynch mob crossed Bunche's mind on more than one occasion."[39] Charles S. Johnson (1893–1956), who, though ambivalent about some of Myrdal's interpretations, served in an advisory capacity to the latter's investigations, suffered throughout his life from the ambiguities entailed in his status and identity as a black sociologist and university president living in and forced to accommodate to the demeaning racial mores of the South.[40] It was just these mores that Myrdal and his colleagues hoped the American Creed would overcome.

The more radically inclined researchers employed by Myrdal, as well as those of a similar persuasion who critically appraised the book after it had been published, however, were suspicious of its sponsor's intent, opposed to its main thesis, and rejecting of its melioristic proposals. Thus, Bernhard J. Stern angrily complained to Richard Robbins that "Myrdal at first took a tough-minded conflict-power approach to the Negro problem but changed it to the 'softer' conception in accord with the moral values of the white middle class because of Carnegie Corporation sponsorship."[41] Like Stern, who had at one time been a consultant to Myrdal's group, Doxey A. Wilkerson, who had been one of Myrdal's researchers, objected to the excision of questions on interracial marriage from his survey and was chagrined to find that his findings, conclusions, and proposals on the limited role of education had also been excised from the final report.[42] In his introduction to Marxist historian Herbert Aptheker's booklet-length critique of *An American Dilemma,* Wilkerson reiterated his assault on the "long, gradual, never ending process of education" that was supposed to bring about an eradication of race prejudice from the hearts and minds of the American people. In place of such a thesis he asserted, "If there is anything which the history and contemporary life of America clearly reveal about the Negro question, it is the stark material, profit-seeking core from which all of the varied forms of anti-Negro discrimination and oppression emerge."[43] Aptheker (1915–) had concluded his own critique on an even more devastating note: "In summary," he wrote, "we find Myrdal's philosophy to be superficial and erroneous, his historiography demonstrably false, his ethics vicious and, therefore, his analysis weak, mystical, and dangerous."[44] Conceding that *An American Dilemma,* "[a]s a source of information and brilliant interpretation of information on race relations in the United States, . . . is probably unsurpassed," Marxist sociologist Oliver Cromwell Cox (1901–1974) argued that, at bottom, Myrdal had employed a "mystical" approach that vitiates any sound understanding of the dynamics of caste structures and their relation to racial hierarchies in America; that the study also fails to see the subtle and complex connections of race prejudice to class positioning; and, in fine, that Myrdal's study "contributes virtually nothing to a clarification of the many spurious social theories of race relations . . . , but, like the fatalists whom he criticizes, relies finally upon time as the great corrector of all evil."[45] The black radical tradition in America would take its point of departure from an altogether different outlook than that enunciated by Myrdal.[46] If to supporters of the status quo or accommodationist-oriented gradualists, Myrdal's ameliorative proposals seemed to be formulated to proceed too fast, to Marxists, as well as to other activist civil rights advocates, they appeared to move too slowly or not at all.[47]

Nor did the drive to secure the civil rights of African Americans enjoy the support of J. Edgar Hoover (1895–1972) during his directorship of the Federal Bureau of Investigation (FBI). Hoover's outlook appears to have turned on the extent to which he believed that alien ideologies and outside forces were influencing the attitudes and actions of America's black population. Thus, a quarter century before the publication of *An American Dilemma,* he had sent a memo to his special agent in New York City, suggesting that Universal Negro

Improvement Association founder, Marcus Garvey (1887–1940)—whom he called "one of the most prominent Negro agitators in New York; . . . an exceptionally fine orator, creating much excitement among the negroes . . . ; [in whose] paper the 'Negro World' the Soviet Union is upheld and there is open advocation of Bolshevism"—might be prosecuted for fraud with respect to his proposed steamship venture and then deported to his colony of origin, Jamaica.[48] With the United States at war from 1941 through 1945, at the very time that critical pressures from Northern liberals and progressives,[49] as well as from such mainstream sociologists as Robert E. Park (1864–1944),[50] were being put on the South's system of race segregation, and Myrdal and his researchers were conducting surveys and gathering all manner of data for *An American Dilemma,* "Hoover's distaste for foreign ideologies, particularly communism, guaranteed that blacks and the black press would be watched closely."[51] On August 15, 1942, the FBI's clandestine investigation of "Racial Conditions in the United States during World War II"—not made public until 1995—reported that, "For a period in excess of two years the Federal Bureau of Investigation has received reports and allegations of forces with foreign influences and with anti-American ideology working among the Negro people of the country as well as exploiting them."[52]

When the Montgomery bus boycott of 1955 threatened to undermine the urban South's tradition of segregated transportation, Hoover, in the spring of 1956, "sent President Eisenhower a series of reports detailing Communist influence in the civil rights movement. At the president's invitation, Hoover briefed the cabinet on the southern racial tradition, emphasizing the Communists' role in lobbying for civil rights."[53] Hoover would maintain his surveillance over African Americans, civil rights advocacy groups, and various nationalist, revolutionary, and militant movements among blacks for the balance of his tenure with the FBI. He targeted such organizations as the National Association for the Advancement of Colored People (NAACP), the Urban League (UL), the Congress of Racial Equality (CORE), the Southern Christian Leadership Conference (SCLC), the Student Non-violent Coordinating Committee (SNCC), the Black Panther Party, and the Nation of Islam ("Black Muslims"), to name but the most significant organizations that he placed under suspicion during his long reign of internal espionage.[54] He assigned agents to report on such leaders as W. E. B. DuBois, Medgar Evers, and Bayard Rustin.[55] The FBI's interest in Martin Luther King Jr. (1929–1968) remained desultory until 1961, when the SCLC member took a leadership role in the "Freedom Rides," a protest tactic devised by CORE to desegregate the South's interstate bus transportation system, and became even more intensive after 1967 when the FBI extended its COINTELPRO operation to include the SCLC; thereafter, the Bureau infiltrated, spied on, and attempted to demoralize King until he was assassinated on April 4, 1968.[56] Malcolm X (1925–1965) also became a target of more intensive FBI surveillance after he returned from Mecca in 1964—his earlier association with Elijah Muhammad (1897–1975) and the Nation of Islam[57] having branded him in the eyes of the Bureau as a cult figure and merely a minor irritant—and announced his public rejection of Elijah Muhammad's separatist ideology in favor of an internationalist, nonracial, Muslim, and pan-African outlook that most probably led to his assassination the following year.[58]

Although there was opposition to Myrdal's more gradualist theses, emanating, for different reasons of course, from left, right, nationalist, and government sources, the resistance offered by defenders of segregation proved to be most aggressive. It is not surprising that, as Myrdal pointed out then, and historian Adam Fairclough would observe many years later, "the South's white liberals were few in number and bereft of popular support, and their political isolation bred a caution that verged on timidity, especially over the issue of segregation."[59] Nevertheless, these supposedly timid souls, together with local black leaders and joined by progressive Northerners, white and black, worked in earnest to effect civil rights, to keep their "eyes on the prize" so long denied to the South's Negroes.[60]

The "prize" was at first those civil rights that could be secured through court decisions, enforced by special commissions, or enacted by the federal congress.[61] But the price for these victories would be high. In the mind of the South's white supremacist supporters, Myrdal's name would forever be associated with those who sought to tear apart the skein of racism that had wrapped itself so tightly around the entire institutional structure of the South. In one infamous instance, in Mississippi in 1959, in his charge to the all-white grand jury that would soon refuse to indict some members of a white mob alleged to have "abducted Mack Parker from his jail cell, beat him, [driven] him to the Louisiana border, shot him twice in the chest, and dumped his body into the Pearl River,"[62] Judge Sebe Dale urged that "we should have the backbone to stand against any tyranny, whether . . . on the national level or [coming from] the reformers that would make us over, . . . and, yes [against] The Board of Sociology setting [sic] in Washington, garbed in Judicial Robes, and 'dishing out' the 'legal precedents' of Gunnar Myrdal."[63]

Sex and the Rank-Order Thesis

Myrdal had in fact pointed out that in the most popular valuation matrix of the traditional South "sex becomes . . . the principle around which the whole structure of segregation of the Negroes—down to disfranchisement and denial of equal opportunities on the labor market—is organized."[64] The validity of his thesis was demonstrated not only by the official response to the lynching of Mack Charles Parker, who had been accused of raping a white woman,[65] but also, four years earlier, and in the same state, by the acquittal of those who had been charged with the brutal slaying of Emmett Till, a fourteen-year-old black youth from Chicago who had dared to whistle at a white woman.[66] As if to prove Myrdal's argument, a Southern senator from Georgia, Herman Talmadge, explained that "the ultimate aim and goal of NAACP leaders in the present segregation fight is the complete intermingling of the races in housing, schools, churches, public parks, public swimming pools and even in marriage."[67] Myrdal had linked the color-caste system of the South to the "aversion to amalgamation," and gone on to argue that in the south law, law enforcement, custom and the region's special race-based codes of everyday conduct are directed at upholding "the ban on intermarriage and other sex relations involving white women and colored men . . . , [an imperative that] takes precedence before everything else."[68] From which it followed, he went on to argue, that there were "all sorts of taboos and etiquettes in personal contacts; . . . segregation in schools and churches; . . . segregation in hotels, restaurants, and theaters, and other public places where people meet socially; . . . segregation in public conveyances; . . . discrimination in public services; and finally, inequality in . . . politics, . . . justice and bread-winning and relief."[69]

In effect then, the postwar[70] civil rights movement in the South, in terms of Myrdal's thesis, would have to pit the values of the American Creed against all those forms of racist practice designed to protect the "sanctity" of white womanhood and the "purity" of the white race. "Gunnar Myrdal proved to be right after all," writes Stephen J. Whitfield, the historian of the Emmett Till affair. "Jim Crow could not ultimately be reconciled with the aspirations of democracy itself."[71] And the American system of court-implemented justice would be the place where those aspirations might be realized. However, as Rhoda Lois Blumberg observes in her sociological account of the struggle for civil rights in the South in the 1960s, "The unequal justice system in the American South . . . , documented in 1944 by Swedish social scientist Gunnar Myrdal . . . , continued during the civil rights movement, as unsolved bombings of black homes and churches and murders of activists proliferated."[72] When, in 1964, the Mississippi Summer Project, seeking to overturn the institutional basis of Southern racism—that is, to register black voters, build a new political party and open "Freedom Schools"—involved thousands of white Northern students working with local blacks, white supremacists murdered the interracial team of Andrew Goodman, James Earl Chaney, and Michael Henry

Schwerner, arousing new tensions among black and white activists and giving impetus to the black power/black culture movement.[73] The assassination of the black civil rights worker, Medgar Evers, on June 11, 1963, by an ordained minister in the Christian Identity Movement, an offshoot of the British Israelites, and soon to become the Aryan Nation, indicated that the resistance to civil rights had organized at both the national and international levels.[74]

The issue of "miscegenation"[75]—on which Myrdal had shown that the white man's rank order of justifications for racial discriminations was based on the belief that having sexual access to a white woman was the first and foremost desideratum of the Negro males; while showing that precisely the inverse constituted the ranking of wants by Negroes, who placed the securing of jobs, land, and credit, and the ending of racial discrimination in public relief and welfare programs at the top of their own list of group and individual concerns[76]—would cease to be the basis of a criminal offense after 1967, when the decision in an aptly named United States Supreme Court case, *Loving vs. Virginia,*[77] nullified laws prohibiting interracial marriage.[78] Although the number of black-white marriages rose slightly, in the next two decades intermarriage was lowest in the South, and in eastern cities was vociferously opposed by African American cultural nationalists, and largely confined to matrimonial unions of black and white persons of the same—that is, the middle—class.[79] Thus, it would appear that Myrdal's rank-order thesis was for the most part correct in its report on how African Americans had actually prioritized their interests.

However, the recognized implications of marriage across the color line in America have changed since Myrdal wrote his *magnum opus,* acquiring new valences. Whereas in Myrdal's day court rulings and conventional sociological studies[80] treated the offspring and descendants of such marriages as *mulattoes,*[81] *quadroons, octoroons,* and *griffes,*[82] evoking painfully ambiguous answers to the question "who is black?"[83] and scholars and outsiders continued to confound such matters as the everyday life of locals in Louisiana by their mutual misreadings of *creole-cajun* and *cajun-creole* terms of reference and descent,[84] matters had "been made even more confused by the varying and unstable juridical definitions of the term *white* as it applied to both immigrants and citizens of the United States.[85] In the aftermath of the successful assault on miscegenation laws, at least two quite different outlooks have emerged. On the one hand is the renewal of the age-old proposal—and hope—that a more intensified and, of course, voluntary program cross-breeding the races will bring about not only a handsomer people, an increase in worker efficiency, and an enhancement of brain power, but also an end to the race problem itself. Negroes and whites are to be amalgamated, becoming a single peoplehood undistinguished from one another by either color or culture.[86] In fact, Lester F. Ward (1841–1913) not only invented the term *social karyokinesis* to refer to the cross fertilization of races arising out of cycles of conquest and reconquest, but also put forward what he called a "philosophy of rape" both to excuse black men's attempts to improve their genetic stock by cohabiting with white women and justify whites' lynching of blacks in order to preserve the purity of their racial line. Ultimately, Ward prophesied the coming of a "gynandrocratic" age in which the sexes will have achieved equality and races will be dissolved in the flux of a global cosmopolis.[87]

In 1963, fifty years after Ward's death, and in the midst of the raging civil rights movement, miscegenation once again was presented as the only effective solution to America's race problem, this time in an essay by Norman Podhoretz, editor of a formerly liberal Jewish magazine, and a rising spokesperson for the burgeoning intellectual movement known as neoconservatism.[88] Acknowledging that his own irrational antipathy toward Negroes had had its origins in childhood encounters with black bullies who picked on him and his coreligionists, as well as on white Catholic boys in a Brooklyn neighborhood, Podhoretz admitted that he not only hates blacks but secretly envies Negroes "for what seems to me to be their superior physical grace and beauty."[89] With this essay Podhoretz in effect reveals that he had learned nothing from the researches carried out by Myrdal two decades earlier.[90] Indeed, Podhoretz asserts that the Negro, unlike the Jew, has no heritage from which he might draw moral sustenance and psychic strength: "His past is a stigma, his color is a stigma, and his vision of the future is the hope of making color irrelevant, by making it disappear as a fact of consciousness."[91] And precisely because he truly believes all of this, Podhoretz proposes that white men like himself cease opposing and in fact actively encourage their daughters' wishes to marry black men, serving by their approval of such marriages as a deterrent to the ideology and practices of the black Muslims. The latter, opponents of black-white marriage, constituted, according to Podhoretz, "the most numerous, influential, and dangerous movement that has grown out of Negro despair with the goal of integration."[92] Hence, for him, intermarriage as a praxis transcends the institutional aims of the civil rights advocates, for it entails "not integration, . . . [but] assimilation, it means—let the brutal word come out—miscegenation . . . , for I believe that the wholesale merging of the two races is the most desirable alternative for everyone concerned."[93] Before offering, hypothetically, it is made clear, but with what he regards as great personal "courage," to give his "blessing" to a daughter of his should she wish to marry a Negro, Podhoretz prefaces his promise of approval for the marriage with the statement, "What I am saying, however, is that in my opinion the Negro problem can be solved in this country in no other way."[94]

Thirty-five years later, in 1998, with Myrdal's thesis about America's racial dilemma again a matter of public as well as academic debate, a widely publicized Hollywood film, *Bulworth,* proffers black-white cohabitation as the panacea for America's racial troubles.[95] The movie tells the story of the last few days of a senatorial campaign for reelection of its eponymous hero (played by Warren Beatty, who also directed the film and had a hand in writing the screenplay), an erstwhile liberal who is suffering what appears to be the onset of a nervous collapse. The senator is ridden with guilt not only over his betrayal of the progressive principles which were the hallmark of his rise to power in the sixties but also of his abandonment of the inner-city blacks with whom he once identified so strongly. In his overwrought state of mind, Senator Bulworth is suddenly gifted with the power to "rap," suggesting, perhaps, that he has assumed the status of Norman Mailer's "White Negro,"[96] and, at the same time to speak in the language of postmodernism. He employs the latter idiom to assert that interracial marriage and interracial cohabitation are likely to be the most effective ways to realize the dream of a united and egalitarian America: "All we need," Senator Bulworth tells his television audience, "is a voluntary, free-spirited, open-ended program of procreative racial deconstruction."[97]

By contrast, in the first major film production in behalf of black-white intermarriage,[98] *Guess Who's Coming to Dinner* (released in 1967, the year that the *Loving vs. Virginia* decision ended the prohibition on cross-racial marriages), Hollywood filmmaker Stanley Kramer was careful to have the one on-screen kiss between the African American doctor (Sidney Poitier) and his fiancee (Katharine Houghton) seen only through the rearview mirror of a taxi; and to have its taboo-defying couple assure her parents (Spencer Tracy and Katharine Hepburn) that they would leave the country right after the wedding, their upper-middle-class status and his position with the World Health Organization firmly secured. Moreover, lest anyone suppose that members of the black domestic and working classes really sought white women as a civil right, it was given to the white parents' black maid (Isabelle Sanford) not only to be the sole opponent of her employers' daughter's marriage to an African American but, more significantly, to couch her disapproval in the very terms of Myrdal's rank-order thesis: "Civil rights is one thing," she asserts, "but this here is another."[99] Indeed, according to William E. Cross Jr., the decade following the release of *Guess Who's Coming to Dinner* was characterized by the development of "Nigrescence" processes, that is, psychological reorientations that culminate in one becoming confident in his or her "personal standards of Blackness . . . [having internalized] feelings [of] Black pride, self-love and a deep sense of Black communalism."[100] Those blacks caught up in their new nigrescence were not likely to seek marriages or protracted sexual liaisons across the color line.

In *Bulworth* all is changed once again. The members of the African American extended family with whom the drug-ridden, manic-depressive senator gets involved are impoverished ghetto dwellers, one of whom (Don Cheadle) is a pimp who exploits his own children as crack dealers, while the black woman (Halle Berry) who becomes the senator's love-interest—it is revealed that his wife (Christine Baranski) is cheating on him—is a prostitute and a hired assassin. When the senator's bizarre rap on the capitalist corruption of the electoral process—he tells both poor blacks and wealthy Jewish moguls of Hollywood[101] that his own speeches are nothing more than misleading propaganda and that his vote is for sale—pays off and he is reelected, the pimp loan-shark forgives the debt of one of his deadbeat clients, a drug addict, and hires the latter to reform—though in what manner is not revealed—his crack cocaine operation. More to the film's point about racial redemption, with but a moment's hesitation, the senator's African American inamorata elects to join him in his return to public life. Their kiss is seen on television by millions. But, as if to say that even this approach to resolving the race problem is doomed to failure, the senator is gunned down in the final scene, a victim of the forces of the corrupt "establishment" that his campaign has dared to expose. He is left to the ministrations of a strange "Rastaman" (Amiri Baraka), whose frequently repeated mantra is that the senator must become a "spirit," not a "ghost." Asked to justify[102] his reintroduction of interracial coupling as a political tool to effect a racially undifferentiated society, in effect, to picture a future of American racelessness, Beatty replied, "If you're doing a movie about race, and you want to offer any kind of conclusive suggestion, that would be it. It's called love."

Despite the continuing popular interest in seeing the mixed-race offspring of intermarriage as either a tragic consequence of, or a promising cure for, America's negrophobia,[103] more and more of the bi- or multiracial offspring of such unions are selecting their own identities and choosing not to be consigned to either of the two aforementioned roles. Calling themselves (or sometimes being called by others) *mestizaje*[104] or *hapa*[105] or *rainbow people*[106] or *mixed-race people*[107] or *multiracial people*[108] or referred to by such older designations as *mulatto*[109] or *mestizo,*[110] or in accordance with locally disputed nomenclatures that do not enjoy national recognition—the so-called Lumbees[111] and the Jackson Whites[112] are good examples—such peoples, in an earlier era, would have been for the most part assigned an ethnoracial identity in accordance with which of their biological ancestry groups had the lower social status.[113] In those days, unless they were able to "pass" as whites or,[114] as in the cases of the Lumbees and Jackson Whites, as well as some two hundred other peoples, they resisted assignment, refusing to be designated as "blacks," sometimes seeking "Indian" identities, [115] their designations became mired in ambiguity. Often, however, they were not successful and were relegated to the ambiguous nonidentity of "other non-whites."[116] The independent and self-identifying interests among today's American mixed bloods gained a new and widespread support when, in 1997, Tiger Woods, a young professional golf champion, rejected identification as an African American and called himself a "Cablinasian," a term derived by combining into a single word the components of his racial ancestry, namely, Caucasian, black, Native American, and Asian.[117] Organized activity by autonomy-seeking mixed bloods finds one expression in the "census movement": "The aim of the 'census movement' of the multiracialists," Jon Michael Spencer observes, "is to convince the federal government to identify mixed-race people correctly as 'multiracial' rather than forcing them into choosing monoracial categories."[118]

The postmodern revolution in thought and practice[119] brought an entirely new outlook to the question of interracial sex and its biosocial aftereffects. Holding to the older ideas about the racial classification assigned to mixed-race persons with Negro ancestry, John P. Pittman—writing six decades after John Dollard (1900–1980) had described both the dangers and the "gains" attending the illicit, and sometimes forced, sexual intercourse of white and blacks in a segregated Southern town[120]—observed: "If the black man's desire for the white woman is a symptom of racial flight, it assumes the character of a self-frustrating and inherently un-satisfying project . . . Race mixing . . . contributes to the degradation of the black race: any mixed-race person is juridically marked as 'Negro' and so in principle, if not actually, chattel."[121] However, in the discourse of such postmodernists as Donna J. Haraway—employing the examples of the idealized mixed-race computer-generated person said, in the fall 1993 issue of *Time* magazine in its special issue on immigration, to be the representative image of the twenty-first-century American, and, more to the point, in the epidermal-illness-and-technology-induced racial reconstruction of the noticeably androgynous popular culture figure, Michael Jackson, about each of which she writes—the "one-drop" rule has clearly been revoked.[122] But the result is not the utopian racelessness[123] that neoconservatives like Podhoretz wished for, or that romantic liberals like Beatty's *Bulworth* proposed, but rather, according to Haraway, there is a "morphing" of a new identity that challenges without resolving each of the either/or dilemmas of race, ethnicity, and gender:

> The sense of utter homogeneity that emanates from *Time's* matrix of diversity is numbing. The blacks are not very black; the blonds are not very blond; the

> range of skin color would require the best chromatography to distinguish one promising golden hue from another.[124]

And Haraway draws on Hollywood films to illustrate her point:

> These figures of the new humanity look like I imagine a catalog of replicants for sale off-world in *Blade Runner* might look—young, beautiful, talented, diverse, and programmed to fulfill the buyer's wishes and then self-destruct. Unlike the terrible white-supremacist scenes of *Birth of a Nation* in 1915, nothing about race and ethnicity in *Time's* "Rebirthing of a Nation" speaks about racial domination, guilt, and hatred.[125]

Yet Haraway is troubled. In the real as well as video world of Michael Jackson's color and lifestyle metamorphoses, as opposed to the cyber-created figures of *Time's* computer-savvy writers, there is presented what biologist Scott Gilbert calls the "intermediate morph of race, gender, and class . . . , a science fiction 'representative' of humanity."[126] But Haraway disagrees. "This," she says in reference to Gilbert's commentary on *Captain E/O,* Michael Jackson's video shown exclusively at the Disney corporation's Epcot Center, "is humanity according to Epcot, where a potent trickster slipped into the monument to a clean and healthy America."[127]

And of what race/gender/class composition is this exception to clean and healthy America? Only a few possess the power or wealth to become real-life color-and-shape shifters. Michael Jackson's own self-chosen shifts in skin color, sex preferences, and real as well as reel imagery—

> Beginning unambiguously as an African American boy with a striking talent, Jackson became neither black nor white, male nor female, man nor woman, old nor young, human nor animal, historical person nor mythological figure, homosexual nor heterosexual. These shape changes were effected through his art, the medical and computer technology of his culture, and the quirks of his body . . . Science and fiction implode with special force in Jackson's iconic body, which is a national treasure of the first order.[128]

—are not such as are likely to be emulated by ordinary people, black, white, or "other." It is not only that, as Michael Omi and Howard Winant remind us, "skin color 'differences' continue to rationalize distinct treatment of racially identified individuals and groups,"[129] but also that, in the 1990s, which racial identity will be chosen, convoked, or provoked by general developments or situational conditions is no longer clear. The race-free or color-blind society that was sometimes associated with Myrdal's discussion of the inverse rank-order perspective[130] has been set aside either in the name of race pride, a proclaimed freedom of ethnoracial choice demanded by mixed-race people, or a postponement until the kind of future envisioned by Joel Williamson, a historian of mulattoes and miscegenation in the United States, has come to pass. Williamson imagined what the mixed-race "Negro" children born in 1975 would be like in the year 2000 and thereafter:

> [T]he next generation, the third generation after the [Harlem] Renaissance, might well be a cultural mutation, a new stage in a long and significant line that has struggled to join black and white comfortably together in America. He and she might well be, in fact, the first fully evolved, smoothly functioning model of a people who have transcended an exclusive whiteness and an exclusive blackness and moved into a world in which they accept and value themselves for themselves alone—as new and unique, as, indeed, a new people in the human universe.[131]

Caught between an era that forbade their coming into being and a future which consigned them to blissful raceless oblivion, the children of those who after 1967 married across the color line currently dwell in an "environment which has offered no positive, viable option of being multiracial, . . . [and still makes it] difficult for people of mixed race to accept and to assert a multiracial identity."[132]

Racial Prejudice and Institutional Racism: An Unresolved Dilemma

Barely twenty years after its publication, "the Myrdal thesis," as it has come to be called, was reconsidered in light of a number of urban uprisings. "In 1963," the National Advisory Commission on Civil Disorders would later report, "serious disorders, involving both whites and Negroes, broke out in Birmingham, Savannah, Cambridge, Md., Chicago and Philadelphia."[133] Over the next four years other outbursts—earlier uprisings had been responses to police-supported, state-and-local organized resistance to the implementation of school desegregation orders; to demonstrations against "separate but equal" seating on city buses and streetcars; to the serving of blacks "sitting-in" at "white-only" lunch counters; and to marches protesting Jim Crow ordinances and customs—would begin as blacks revolted against their all too common confinement to racial ghettoes in such northern and western cities as Chicago, Cincinnati, Newark, and Los Angeles.[134]

In a celebratory address on the occasion of the centenary of the Emancipation Proclamation of 1863, Vice-President Lyndon Johnson took note of how little progress had been made in the one hundred years following the abolition of slavery. He began his remarks with an accusation that suggested most eloquently that the American Creed, upon which Myrdal had pinned his optimistic outlook of 1944,[135] had not yet overcome the forces of racist bigotry:

> To strike the chains of a slave is noble. To leave him the captive of the color of his skin is hypocrisy. While we in America have freed the slave of his chains we have not freed his heirs of their color. Until justice is blind to color, until education is unaware of race, until opportunity ceases to squint its eyes at pigmentation of human complexions, emancipation will be a proclamation—but it will not be a fact. To the extent that the proclamation of emancipation is not fulfilled in fact, to that extent we shall have fallen short of assuring freedom to the free.[136]

Four years later, on July 27, 1967, President Johnson addressed the nation on the subject of the previous week's uprisings.[137] "We have endured a week such as no Nation should live through: a time of violence and tragedy." Announcing that he had appointed a "Special Advisory Commission on Civil Disorders," chaired by Otto Kerner, governor of Illinois, Johnson warned, "There is a danger that the worst toll of this tragedy will be counted in the hearts of Americans; in hatred, in insecurity, in fear, in heated words, which will not end the conflict, but prolong it." However, in addition to the new laws that he suggested might be needed to quell future disturbances, the president, still echoing the Myrdalian theme, called "upon every American to search his own heart," and in place of the racial hatred that might be found there, he offered, "[L]et us build something more lasting; faith between man and man, faith between race and race. Faith in each other—and faith in the promise of beautiful America." And, once again, he combined his request for legislative action on education, jobs, and housing with a general call to prayer:

> Let us pray for the day when "mercy and truth are met together; righteousness and peace have kissed each other." Let us pray—and let us work for better jobs and better housing and better education that so many millions of our own fellow Americans need so much.
>
> Let us then act in the Congress, in the City halls, and in every community, so that this great land of ours may truly be one Nation under God—with liberty and justice for all.

Myrdalian hopes still held. However, one year after the Kerner Commission had delivered its report—its conclusion admonishing Americans that unless policy-makers instituted a program combining enrichment of the life of ghettoized inner-city blacks with active efforts at racial and class integration, the trend, toward which "the nation is rapidly moving . . . , [becoming] two increasingly separate nations,"[138] would be accelerated—the Urban Coalition and Urban America, Inc., two independent nonprofit organizations, examined what had been the national response to the commission's dire warning.[139] Had the lives of black men, women, and children improved? Had the deepening racial division been reversed, or, at least halted in its pace? The answer to each of these questions was a resounding "No":

> The nation has not reversed the movement . . . The black neighborhoods in the cities remain slums, marked by poverty and decay; they remain ghettos, marked by racial concentration and confinement. The nation has not yet made available—to the cities or the blacks themselves—the resources to improve these neighborhoods enough to make a significant change in their residents' lives. Nor has it offered those who might want it the alternative of escape.[140]

And, what had happened to the reshaping of the whites' hearts and minds, the much-vaunted growth of the "American Creed," the empathy and identification with the Negro's aim, presented in 1949 by Arnold Rose (the researcher listed on the title page, together with Richard Sterner as an assistant in the writing of *An American Dilemma*) as "full achievement of democracy and its concomitants—liberty, equality, and fraternity?"[141] Two decades later, the report of the evaluators of the Kerner Commission's effects was not promising:

> Blacks and whites remain deeply divided in their perceptions and experiences of American society. The deepening concern about conditions in the slums and ghettos on the part of some white persons and institutions has been counter-balanced—perhaps overbalanced—by a deepening aversion and resistance on the part of others. The mood of the blacks, wherever it stands precisely in the spectrum between militancy and submission, is not moving in the direction of patience.[142]

During the decade of Negro uprisings, Myrdal, on three separate occasions, addressed the issues raised by the failure of the American Creed to have yet triumphed over its internal enemies. Writing in 1972, to take the last of these commentaries first in this discussion, Myrdal severely criticized the era of anti-communist repression in the 1950s, the Cold War foreign policy, and the unwarranted prosecution of the Vietnam War as major factors inhibiting the fulfillment of the Creed's promise. Without these impediments to interracial progress, the ideals of the American Creed might have been translated into an effective reconstruction of America's poverty-ridden enclaves, eliminating not only prejudice but also the horrible havens of the poor of all races. Noting that "the living conditions for the desperately poor in the rural and urban slums—of whom only a third at most are Negroes—are for the time being nowhere substantially improving . . . [and in] some respects and in some localities . . . are even deteriorating . . . further," he asserted that there "is an urgent need for rationally coordinated reforms in many fields, including the almost complete rebuilding of the cities and the provision there of parks and open spaces, the break-up of residential segregation, and a radical change in transportation policies."[143] Not neglecting the hearts and minds issue, Myrdal spoke not of a need to invigorate the proper mental outlook of the whites, but, instead, turned his ameliorative attention to the *mentalité* of the blacks: "Most important is the curative remolding of the human beings inside the slums, and the integration of slum dwellers as productive and self-confident citizens into modern industrial society."[144]

Such a vast and multifaceted program would not only be expensive ("The costs of these radical reforms are in the order of trillions of dollars . . . The estimates now and then publicized, that the problem of poverty and its effects on human beings can swiftly be solved by some $10 or $20 billion a year, are ridiculously inexpert"),[145] but also long term by way of complete accomplishment ("And the healing process will take at least a generation, even if begun with courage and determination and pursued persistently").[146] Calling attention to the fact that his proposals would "require sacrifices by the majority of Americans who are well off, and also the abstention from expensive conspicuous public consumption," as well as admitting his awareness of "the many vested interests working to prohibit the needed reforms"—interests, that is, that are "rooted in . . . the selfishness of broad strata of the American people and their distorted feelings of priorities, which are reflected in the decisions of Congress"[147]—Myrdal nevertheless refused to succumb to what he called "defeatism."[148] Taking heart from, and consigning the burdensome task entailed by his argument to, America's young people—("It is on America's youth that we must pin our hopes . . . It [would be their] duty, individually and collectively, to strive *against* further deterioration and *for* initiating reforms, . . . [taking their] stand on those ideals of justice, liberty, equality, and brotherhood . . . that is their spiritual legacy . . .")[149]—Myrdal also looked to America's "puritan legacy," which, while "not always productive of wholesome effects," had as part of its tradition in the United States the tendency, when aroused, to induce "radical conversions."[150] The "self-examination that the American nation now needs to undertake," he concluded, once more on a sanguine note, "will soon, I hope, acquire momentum and strength and have a . . . result in changed opinions."[151]

Myrdal, then, placed his confidence for putting the American Creed into everyday practice in "the coming generation [that would] more devotedly and effectively than their [sic] elders, see the light and do their moral duty."[152] It simply was "not a tenable position," he asserted, "for the United States to be that country among the rich countries that has the most and the worst slums, the highest rate of unemployed and unemployables, and the least developed health services, and that is most niggardly toward its old people and its poor children who are so many, as well as being the country that leads the world in violence, crime, and corruption in high places."[153] The "conversion" in thought on which his thesis battened would have to come soon, but, he reminded his readers, "it will have to go deeper and extend over a wider field."[154]

What, in 1972, Myrdal had asked from white Americans in general and from U.S. public policy in particular as part of a major effort to find a solution to America's racial dilemma, in 1963, he would request in behalf of the countries then being released from Europe's colonial oppression:

> I believe [he told the Conference on "The Negro in a Changing Society," holding an "Anniversary Celebration of the Emancipation Proclamation" at Wayne State University in Detroit, May 2–8, 1963] we are on the point of an awakening to dangers implied in present trends but not yet realized by most people, even among those specializing in development problems. What we should then hope is that the rich countries in the world will rise to the challenge and be prepared to accept real sacrifices in order to make possible a change in the discouraging trends.[155]

In that essay, Myrdal sought to show that since the end of the Second World War the responses of the formerly colonial countries to their erstwhile and for the most part dark-skinned subjects had been—here I borrow a metaphor from Haeckel's discredited evolutionary biology[156]—running the risk of ensuring that a global ex-colonial phylogeny would recapitulate America's mistake-ridden, slave-emancipating ontogeny. In plainer words, America would repeat the errors that continue to arise from the as yet unlearned lesson that one cannot emancipate a people without having, concomitant with that liberation, a rational plan for fitting the newly freed men and women into their new and hardly established status.[157] In so doing, Myrdal added a historical understanding to his explanation for the development of America's persistent race problem. The particular error made after 1865, he pointed out, was the failure to institute a vast and comprehensive land reform, distributing land to the Freedmen and -women and thus providing them with an independent economic base, and a sound basis, for making a life for themselves:

> In the wake of the abolition of slavery in the United States there were high hopes expressed, far-reaching declarations made, and political decisions taken, some of these latter in the form of changes in the constitutional law of the country, all aimed at rapidly establishing real social, political, and economic liberty and equality of opportunity for the Negroes now no longer held in slavery. After a few confused years of Reconstruction, however, these attempts were given up almost entirely . . . For sixty years thereafter, until about the

time when I happened to be finishing my study of the Negro problem in America, the status of the Negroes remained almost unchanged.[158]

The real cause for the mistakes made in the years 1865–1877, that is, the post–Civil War era of Reconstruction, was, according to Myrdal, rooted in the fact that "there was no real preparedness to undertake large-scale social and economic reform, which would have had to imply, among other things, redistributional intervention and, in particular, . . . land reform."[159] Although, in 1963, he allowed that "only during the last twenty years has there been again a consistent trend upwards that gradually has begun to give more reality to the hopes, declarations, and decisions following the Civil War,"[160] in 1972, Myrdal would reprove his critics, impatient for the changes he had proposed to be implemented and have their beneficent effects realized, observing that "it is . . . an absurd idea [to imagine] that an issue like that of the Negro problem in America, rooted in centuries of a tragic and often even hideous history and still injecting its peculiar effects into all social, economic, and political relations in the country, could be 'resolved' like a mathematical problem or an engineering project."[161] Noting how what he now called "the Negro rebellion" had changed as it moved into the northern cities, Myrdal had to concede that once again those who longed for the full emancipation of the African Americans would have to wait:

> Even after another thirty years we shall still live with it [i.e., the Negro problem], though it will have altered. I do hope that the changes will proceed more rapidly than in the last five to eight years, and that they will go more consistently in the direction of an ever better fulfillment of American ideals and aspirations. But this will depend upon what policies the American people will come to follow, individually and collectively.[162]

Less than one year after he had addressed the centenary celebration of the Emancipation Proclamation, Myrdal participated in a wide-ranging and rather rambling round table discussion of America's race problem, moderated by Norman Podhoretz, author of "My Negro Problem—and Ours" and editor of *Commentary,* and including James Baldwin, Nathan Glazer, and Sidney Hook, with additional comments and queries from such members of the audience as Charles Silberman and Kenneth Clark.[163] Myrdal championed a synthetic approach to the debate over whether the American people's ethics or America's public policies should take precedence in both understanding and taking action on that problem. However, in his few moments of conversation with his colleagues, Myrdal spoke to two emerging issues in the civil rights struggle, issues that would become most controversial during the next three decades: the implications of the multiracial composition of America's minority population for the movement to secure civil rights; and, what would come to be called affirmative action, that is, the manner and form by which the much-desired equality might be extended to America's blacks.

In *An American Dilemma,* Myrdal had put great emphasis on the unique conditions that rendered the American Negro's situation so different from that of America's Chinese, Japanese, Filipinos, and Mexicans on the one hand, and immigrants and the descendants of immigrants from Europe on the other.[164] He had also suggested a parallel of the problems of women to those of the Negro, both groups' dilemmas arising out of the "paternalistic order of [American] society," the former hindered in their emancipation by their role in the "more eternally inexorable" function of procreation; the latter by having to labor "under the yoke of the doctrine of their unassimilability."[165] At the 1964 round table, however, Myrdal shifted from his earlier emphasis on the singular character of the Negro question to voice his more general concern for all of America's minorities. He introduced the term *underclass* to refer to "so many other groups—the Puerto Ricans, the Mexicans, and the poor whites in all the big slums in the big cities, and the small slums in the small cities and the rural slums in the country."[166]

Moreover, his faith in the American Creed's ability to overcome prejudiced attitudes and discriminatory policies toward blacks seemed to have been chastened by the realities of power: "As to white attitudes toward Negroes, yes, I do believe that there have been changes. But you know, no upper class ever gave up its monopoly or its privileges out of ethical principles; the submerged group needs power to force its way in, and it is this that makes the ethical principles prevail."[167] On this point Myrdal spoke more as a political and sociological economist:

> Improving the lot of this whole submerged group has become a very acute problem for America, and it is only in that larger setting that the Negroes will be able to achieve anything more than formal equality.[168]

Moreover, he indicated that, however much America's whites had learned to be sympathetic to the Negro's plight, the progressive element of that learning did not extend to any widespread support for investing significant amounts of the nation's economic resources in programs that would benefit Negroes alone. Myrdal cast doubt about the likelihood of implementing Sidney Hook's suggestion—namely, that preferential treatment for Negroes might be a necessary if only temporary element facilitating that people's liberation.[169]

By 1964, Myrdal's proposed program for rectifying America required a wholesale reconstruction of its economic, educational, and social institutions: "[O]n the whole what is needed . . . is to lift *all* the poor people at the bottom, the people I call the "underclass" or the submerged group, out of poverty and everything that poverty implies. And this means . . . remaking American society."[170] Alas, for all of Myrdal's cautious optimism, such a program did not emerge.[171]

Myrdal at the Millennium: Faith versus Works

In 1988, the Kerner Report, the National Advisory Commission on Civil Disorders' account of the long hot summer of urban uprisings in 1967, was reissued with a doleful preface by Fred R. Harris, one of the commission's original members. Reiterating, for the benefit of those who still subscribed to the kind of thinking that the FBI's J. Edgar Hoover represented, the commission's finding that "the urban disorders of the summer of 1967 were not caused by, nor were they the consequence of any organized plan or 'conspiracy,'" Harris reminded his readers that the commission had shown that "segregation and poverty have created in the racial ghettos a destructive environment totally unknown to most white Americans."[172] He acknowledged that "for a time after the [release of] the Kerner Report, through the mid-1970s, America made progress on almost all fronts that the report had covered."[173] But then a counter-reaction had set in: "a series of recessions and other economic blows that were most severe for poor people and minorities . . . were accompanied by federal cutbacks in jobs, training and other social programs most important to the poor." And then came a more resounding blow, one, although Harris didn't put it that way, that seemed like a rebuke both to Myrdal's original proposals as well as his later urgings that immediate official action be undertaken to forestall America's racial powder keg from exploding: "Just a few years after the bitter lessons of the sixties, the government lost interest in, and even became hostile towards, affirmative-action programs and civil-rights laws."[174]

In the face of this backlash, Harris and Roger W. Wilkins "set up a non-governmental 1988 Commission on the Cities"[175] to review the matter and, more important, to "bring the problems of race, unemployment, and poverty back into the public consciousness, [and] put them back on the public agenda."[176] Invoking Myrdal's terminology, the report of the Commission on Cities pointed to the conclusion of Professor Gary Orfield that "the condition of inner-city black families and communities is even more precarious and more separated from mainstream American society than it was [in 1968],"[177] and, in the face of the facts as gathered by their commission—and other researchers who then and later reported equally disheartening findings—the commissioners summarized the continuing advances of race and class segregation in schools,[178] neighborhoods,[179] and jobs,[180] concluding, "The result of these trends is the existence of a persistent, large, and growing American urban underclass."[181] A renewed onslaught on poverty and racism was necessary,[182] so the commissioners believed, but, unlike President Lyndon Johnson's earlier response to the same issue, this time the war on poverty was not even declared.

By the mid-1990s another reexamination of *An American Dilemma* seemed to be called for. The outbreak of yet another urban rebellion in Los Angeles, in 1992, accompanied by disorders in other urban areas of the United States, set off when the first trial of four white police officers—who had been videotaped applying fifty-six blows to the body of Rodney King, a black man who the policemen said was resisting arrest—ended in their acquittal, called for an explanation. As before, the responses were not unlike that of poet, author, and publisher Haki R. Madhubuti, who observed "The rebellions in L.A. and other cities in the country were not aberrations but unsophisticated and uncoordinated reactions to injustice and political/economic frustrations."[183] Andrew Hacker, whose analysis of America's race problem concludes with a critique of Myrdal, treated the violent activities in Los Angeles that year as one more incident in the persistent nationwide betrayal of the "American dream" as it was supposed to apply to blacks and other minorities:

> Los Angeles's South Central section is part of inner-city America, in which millions of black men, women, and children know a poverty and a despair unmatched elsewhere in the advanced world. Seen as subordinate citizens, they know they are scorned by mainstream society and few see hope for a change in their fortunes . . . yet despite exhortations to action and political promises, the festering conditions remained in place. . . . Discontent like that which surfaced in Los Angeles will not easily be assuaged.[184]

David K. Shipler, whose Pulitzer-Prize–winning study, *A Country of Strangers: Blacks and Whites in America,*[185] has no index reference to Myrdal, treated the eruption in the South Central District of Los Angeles neither as a "rebellion" nor an "uprising." "[I]t was just a riot," he asserts. However, he goes on to describe it in terms not dissimilar from those of Hacker, or that would be recognized by readers of the Kerner Report, the Report of the Urban Commission, or by Myrdal himself: "It was a convulsion in a simmering fever of rage among people too abused by the police, too impoverished by the economy, too marginalized by the society to have much stake in the preservation of neighborhood or system."[186]

When, in 1996, with a "Foreword" by Myrdal's daughter, Sissela Bok, the Russell Sage Foundation published Obie Clayton Jr.'s anthology, *An American Dilemma Revisited,*[187] its eighteen contributors focused their critiques on whether and to what extent Myrdal's sanguine hopes, and positive predictions—

about the extension of the franchise; the end of residential segregation; black economic development; the future of America's Negro underclass; the rise of nonwhite business opportunities, advancement of black professional life, and improvement of Negro education; enhanced role for religious institutions; establishment of true justice, positive relations with agencies of law enforcement, lawful criminal court procedures, equality of women, and a normatively eufunctional African American birth and death rate—had been realized. For the most part their reports did not rejoice over the "progress" that Myrdal's great effort was supposed to have engendered. Each contribution to this reconsideration presented its author's specific misgivings: "Political power to define and establish domestic social policies has not kept step with levels and quality of participation among African Americans," observed Robert A. Dentler.[188] "Social and economic trends may encourage . . . more residential integration in the future," Reynolds Farley conceded "but it is highly unlikely that the next census will report that segregation of blacks declined to the much lower levels now observed for Latinos and Asians."[189] Nor, according to the analysis of wage differentials by Ronald F. Ferguson, "had the dream that inspired [the civil rights and Black Power] movements . . . , that African Americans might lead more healthy, happy, and productive lives, free from the hardships and degradations of social and economic subordination . . . , fully come true."[190] Indeed, the foreboding comparative historical study carried out by William Darity Jr. argued that African American "migrants came to the North without the advantages of say, Jewish immigrants to the United States in the 1890s or Asian immigrants to the United States in the 1960s . . . , [and the] lack of those advantages would harden their status and their children's and their grandchildren's status at the bottom of the nation's hierarchy."[191] John Sibley Butler conceived of today's members of what used to be called the Negro professional class as "a segment of black America, which because of segregation, can be called a sort of truncated middleman . . . [utterly dependent on] the values that made blacks successful as professionals in the early days . . . , [e.g.,] the importance of [an] education . . . [that is] more likely to produce a [small] professional class . . . [whether] there is integration or segregation."[192] However, even that status and its eufunctional concomitants have been limited by the fact that, as urged by Walter R. Allen and Joseph O. Jewell, the "dilemma of which Myrdal spoke is very much still with us in the area of black educational opportunity and achievement."[193] The education impasse was made even more visible in 1998 when, as a result of actions taken by the Regents of the prestigious and public University of California and in behalf of an initiative approved by the state's electorate revoking the affirmative action benefits available to minority students, the number of blacks accepted to the Berkeley campus's freshman class dropped from the previous year's 547 to 224, with only 98 of the latter having accepted their selection by mid-year.[194] Institutions serving the African American community exclusively fared even worse: "The conditions that made the black [religious] ministry less attractive in Myrdal's day have become even more powerful since," writes Obie Clayton Jr., explaining that "the brightest and the most ambitious have no thought to become preachers and the consequences for the black churches have been what Myrdal most feared—a loss of influence in the black communities."[195] Testimony to the persistence of racial inequities was more powerfully represented in three reports on criminal law and sentencing. An examination of the lower courts in Detroit led researchers to conclude that "differential patterns of justice remain. Bringing about a justice system that is truly just remains an American dilemma."[196] Another study, focusing on changes in policing in the South a half century after Myrdal's own analysis of the same phenomenon, pointed out that, although "the racial caste system of which it was a part has been abolished . . . racial discrimination in policing remains." By way of elaboration, its author, Samuel Walker, observed, "The problems that exist today are far more subtle and intractable than those described by Gunnar Myrdal."[197] In yet another research project on the racial situation with respect to courts, sentences, and prisons, the investigators found that "while the reforms envisioned by Myrdal may have eliminated the more obvious examples of racial discrimination in the criminal justice system, they have not produced an equitable, or color blind, system of justice."[198] And, when Antonio McDaniel insisted in effect that the much-vaunted egalitarian individualism that is said to be central to the American Creed is vitiated by both the scientific and the everyday uses of racial classifications, the modes of human aggregate assignment that "help to reconfirm [the] social inequality of different populations within . . . [American] society,"[199] Doris Wilkerson virtually affirmed his argument with a statement that, while "gender discrimination is [definitely] a source of structural inequities . . . , we live in a social system where race endures as a politically defined attribute and where racism is a paramount ideology along with class domination and economic oppression."[200] According to the researches reported in *An American Dilemma Revisited,* then, the American Creed has not yet driven the racist orientation out of the hearts, minds, politics, and socioeconomic institutions of the people of the United States. Nevertheless, the writers of the introduction to this volume are not moved to surrender to this powerful enemy of societal advance. Like Myrdal fifty years earlier, Obie Clayton Jr. and Wilbur Watson assert, "America cannot afford to allow significant numbers of its citizens to lose hope, to give up on the myriad opportunities of American life." Myrdal's proposals for solving the American race problem might not yet have proved effective, but he is still a model and a goad and his book still a source of inspiration: "Somehow," they conclude on a less than optimistic note, "we must find workable solutions to an American dilemma."

Virtually all the critics of Myrdal focus on the material, that is, institutional, economic, and political, aspects of his argument, failing to give sufficient attention to its spiritual component. For Myrdal, who was moved as much by religious as by secular perspectives, the "American Creed," as his biographer Walter A. Jackson points out, "was not simply a vague set of social norms . . . It was deeply rooted in the ideas of the Enlightenment, anchored in the Constitution, and powerfully conveyed through the public school system and the pervasive moralism of the Protestant churches."[201] It is the pervasive moralism of the Protestant churches, energizing an interracial movement for civil rights and influencing a responsive, liberally minded Congress and president, that Myrdal seems to have counted on most. "Perhaps because he identified with the dominant Anglo-Protestant political culture," Michael W. Hughey has suggested, "Myrdal did not see that the intolerant and exclusive values and practices he disdained were not simply anomalies in that culture, but fundamental and endemic features of it."[202] His fidelity to the Christian concepts adumbrating the American Creed was such that he could not "imagine that . . . racism and intolerance . . . might also be grounded in America's religious heritage."[203]

His was, in effect, if unacknowledged as such, a faith in a variant of the Arminian form of the Protestant theodicy, that is, that sectarian view, most popular in Holland and the United States,[204] that had been put forward by Jacobus Arminius (1560–1609) and condemned by the Synod of Dort (1618–1619). "Arminianism," according to Sidney E. Ahlstrom, "was a term used to designate almost any form of Reformed theology that modified the traditional doctrines of total depravity, limited atonement, or unconditional election and accentuated man's role in salvation . . . In America the term often was a synonym for 'liberal' or 'broad' and 'catholic.'"[205] American adherents of Arminianism, hence, might be expected to make room for the "doctrines of free will, free grace, and unlimited hope for the conversion of all men"[206] not only in their churches but in their society as well. Moreover, Arminian praxes, as derived from the Humanist Rationalism of Desiderius Erasmus (1466?-1536), as well as the largely secular statist doctrine of Hugo Grotius (1583–1645), encouraged government to employ its powers of control and administration in service to the common good.[207] As Seymour Martin Lipset sums up American versions of the Arminian outlook, "Men were expected to be righteous, hardworking, and ambitious. Righteousness was to be rewarded both in the present and hereafter, *and the successful had an obligation to engage in good works and to share the bounty they had attained.*"[208] Indeed, Lipset goes on to insist that "the strong commitment to a voluntaristic denominational Protestantism [in the United States] reinforced the support for minority rights even in the religious sphere itself."[209]

For Myrdal, the American Creed found its most effective mode of expression as a civil religion.[210] It was "alive deep down in every American, although often in conflict with other norms."[211] According to this perspective, the wickedness of Southern racists arose not because their own interests ran counter to those of the Negro; rather, "the wicked did wrong either because they could not see their own true interest, or because legal barriers prevented the free play of their natural goodness."[212] To Myrdal, belief in the natural goodness of even the worst racists and, even more important, faith in America's ability to reform itself without a violent revolution were necessary, but not sufficient bases for solving the race problem.[213] Myrdal would hang on to this faith even when some of his own researchers had despaired of the possibility of achieving the full complement of justice, equality, and freedom for African Americans. "I do not despair about America . . . ," he pointed out in 1972; "[no other nation] is more prepared and accustomed to revise and change its views and policies. Americans are . . . more dynamic than any other nation." To Myrdal, America's Protestant origins ensured its progress in matters of racial justice: "I see this distinctive character of American thinking and acting as part of its puritan legacy."[214]

"The accidents of my life and work," Myrdal observed in the early 1970s, "have led me to a deep identification with the inherited ideals and aspirations of the American nation—what I once called the 'American Creed.'"[215] Others, however, including Kenneth B. Clark, the psychologist whose studies of the demoralizing effects of segregation on black children, together with Myrdal's *American Dilemma,* contributed to the Supreme Court's decision to end school segregation in the United States,[216] succumbed to the very despair that Myrdal had warned against;[217] or, like Doxey A. Wilkerson, no doubt disgruntled over the censorship and virtual nonuse made of his left-oriented contribution to Myrdal's original research project,[218] became outright critics.[219] Among the harshest critics is the historian Joel Williamson, who challenged Myrdal's imputation of the Southern whites' adherence to the American Creed: "If idealized research could have looked into the hearts of its Southern white subjects in those years, it would have found them bleeding hardly one drop for the oppressed blacks . . . In fact, Southerners felt that blacks were in their appointed place, and that they, the Southern whites themselves, were the most democratic of Americans."[220] But even when some of Myrdal's proposals were adopted, their effectiveness was called into question. Thus, to

Berman E. Johnson, despite the fact that since the 1960s historians had "done much to correct unsubstantiated beliefs about African Americans, . . . the American Dream remains deferred, and the gauntlet is laid down for yet another generation—perhaps in additional media—to rekindle its vital messages."[221] Writing in the midst of the crisis-ridden sixties, Charles E. Silberman denied that there was a problem in the hearts and minds of Americans of the kind described two decades earlier by Myrdal: "The tragedy of race relations in the United States is that there is no American Dilemma. White Americans are not torn and tortured by the conflict between their devotion to the American Creed and their actual behavior. They are upset by the current state of race relations, to be sure. But what troubles them is not that justice is being denied but that their peace is being shattered and their business interrupted."[222] In effect, the higher transcendence that Myrdal attributed to the branch of Protestantism that had been brought from England via Holland to America[223]—the moral perspective that would unite self-aggrandizement with public altruism, private interest with civic virtue,[224] social science with civil rights[225]—had not emerged in all its much-vaunted egalitarian glory. Indeed, by the 1990s, the American Creed had become like the salt that lost its savour; it could neither season nor sharpen American thought on the race question.

In a general sense, this might have been foreseen. During the first decades of the twentieth century both Georg Simmel[226] and Ernst Troeltsch[227] had warned of the decline of Christianity's inner worldly asceticism as a moral force encouraging social progress, while at the same time Max Weber had observed, "Insofar as the modern proletariat has a distinctive religious position, it is characterized by indifference to or rejection of religions common to large groups of the modern bourgeoisie . . . [I]n the sphere of proletarian rationalism, religion is generally supplanted by other ideological surrogates."[228] In America these ideological surrogates have included only occasional and short-lived programmatics of interracial solidarity with what Myrdal called the black "underclass." More often they are formulated in terms of a race-based pseudo-Marxism that either segregated within or excluded altogether from the ranks of organized labor those African Americans and other nonwhite minority workers who, absent these restrictions, might have gained much from interracial collective bargaining.[229] Such practices fostered the idea that the American political economy serves only a "white republic."[230] Still other Americans found versions of a white, Negrophobic, and antisemitic orientation in the various associations built around "Christian Identity" (that soon evolved into the militia movement supporting the Aryan Nation).[231]

But not only right- and left-wing ideologies and the American labor movement turned away from the promise of *An American Dilemma.* By the 1980s, although the advances made possible by the civil rights movement had facilitated the growth and development of a substantial black middle class, that seemingly positive development had also "contributed to a distillation of ever more concentrated pools of poverty and despair in the inner cities—a process greatly worsened by the catastrophic decline of decent manufacturing jobs and the growing hardheartedness and insolvency of social policy at every level of government."[232] Myrdal's underclass[233] was now all too visible: "Half of all African American children live in poverty. A third of all black men between the ages of twenty and twenty-nine are entangled in the criminal justice system. The leading cause of death among young black men is gunshot wounds."[234] And, in the face of these developments, both liberal and conservative leaders turned against the two ameliorative proposals put forward as educational, economic, and sociocultural remedies: affirmative action[235] and multiculturalism.[236] The new antiparadigm of postmodernism would go even further,[237] fragmenting both the nearly dead civil rights coalition,[238] treating identity crises and the marginalization of nonwhite peoples, women, homosexuals, and the physically and emotionally handicapped as features of an emerging global chaos,[239] and, in the words of one sociologist, promoting "the 'politics of difference'; [in which identity] is not unitary or essential, [but] . . . is fluid and shifting, fed by multiple sources and taking multiple forms ([hence,] there is no such thing as 'woman' or 'black')."[240]

In 1972, conceding only in part to those of his critics who had labeled his commitment to the American Creed the sure sign of his having become an unreconstructed idealist, Myrdal retorted: "Ideals, when they are rooted in institutions like the Constitution, and have a place also in people's hearts, are real forces, though not the only ones, sometimes not even the most powerful ones."[241] By the 1990s, the very existence of those ideals would be called into question as a new malaise settled over the United States.

Counsels of Despair and Their Counters

Myrdal's methodological approach to understanding the American race problem through a scientific examination of American values sought among other things to "avoid the collapse into simplistic relativism and its by-products: irrationality, obscurantism, and, too often, the fatalism and intellectual defeatism of so many social scientists."[242] More to the point, his theory of "cumulative causation," holding with respect to the race problem "there is not one factor at play but many interlocking ones," was designed as "a counter to the counsels of despair," since "so long as it is possible to break in at any one point and begin to set in motion more generalized effects for the better throughout the system, there can be no room for defeatism."[243] Nevertheless, such counsels of despair did arise. These have taken three distinct forms: A melancholy retrospective, best presented in the post-Myrdal writings of Kenneth B. Clark; a rejection of Myrdal's fundamental perspective, best illustrated by the "two nations" thesis of Andrew Hacker; and a resigned acceptance of previously opposed alternatives to assimilation and monoculturalism, exhibited most noticeably in the turnabout in the thought of Nathan Glazer. In opposition to these pessimistic perspectives, such neoliberal and neoconservative social scientists as Alan Wolfe and Stephan and Abigail Thernstrom have celebrated Myrdal's prescience, revived his argument against defeatism, and opposed those favoring affirmative action and multiculturalism.

Kenneth B. Clark

Kenneth Bancroft Clark began to grow skeptical about the ubiquity and force of the American Creed when he discovered to his dismay that some fellow social scientists regarded his own ethic for social research—"the use of disciplined intelligence in achieving social justice"[244]—as outside the purview of objective social science and improper for use as such in the Supreme Court's decision of 1954, *Brown vs. Board of Education.*[245] In the now famous footnote number 11 in that decision, Clark's researches on the deleterious effects of segregation on the hearts and minds of the pupils, together with Myrdal's *An American Dilemma,* had been cited.[246] Addressing the Society for the Psychological Study of Social Issues six years later, Clark described in detail the character of his researches, their relation to the court cases brought by the NAACP to end public school segregation, and concluded by urging his colleagues to recognize that the "magnitude and implications of the desegregation problem make it imperative that American social scientists assume the responsibility inherent in their role as objective students of our society and attempt to understand the dynamics and complexities of this aspect of social change."[247] Moreover, he insisted, "This obligation must be fulfilled in spite of the fact that the desegregation problem in America and the contextual problem of the changing status of racial groups throughout the world are issues fraught with subtle and flagrant biases, intensified by emotional entanglements, and confused by historical, economic, political, and international factors and practical power considerations."[248] More and more, however, Clark came to believe that the successful completion of school desegregation not only in the South but in the North as well was dependent on the actual amount and effective usage of social power in behalf of the extension of civil rights: "The problem posed for Negroes and those whites who are committed to actual social change as a reality and not a mere social posture," he observed in 1965, "is that of identifying, mobilizing, and using that power necessary to translate laws into meaningful changes in the day-to-day lives of those whom the laws are intended to protect."[249] Myrdal had written the foreword to the book in which Clark made this statement, and the Swedish scholar had noted that Dr. Clark was demanding "large reforms, far beyond the formal enactment of civil rights, [and he pointed out that these reforms] have become necessary and urgent."[250] But, in the next few years, Clark's disappointment with several fellow social scientists' repudiation of the engagé research projects of earlier decades increased. Their failure to continue social scientific work in pursuit of America's unfulfilled promise caused him to become angry: "Within the past decade," he complained in 1974, "it has become fashionable for a group of social scientists, fortified by their training and trappings and jargon and methodological pretensions, to reverse the direction of the Allport, Boas, Bunche, Klineberg, Myrdal models of social science and express as a virtue their alliance with the present controllers of social and political power."[251] Further, he charged that the "present group of neo-conservative social scientists are well-publicized defenders of the political, social, racial, and economic status quo."[252] Moreover, he confirmed that "social scientists, who by their glib, fatuous willingness to compromise the fundamental humanity of dark-skinned children and who by doing so provide pubic officials with rationalizations for regressive policies of malignant neglect, are not only accessories to the perpetuation of injustices, [but also] they become indistinguishable from the active agents of injustice."[253] And, in 1966, referring to Myrdal's *An American Dilemma,* Clark observed, "Ideals, alone, . . . do not bring justice. Ideals, combined with necessity, may."[254]

"The new American Dilemma," Clark wrote in that same essay, "is one of power . . . The fact is that man has never effectively resolved the issue of power versus ideals, or of power as an instrument of the maintenance of ideals, or of ideals themselves as a form of power, or of fundamental emotions, such as love and hatred, as primary sources of power."[255] Insofar as blacks employed some element of power in their quest for the recognition and implementation of their civil rights, Clark pointed out, they acted through the civil rights movement and more specifically through the several organizations—the National Association for the Advancement of Colored People, the National Urban League, the Congress of Racial Equality, the Southern Christian Leadership Conference, and the Student Nonviolent Coordinating Committee—using a variety of methods to achieve the common goal.[256] However, he showed that each organization had its own organizational weakness, leadership problems, or ideological shortcomings. Which means was most effective? Clark's answer suggested that none by itself could succeed: "The ultimate test of a given approach or pattern of approaches will be in the demonstration of observable and sustained changes in the status of Negroes—the evidence that the Negroes are included in all aspects of American life with the equal protection of laws and governmental power."[257] Such an accomplishment has not yet been realized.

Nor would it be realized when, in his seventy-sixth year, Clark looked back on the decades-long era of civil rights struggle to which he had devoted virtually the whole of his professional and personal life. More than a quarter century earlier, when addressing from the audience Norman Podhoretz's *Commentary* round table on America's racial situation, Clark had broken away from Myrdal's belief in the ameliorative function of the American Creed: "With all due respect to my friend and former colleague and boss, Professor Myrdal, I have come to the conclusion that so far as the Negro is concerned, the ethical aspect of American liberalism or the American Creed is primarily verbal. There is a peculiar kind of ambivalence in American liberalism, a persistent verbal liberalism that is never capable of overcoming an equally persistent illiberalism of action, . . . [L]iberalism as it is practiced . . . *is* an affliction. It is an insidious type of affliction because it attempts to impose guilt upon the Negro when he has to face the hypocrisy of the liberal."[258] In 1990, in his memoir, published in the proceedings of the University of Wisconsin at Madison's conference to memorialize and appraise thirty-five years of post-*Brown* school desegregation efforts and twenty-five years of legislation and litigation in support of (or opposition to) the Civil Rights Act of 1964, Clark presented a most disillusioning picture.

> Attempts to desegregate northern public schools elicited an intense and sustained antibusing campaign in deference to de facto segregated schools. Curiously, after the *Brown* decision more students were attending segregated schools in northern cities, such as New York City, Chicago, Los Angeles, and Detroit, than in many southern communities . . .
>
> At the same time that progress in economic, political, and social equality was being observed . . . [s]ome whites argued that the process of social justice for blacks resulted in injustice for whites. They maintained that obtaining equality for blacks could only be done at the expense of whites—especially the white males . . .
>
> At the time that this form of reasoning by white supremacists was gaining favor with decision makers, it was being paralleled by complex psychological reasoning on the part of black separatists. These black nationalists openly renounced racial desegregation, arguing that racial justice could be obtained only by their form of isolation and inverse racism . . .

> [Despite the fact that the] number of black elected officials has increased in the years since the Voting Rights Act [was passed], . . . the status of inner-city blacks has deteriorated. A small number of blacks have benefited from affirmative action and have moved into the middle class. But an increasing number have remained in the inner-city underclass . . .
>
> The existing total pattern and the cycle of pathology now inflicted upon the nonwhite underclass in our deteriorating inner cities are found in the buildings that are abandoned and in the human beings who are also abandoned. These are the symptoms of a deep and pervasive racism.[259]

Clark attributed the optimistic enthusiasm that had accompanied the *Brown* decision and Myrdal's analyses to the fact that at the time "it was not so clear to many of us that racism was not limited to its flagrant forms found in the southern states . . . In such large urban communities as Los Angeles, Boston, Detroit, Philadelphia, and New York City, patterns of racial injustice were deeply imbedded in the social structure, and whites bitterly resisted change."[260] Although he believed that "more appropriate and effective methods must now be developed and used to obtain observable progress at this stage of the continuing struggle for racial justice," Clark dolefully concluded his memoir with a decidedly un-Myrdalian announcement: "I am forced to face the likely possibility that the United States will never rid itself of racism and reach true integration . . . and . . . that my life has, in fact, been a series of glorious defeats."[261]

Andrew Hacker

The political scientist Andrew Hacker has cast a discerning eye on the statistical facts of the black-white divide in America and believes they demonstrate not the prejudiced contradictions to creed and conscience that moved Myrdal to make his proposals for resolving what he perceived as an only apparent impasse, but, rather, a society like that described by the nineteenth-century Anglo-Jewish British prime minister, Benjamin Disraeli (1804–1881): "Two nations, between whom there is no intercourse and no sympathy; who are as ignorant of each other's habits, thoughts, and feelings, as if they were dwellers in different zones, or inhabitants of different planets."[262] If more data[263] are needed to buttress his thesis, Hacker interprets the disparity in black and white reactions to the jury's "not guilty" verdict in the trial of Orenthal James ("O.J.") Simpson as a powerful as well as prescient illustration of the gulf dividing the African American "nation" from that of the whites. With stunning accuracy, Hacker predicted that the white-dominated institutions of policy and the California electorate would dismantle affirmative action, reduce support for or close down altogether inner-city hospitals, and seek to unseat blacks elected from voter districts that had been redesigned to secure the latter's chances for becoming fully enfranchised participants in the democratic process.[264] The nearly all-black jury's nullification of what seemed to the thousands of whites who had followed "the trial of the century" day by day as a clear instance wherein a popular sports celebrity had murdered his ex-wife and her white male friend had been interpreted, so Hacker believes, as a "defeat" for the white race. "This is not to say that whites will consciously impose punishments for what one jury did," Hacker concludes. "But minds and actions shift by degrees, and white Americans are not apt to forget that they have a defeat to make up."[265]

Hacker's vision of an America bifurcated by two warring racial nations cannot be harmonized with Myrdal's view, as summarized by Hacker, that the country is "beset by a social and moral paradox." It "may have been," Hacker suggests, "that Myrdal misread America's ideals."[266] In contradistinction to Myrdal's thesis, Hacker offers that of Alexis Charles Henri Maurice Clerel de Tocqueville (1805–1859). Tocqueville's *Democracy in America,* 1835),[267] based on his nine months of travels in the United States in 1831–1832,[268] has remained a classic as well as an influential account of the exceptional society that would emerge out of America's political and sociocultural separation from Europe.[269] From his writings Hacker selects quotations in which Tocqueville indicts Europeans for choosing "their slaves from a race differing from their own, which many of them considered as inferior to the other races of mankind"; condemns "White Americans . . . [for violating] every right of humanity by their treatment of the Negro"; argues that the "most formidable of all the ills that threaten the future of the Union arises from the presence of a black population upon its territory"; supposes that if the enslaved Negroes "are to be raised to the level of freemen they will soon revolt at being deprived of almost all their civil rights"; describes the relations between the races as two peoples "placed in the situation of two foreign communities . . . fastened to each other without intermingling . . . , unable to separate entirely or to combine"; and predicts "that the abolition of slavery will, in the common course of things, increase the repugnance of the white population for the blacks."[270]

Toccqueville, who actively opposed both slavery[271] and racism[272] (but, in his later years, lent support to French colonial rule over Algeria),[273] concluded that the "danger of a conflict between the white and the black inhabitants haunts the imagination of the Americans, like a painful dream."[274] Hacker would have found even more evidence for his own thesis in the form of the appendices that Tocqueville's traveling companion, Gustave Auguste de Beaumont de la Bonniniere (1802–1866), attached to *Marie or Slavery in the*

United States: A Novel of Jacksonian America. One was entitled "Note on the Social and Political Condition of the Negro Slaves and of Free People of Color"[275] and provided a detailed critical political ethnography; another, entitled "Note on Equality in American Society" reported on the one exception to the country's commitment to egalitarianism: "Social and political equality in the United States is never seriously infringed except with regard to the black race . . . [A]mong the whites . . . a white skin is the mark of nobility . . . , and they treat each other with the regard and honor habitual among the members of a privileged class."[276] To Hacker, America's race problem did not arise out of an as-yet-unresolved dilemma, but rather as a major institutional default: "A century and a quarter after slavery, white America continues to ask of its black citizens an extra patience and perseverance that whites have never required of themselves."[277] Myrdal's American Creed, if it operated to any extent as all, had not driven its racist adversary out of the organizational structures or the hearts and minds of the dominant majority. Instead, Hacker warned, a "huge racial chasm remains, and there are few signs that the coming century will see it closed."[278]

Nathan Glazer

Whereas Hacker sees no cause for optimism in the statistical disparities and public opinion polls that illustrate the depth and fervor of his two nations' thesis, Nathan Glazer, a sociologist at Harvard University who, until April 1998, had been a leading opponent of affirmative action[279] and a critic of multiculturalism,[280] and who had argued against the possibility of achieving integration in New York City's public schools,[281] has recently reversed himself and turned away from the position on the race question that he had held for over a quarter of a century.[282] However, Glazer's renunciation of the outlook that Richard Rorty calls that of "the pre-Sixties reformist Left"—namely, that "insofar as it concerned itself with oppressed minorities, did so by proclaiming that all of us—black, white, and brown—are Americans, and that we should respect one another as such"—in favor of one seemingly closer to that which Rorty designates "the contemporary cultural Left"—that is, one that "urges that America . . . not be a melting pot . . . [and] wants to preserve otherness rather than ignore it"[283]—is upon closer inspection a counsel of disappointment and resignation over the failure of Myrdal's thesis to become fact.[284]

To Glazer, multiculturalism arises as the narrative that replaces the older but no longer viable "American Epic." The latter had celebrated the expanding frontier, free land, and free institutions; lauded such pioneers, explorers, and discoverers as Daniel Boone, Lewis and Clark, and Columbus; and taken pride in such presidents as Washington, Jackson, Lincoln, and Theodore Roosevelt.[285] A new epic, Glazer observes, seems to have appeared as part of the post-sixties era, emphasizing ethnoracial and gender diversity in moods that swing from otherness-celebrating optimism to a harsh critique of racism, patriarchy, and sexism. When, in 1973, the historian of American immigration Oscar Handlin published a new edition of his classic work *The Uprooted,* the cover added a subtitle, *The Epic Story of the Great Migrations That Made the American People,* and the author's introductory paragraph consisted of only two sentences: "Once I thought to write a history of the immigrants in America. Then I discovered that the immigrants *were* American history."[286] However, Glazer points out, by this time the type of epic that is represented in Handlin's studies was being displaced by one that was simultaneously more pluralistic and less patriotic.[287] "[D]esperate efforts," he says, "were being made to induct the non-immigrants—Native Americans, as the Indians had become, and the African-American descendants of slaves—into American epics that had ignored or disdained them . . . Black studies at the time were spreading rapidly and were soon to become a fixture in the academy, along with Latino, Asian-American, and Native-American studies."[288] The net result, to which Glazer's most recent writings grudgingly acquiesce, is the replacement of the one usable past with another quite different, one that produces skepticism and uncertainty. "We are now doubtful about our capacity to improve the lives of other peoples."[289] But even if that capacity were to be restored, Glazer doubts "whether the improving of group relations can replace the conquest of a continent as the subject of epic."[290] Glazer points out that Myrdal's *An American Dilemma* belongs to the era when inclusion was the theme of the American epic and assimilation was regarded as the sure solution to America's race problem.[291] Today "[w]hatever the causes, the apartness of blacks is real . . . ; [moreover,] the difference that separates blacks from whites, and even from other groups 'of color' that have undergone a history of discrimination and prejudice in this country, is not to be denied."[292] And, Glazer concludes on a note of regret, "this separation . . . is the most powerful force arguing for multiculturalism and for resistance to the assimilatory trends of American education and American society."[293]

Glazer's about-face on affirmative action in higher education comes on the heels of California's triple-threat revocation—of affirmative action,[294] bilingual education,[295] and race-conscious admissions to its state university[296]—and the University of Texas Law School's Regents' plaintive appeal of the March 1996 decision in *Hopwood vs. Texas,* the Fifth Circuit Court's ruling that virtually halted altogether the use of race or color in the crafting of diversity-oriented school admissions' policies.[297] However, Glazer's new position is not one that is aimed at resolving the debate over affirmative action that currently divides the ranks of the post–Cold War left,[298] nor is it a concession to the civil rights advocates who see in affirmative action a revival and continuation of the egalitarianism of the Reconstruction era.[299] Nor does Glazer directly repudiate the arguments put forward by such African American neoconservative opponents of affirmative action as Stephen L. Carter,[300] Glenn C. Loury,[301] or Thomas Sowell.[302] Rather, his position is in effect an abandonment of Myrdal's "faith" in the effects of "good works"—for example, tearing down the wall of Jim Crow racial separation, outlawing segregation, and, perhaps most important to Glazer in the four decades after *An American Dilemma* was published, encouraging African American youth to take advantage of the opportunities that the civil rights movement had opened up—to stay in school, work hard, refrain from having children until marriage has ensured a two-parent family, and, in general, actively seek the successes that are promised to those who believe in the American Dream and emulate America's Asian and European immigrants.[303]

In fact, Glazer's description of the actual plight of African Americans in 1998 is not substantially different from their own perspective on the racial situation, one that he reported to Norman Podhoretz's *Commentary* round table in 1964. In the latter year, Glazer told his fellow discussants that, Negro protestations to the contrary notwithstanding, "the American Creed does prevail in the North."[304] Although he was able to point to the facts that "bills can be passed; whites and Negroes can confer together on what ought to be done about discrimination; you can get a Fair Employment Practices Law; you can get a Fair Housing Law . . . And they get results—Negroes *do* get jobs . . . , [he nevertheless had been forced to concede that] the results aren't good enough—at least not good enough to make the Negroes feel that the political order is responsive to their real situation."[305] Thirty-four years later, Glazer acknowledged in effect that the protesting blacks had been and continue to be justified in their complaint. Despite the fact that "amid the civil rights revolution of the 1960s, affirmative action had been instituted to compensate for the damage done to black achievement and life chances by almost 400 years of slavery followed by state-sanctioned discrimination and massive prejudice . . . , [there still exists] today a vast gulf of difference . . . between the educational and occupational status of blacks and whites, a gulf that encompasses statistical measures of wealth, residential segregation, and social relationships with other Americans."[306] In 1964 Glazer had argued that "formal equality simply hasn't worked to produce actual equality, or rather it has been working too slowly."[307] Taking one example, Glazer asserted that the New York City public school system produces "tests which for a lot of reasons Negroes find hard to pass."[308] In

1998 Glazer pointed to recent data that showed that "only 1.7 percent of black students scored over 600 on the verbal section [of the Scholastic Aptitude Test] in 1995, and only two percent scored over 650 on the math [portion of the same test]."[309] Although Glazer agreed that these scores indicate "considerable progress over the last 15 years," he felt obliged to acknowledge, with sadness, that "black students still lag distressingly far behind their white counterparts."[310] Whatever was believed to have resulted from the positive response to Myrdal's analysis and to merit-based public policies, Glazer has come to the conclusion that, regardless of the value of "qualifications" tests, affirmative action in behalf of assuring diversity ought to be continued. "We are," he has to admit, "still, though less than in the past, 'two nations,' and one of the nations cannot be excluded so thoroughly from institutions that confer access to the positions of greatest prestige and power."[311] "Fortunately," he closes the essay that disconcerted all those neoconservatives and neoliberals with whom his earlier writings had resonated so closely,[312] "those two nations, by and large, want to become more united."[313] Not everyone would agree.

Abigail and Stephan Thernstrom

An entirely different perspective is found in the writings of Abigail and Stephan Thernstrom, the former, a Harvard Ph.D. currently a senior fellow at New York City's Manhattan Institute; the latter, Winthrop Professor of History at Harvard. Self-proclaimed advocates of race-neutral policies,[314] the Thernstroms, separately and jointly, treat drives to eliminate "tracking" and "competence" groupings in public schools as well as demands for such curricular reforms as racial sensitivity training and culturally appropriate tests as features of an all-embracing preferential race-conscious agenda. That agenda, they believe, seeks to alter or hide rather than eliminate the educational deficiencies of black students.[315] Thus, the Thernstroms severely criticize such current advocates of multiculturalism and affirmative action programs as Derrick Bell;[316] and share with such members of the new black neoconservative vanguard[317] as Glenn C. Loury the belief, in the latter's words, that "there can be no empathy and persuasion across racial lines . . . [unless we understand] that the conditions and feelings of particular human beings are universally shared";[318] and with Thomas Sowell—"the most penetrating critic of affirmative action in higher education"[319]—that it makes little sense to put black "students into fast-paced colleges for which they were so ill-prepared that they required special slower-paced courses."[320] Unlike Clark, who is disillusioned by the interminably slow pace of racial progress in America; or Hacker, who does not see much likelihood that the "two nations" will be reunited, free, and equal in the foreseeable future; or Glazer, who, although he refuses to accept the "defeatist" label that the sociologist Alan Wolfe has hurled at his defection from the neoconservative cause,[321] can no longer put his faith in race-neutral approaches to the American race problem, the Thernstroms have not only kept the Myrdalian faith, they credit the Swedish scholar with true prescience.[322]

The Thernstroms have enlisted the spirit of Myrdal in what the sociologist Stephen Steinberg calls their "attack [on] the logical and empirical premises on which affirmative action is based."[323] However, whether Myrdal would share their animus toward affirmative action today is by no means clear if one examines his ambiguous statement on the matter presented to Podhoretz's *Commentary* discussion group in 1964:[324] "Prejudice will continue to exist even if the legal and institutional basis for it is removed. And . . . , since the Negroes are poor—and since they have a higher proportion of illiteracy, of school dropouts, and the rest of it—other things besides the removal of prejudice are needed to lift the group." A few moments later Myrdal predicted, "I don't think Negroes are going to be given preferential treatment and I think it would be most unfortunate if they were—though . . . there are individual cases in which preferential treatment might work." Returning to massive public policy measures, Myrdal in effect distinguished their morality from their practicality: "I think it would be most unfortunate to try to get a kind of Marshall Plan specifically for the Negro . . . Politically, I doubt that it would be possible to push such a plan through—if only because white people today simply do not have a bad conscience over the fact that Negroes were brought here into slavery a long time ago . . . Furthermore, . . . anyone with any sense knows that it's not possible to solve the Negro housing problem as a *Negro* housing problem. For one thing, you could never get the money; and even if you could . . . , I doubt that it could technically be done . . . [T]he same is true of education: you'll have to get rid of all your black schools and improve the *whole* educational system."

The Thernstroms' specific case against affirmative action has been summarized by Steinberg,[325] its most ardent critic: "Since advocates of affirmative action predicate their argument on the idea that racism is still embedded in American society, compounded by deep social class inequalities along racial lines, the Thernstroms are intent on showing . . . that affirmative action is 1) unwarranted, because America is no longer the racist society that it once was; 2) unnecessary, because blacks have made enormous strides without affirmative action; and 3) counter-productive, because it violates their 'rule of thumb' that anything that is divisive is bad."[326] Steinberg finds all of these reasons fallacious or misleading.[327] However, in a separate essay, Stephan Thernstrom, apparently in the sanguine spirit of what he believes was Myrdal's "sunny optimism—justified by the remarkable change in the status of blacks even before the 1960s and so integral to the success of the subsequent civil-rights movement"[328]—greets the drop in black and Hispanic enrollments, after the universities, law schools, and medical schools of California and Texas had been forced to eliminate affirmative action policies, with equanimity: "[I]t will benefit those with solid qualifications by removing the stigma of having been admitted under different and distinctly lower standards."[329]

And what of the opportunity offered in the final pages of Myrdal's great work? "America," the Swedish scholar had pointed out in 1944, "can demonstrate that justice, equality, and cooperation are possible between white and colored people . . . If America in actual practice could show the world a progressive trend by which the Negro became finally integrated into modern democracy, all mankind would be given faith again—it would have reason to believe that peace, progress and order are feasible."[330] The Thernstroms seem to want Americans to keep the faith but forego what had been thought as the good works: "Myrdal's optimism served his generation well; his voice is needed today."[331] The repudiation of multiculturalism, race-consciousness, and affirmative action is not proposed by the Thernstroms because race is no longer relevant in America. "We are far from being a society in which race is unimportant," they admit.[332] But, for the Thernstroms, the achievement of a non-racist, democratic, free, and equal society is, as so often has occurred before, projected into the future, becoming a hope deferred. As far as education is concerned, Stephan Thernstrom seems pleased to predict that "the change [to race-neutral admissions policies] will produce a far healthier academic environment in which no group of students predictably and consistently ends up with the poorest academic records and with high rates of failure on the bar exams or medical boards."[333] It is doubtful that Clark, Hacker, or Glazer would agree with his assessment.

The Future of *An American Dilemma*

As the twenty-first century beckons, the status of Myrdal's great work on America is not clear. Looking back at his efforts a little more than a quarter century after *An American Dilemma* had been published, Myrdal warned, "There must be equality of opportunity in the pursuit of happiness, or else this nation will disintegrate into factions among which there is no national solidarity."[334] The failure in America to bring about full integration and the rise of multiculturalism in America and on many parts of the globe threaten to make his warning into a fact. At the same time, the "progress" attributable to Myrdal's study, the civil rights movement, and the black and other ethnic insurgencies seems to have reached their points of marginal utility and to have sparked an ongoing backlash of regressive court opinions and policy measures.[335] Yet, much of American life is modified and conditioned by a person's or a group's location in the economy—so that racial progress is all too often measured by comparing occupational "success," financial status, and a people's portion of the national wealth.[336] Still, the moral purpose that stood behind Myrdal's faith in the American Creed, despite the disillusions that have arisen in the hearts and minds of those whose hopes for a better society have been dashed, is not a mere creature held captive in the political economy.

> Its religious underpinnings may have eroded, but these might be transvalued, indeed, transubstantiated, into the rule of—and a revitalized role for—Constitutional law, not only in interpreting broadly those rights embodied in that document's Fourteenth Amendment guarantying each person the equal protections of the laws, but mediating the ongoing struggle between competition and cooperation, assimilation and pluralism, individualist claims and group demands.[337]

For, as economist W. Arthur Lewis has reminded us, "In the end, economics is not enough. People of different races, religions, and cultures have to learn to live peacefully with each other, and to develop pluralistic and federal institutions where this is the only way. Economic progress will help decisively, but racism has its own deep psychological springs that must be drained directly."[338] Lewis believes such learning takes a long time,[339] but Bart Landry holds that "today it is only the initiative and leadership from state and, especially, the federal government, that are up to the task."[340] Moreover, Landry concludes, "Without a massive effort, similar to the Civil Rights era of the 1960s, the racial problems of today will only become worse in the twenty-first century."[341]

From the perspective of America's history, John Higham points out that there have been three "Reconstruction eras" in the nation's past—the first, outlawing the slave trade after 1808; the second, following the abolition of slavery and the adoption of the post–Civil War thirteenth, fourteenth, and fifteenth amendments to the Constitution; the third, occasioned by Myrdal's pathbreaking study, the civil rights movement, the ending of state-sanctioned segregation, and the adoption of Civil Rights and Voting Rights Acts in 1964 and 1965.[342] But, he goes on to point out, each of these "Reconstructions had faltered and came to an end when the economic environment turned decisively unfavorable."[343] At present, the United States is going through a post-Reconstruction era, and there is "indifference at the top of the social scale and bare-knuckle antagonism down below [and these are] again widening the racial chasm."[344] What is to be done?

What is needed in the twenty-first century is yet a fourth "Reconstruction," one that Higham believes will require a three-fold ideational shift: the recognition not of the failure but of the incompleteness of the first three "Reconstructions"; participation of blacks and whites in "some larger identity, some greater loyalty, that connects them without threatening their separate qualities and needs . . . , [one that draws on] the liberal nationalism that was forged in a Christianized Enlightenment and in the twentieth century renamed the American Creed"; and a disavowal of "a 'culture of defeat' [that, since the collapse of "the vaulting expectations of the 1960s,"] has infected attitudes toward national projects among academics, much of the black middle class, and even the public at large.[345] However, whether this new alliance of engagè people and progressive ideas will come about is not assured. "Cynicism has ravaged belief in an inclusive national community and in its reach toward a better world."[346] "The American Creed lives on," Higham concedes, "but only one of its three pillars—the idea of human freedom—remains essentially unchallenged."[347] Hence, the future of the liberal revolution might entail yet another failure in the long march to racial freedom, equality, and dignity.

"As likely as not," Bruce Ackerman warns, "the world of 2020 . . . will contain a Europe of hostile nation-states and an America impoverished by economic nationalism, racked by ethnic division, and the alienation of hopeless slums."[348] Having failed to revitalize the kind of society and the kind of world that Myrdal had hoped to energize, the "self-proclaimed First World will look out upon a larger complex of competing xenophobias and bitter proletariats while it gasps for breath in an environment that all have mindlessly conspired to destroy."[349]

But there is an alternative possibility. Ernst B. Haas argues, "Liberalism allows for open political space, for alternative solutions, because it features rational discourse and compromise, not decisions based on faith and force."[350] For Haas, "Compromise . . . demands the acceptance of a degree of multiculturalism shorn of the features of cultural separatism . . . [and demands] the reassertion of individualism tempered at the margin with concessions to communalism."[351]

Here, then, is an "American dilemma" for the twenty-first century. It is a bequest from Myrdal and the people of the twentieth century to their children. Will a second Myrdal arise who can lead us into the fourth "Reconstruction," show us how, in the words of Ackerman, "to build a liberal state dedicated to our equal right to be different . . . , something more than strangers, if less than friends . . . , a civilized political life that allows each of us to respect the other's quest?"[352]

This is the challenge.

CHAPTER TWO

The "Yellow Peril" Mystique

Origins and Vicissitudes of a Racist Discourse

> The Hearst Press went periodically frantic about an oncoming "Yellow Peril," with the Tong Wars in Chinatown as proof that Chinese were bloodthirsty sneaky, and—as I would learn in one special vaudeville show put on to combat drug addiction—lustful for white women. Many were the front pages with the immense black headlines "TONG WAR!!"—accompanied by drawings of Chinese cutting each other's heads off and holding them up victoriously by their pigtails. It made me wonder why anybody went to Chinatown at all.
>
> —ARTHUR MILLER, *Timebends: A Life*

> The war in the Pacific is the World War, the war of Oriental Races against Occidental Races for the Domination of the World.
>
> —Editorial, *Los Angeles Examiner*, March 23, 1943

> No one knows who's in the shadow of whom. Every cliché comes from someone's perspective.
>
> —WYNTON MARSALIS in Beijing (February 2000)

Introduction

For more than twenty years, since the late 1970s, Paul Spickard, a professor of Asian American Studies at the University of California, Santa Barbara, has asked his undergraduate students to fill in their own ratings on his improvised ethnic social distance test.[1] Each year he asks them to rank the same list of ten American ethnic groups "according to how closely they approximate the core of what it means to be an American."[2] In recent years the students have tended toward the same ethnoracial hierarchy, putting English, Swedish, and Irish, respectively, in the first, second, and third rankings; Polish and Jewish on the fourth and fifth; Black and Indian in the sixth and seventh; and Japanese,

Mexican, and Arab in the eighth, ninth, and tenth places. (Chinese are not included on Spickard's list.) However, Spickard recalls that in the first few years that he tabulated his results, Japanese Americans placed in third or fourth rankings, but then, in the years 1981–1983 and thereafter, when the American economy "took a nosedive and much of that problem was blamed on Japan . . . , the position of Japanese Americans . . . dropped like a stone, from near the top to the bottom."[3] Had he conducted this exercise a half century earlier, he would likely have found both Japanese and the Japanese Americans near the bottom. For this people, as well as other peoples whose ancestry and heritage are Asian in origin, have long been characterized as personifications of a dreaded enemy of and challenge to Western civilization: a fire-breathing dragon that is the "yellow peril." Indeed, the higher place that Japanese briefly occupied in Professor Spickard's students' rankings is exceptional,[4] while the post-1981 rankings announce a return to the older place that Americans reserve for Asians. Moreover, when Japan and the Japanese are not in the lower ranks, it means that China and the Chinese have, for the moment, taken their place. Such, in fact, is the case at the present time.

The present version of the "yellow peril" in the United States has a past. Although it had a point of origin—to be discussed below—it did not arise in its many complexities all at once; rather it developed piecemeal in terms of Asia's place in U.S. public policies. American popular literature regarding Asia and the peoples therefrom contributed mightily to its reinforcement. During the course of its becoming embedded in America's consciousness of itself, America's sense of its own basis for nationhood, and America's establishment of itself as a world power—with each of which it was associated—the yellow peril appeared first as China, then as Japan, then as China and North Korea, then as China and Vietnam, then briefly as a temporarily prosperous Japan again, and, at the moment—once again—as China. What follows is an interpretive history of its place in America's relations with China and Japan and how it got there.

China's Challenge to the Occident

Allegations—so far unproven—that a Chinese scientist might have turned over top secret materials to the People's Republic of China, have evoked American fears of a revived threat from the Far East and moved China and Chinese Americans to the top rung of yellow peril enemies, not only replacing Japan but also for the moment reducing the sense of danger from such other potentially "enemy" states as North Korea.[5] Senator Don Nickles put forward the claim that Wen Ho Lee—(the accused Chinese engineer who had been fired from his position and, later, indicted and held without bail on charges for several months—all but one of which would eventually be dropped—that he had unlawfully removed American nuclear secrets from the Los Alamos National Laboratory[6])—is responsible for the "most serious case of espionage" in United States history.[7] Houston Hawkins, a former Defense Intelligence Agency security officer, who at first did not put much stock in the espionage story,[8] later, when asked whether China was capable of mounting a sophisticated spying operation in the United States, replied, "They've been practicing espionage for 2,000 years."[9] But, an even more insidious interpretation on this matter has been presented by Paul D. Moore, from 1976 to 1988, the FBI's chief analyst for Chinese counterintelligence:

> China does not normally pay an agent for information, request that the agent provide classified documents, use intelligence officers to elicit information from the agent or engage in clandestine activity . . . China prefers to obtain its information a little bit at a time, by having its scientists and experts exploit individuals who are visiting China in the normal course of business. . . . The principle that the Chinese apply is simple: people will almost never commit espionage, but they will often enough be indiscreet—sometimes to the point of making a major mistake—if they can be put in the right circumstances.[10]

Like the Japanese immigrants and their American-born offspring, who in 1942 were accused of having chosen their places of residence on the Pacific coast so that they could report to Japan on American military installations,[11] so today, one might infer from Wen Ho Lee's arrest and Moore's perception on the matter, that Chinese American scientists—and, perhaps, anyone who accepts an invitation to visit China or to entertain visitors to America from China—are to be regarded either as dupes, as potential victims of cleverly trained agents of the People's Republic of China, who, during the course of an ordinary conversation, are able to extract secrets from them, or as spies working for a foreign government.* Thus has there arisen once again an apprehension of a Chinese "yellow peril."

---

*To this story must be added the anecdote distinguishing Soviet from Chinese modes of espionage once told by former FBI assistant director for intelligence, James H. Geer, and published twelve years later in the *Los Angeles Times:* "If a grain of sand were a piece of information, the Soviets would bring a submarine offshore in the dead of night and send a dinghy with men dressed in dark wet suits who would fill a bucket of sand and go back to the submarine and steal away in the dead of night. The Chinese, on the other hand, would send 100,000 bathers to the beach in broad daylight and during the course of the day, each bather would pick up one grain of sand and bring it home with him . . . That's pretty much what's happening." Quoted in Ling-Chi Wang, "China Spy Scandal Taps Reservoir of Racism," on the Internet. URL:http://www.minorities-jb.com/asian/news/spying3.c.html. And, though not stated in the quoted material, it is reasonable to suppose that the "100,000 bathers" would be drawn from the Chinese American population, each one of whom should, hence, be suspected of serving as intelligence agents for the People's Republic of China.

The current shift of China to enemy status has been catalyzed by the following: in 1997, Peter H. Lee, like Wen Ho Lee, a naturalized citizen from Taiwan who also had worked at Los Alamos, pleaded guilty to the charge of orally passing classified information on nuclear weapons to Chinese scientists while attending a conference in Beijing;[12] a book published in late 1999 by Larry Englemann and his wife, Meihong Xu, asserts that attractive Chinese women are trained to go abroad, marry, adopt new identities, get jobs and then, years later, surface as spies for the People's Republic of China;[13] with the help of Japanese smugglers, a number of Chinese, posing as immigrants from Japan, are entering the United States via Hawaii;[14] some working-class Chinese women in America, desperate to keep their low-paying, labor-intensive, and long-hours jobs in the garment shops of New York's, San Francisco's, and Los Angeles's Chinatowns, send their American born children to China to be raised by relatives[15] (that is, put these children in a position similar to that of the *Kibei* Japanese, who, born in America, educated in Japan, and returned to America, were more suspect than other Japanese Americans during World War II);[16] and that the recent victories of pro-independence elements in Taiwan bid fair to heighten tensions in that area of the world. In addition, the Wen Ho Lee matter recalls the case of Chinese scientist Qian Xuesen, accused of being a communist during the McCarthy era, held under house arrest for five years, and then deported to China. Qian, who had participated in developing America's rocket program, became a leader in China's missile and armaments development.[17] In 1999, recalling his own treatment in that earlier era, John Paton Davies, hounded out of the U.S. State Department for "losing" China to the communists, pointed out, "Our infatuation with China—whether it is a potential enemy or a dear friend to be protected and indulged—hasn't changed all that much."[18] However, the manner in which Wen Ho Lee was first fired, then indicted, and, despite protestations of loyalty to the United States, denied bail, but finally released, has had a chilling effect on virtually all persons of Asian, especially Chinese, descent[19] working in American high-tech industries. "In this climate of [suspicion]," observes Chang-Lin Tien, former chancellor of the University of California at Berkeley, "many Chinese [Americans] feel they are being watched all the time, as if they are not full citizens."[20] Like its previous incarnations, this version of the "yellow peril" adversely affects the lives, livelihoods, and civic status of all persons of Asian descent living in the United States.

However, the yellow peril image of Asia has an even longer history. As a foundational, essentialist discourse on an entire geocultural area and its inhabitants, it resembles that element in history that achieves legitimation because—as in Weber's famous analogy of historical events to "loaded" dice[21]—it has been given a privileged place and precedence over all other discursive devices in the understanding of what is meant by such terms as *Asia,* the *Orient,* and the *Far East.* It could be considered a genus of what has been called *Orientalism.* But, if this term is to be applied, it could not be used as a synonym for the "Orientalism" that has been subjected to analysis by Edward Said[22]—the purpose of whose critique, as Bryan S. Turner argues, "appears to be merely recommending an improvement in our account of Islam."[23] Rather, the yellow peril thematic presents itself as a coded ethnomethodological[24] discourse that, under the cover of a guarded defense of the Occident-under-siege, "represents the exotic, erotic, strange Orient as a comprehensible, intelligible phenomenon within a network of categories, tables and concepts by which the Orient is simultaneously defined and controlled."[25] More to the point of this paper, the yellow peril discourse orders the peoples and phenomena of the Far Eastern "Orient" into a praxiologically constituted modal moral "logic."[26] Doing such, it should be properly understood as a variant formation of race prejudice, as Herbert Blumer describes the institutionalization of that social process, that is, as a positioning of Asians and Asian Americans as members of a single conceptual group or abstract category toward whom there is a collective or shared attitude: "The prejudice is manifested against a specific individual [or aggregate thereof] by identifying the individual [or the members of the aggregate] with the conceptualized object and then directing towards him [or her, or them] the attitude that one [or the few, or the many] has toward the conceptualized object."[27] The attitude, in turn, speaks to the "sense of group position" that the prejudiced person or institution holds with respect to the individual or aggregate under consideration. The positioning is "vertical" in character, expressing adherence to a hierarchy of values and morals and arranging the designated aggregates in accordance with presuppositions about their relation to the latter.[28] In the matter of the yellow peril, the Asian aggregate, or some subsegment of it, for example, the Chinese, the Japanese, the Vietnamese, are feared because the dominant group, or, to be more specific, its spokespersons, leaders, officials, intellectuals, opinion makers, and so forth, believes that the particular element of the Asian aggregate under discussion, "is not keeping to its [appropriately subordinated] place but threatens to claim the opportunities and privileges from which it has been excluded;" even more fearsome is the belief "felt [that the Asian aggregate or its subset is] . . . a threat to the status, security, and welfare of the dominant ethnic group."[29]

Like other norms and imperatives that come to hold sway in a given society or civilization, the sense of vertical racial group positioning is a historical product. It has a documentable beginning—the first throwing of the "loaded dice." Although some students of the origin of the "yellow peril" idea would date its beginnings back to Greco-Persian conflicts in antiquity,[30] it seems better to link its modern appearance to certain statements about "Asia," the "Orient," the "Far East," made by leaders, intellectuals, and prestige bearers in the Occident's Enlightenment era and thereafter. However, as Jonathan D. Spence has recently shown, such significant eighteenth-century figures as Leibniz, Montesquieu, Herder, and Voltaire, each of whom sought to find the key to China's culture, civilization, and future through the study of its language, came to different conclusions.[31] Nevertheless, one idea seemed to be common to their outlook—namely, that China's culture had become petrified and immoveable, and that this set of mores and folkways had become so deeply embedded in the fabric of Chinese society that those who conquer China militarily would nonetheless be overcome and absorbed by its inexorably enveloping culture. So long as China remained, in Herder's words, "an embalmed mummy, wrapped in silk, . . . painted with hieroglyphics . . . [and governed by] unalterably childish institutions,"[32] it would be no threat to the West. But, should the "mummy" awaken, throw off its constraining wrappings, and mount its fire-breathing dragon, it seemed to be implied, there would be great danger to Western Christendom.

China as a Military Threat to America, 1880–1907

The idea of an awakened China was given a particular meaning by Kaiser Wilhelm II in 1895.[33] Forerunners of Kaiser Wilhelm's version of a yellow peril did exist of course; they were to be found in those European fears that arose over the depredations of Genghiz Khan [d. 1227 C.E.] who, after 1189, "made the Mongols the greatest power of central Asia";[34] or in an earlier apprehension over Attila's invasion of Europe, finally brought to a halt in 451 C.E., when a combined force of Romans and Visigoths defeated the Hun king at Chalons-sur-Marne; or even earlier, when the spread of Persian culture seemed to threaten the survival of Greek civilization. As one investigator of it concluded, the "Yellow Peril," as a generalized fear of the nations and states of Asia, has "survived with varying intensity and in different forms, . . . [from] the Middle Ages down until the present day."[35] Before Kaiser Wilhelm made his contribution to this mystique, radicals of the left and the right had offered their own frightening visions. At the Geneva Peace Conference convened in 1871, Mikhail Aleksandrovich Bakunin (1814–1876), often called the "father of anarchism," reportedly presented a variant of the yellow peril thesis to his fellow delegates.[36] A decade later, Arthur de Gobineau (1816–1882), regarded as the "father of modern racism," having taken note of the passage of the Chinese Exclusion Act in the United States, the outcries against Chinese settlement in the Dutch colony of Java, and the fears of an Asiatic invasion then being evoked in Australia, refashioned the yellow peril as what he imagined was a well-grounded fear of the Chinese workingman, asserting that "in all these countries the Chinaman—though far from his native China—has become an object of horror and fear, because people do not know how to answer the industry, applications, persistence and, ultimately, the unparalleled cheapness of his labour," and concluding that "these are the concrete reasons why we now know that the Chinese are to be feared."[37]

However, it was a painting by the German artist H. Knackfuss, commissioned in 1895 by Kaiser Wilhelm II, that called onto center stage the present era's romance with the yellow peril.[38] Kaiser Wilhelm caused the painting to be copied in oils and sent to his fellow European monarchs and to U.S. President William McKinley, thus giving a wide scope to *die gelbe Gefahr.* As described in Richard Austin Thompson's comprehensive examination of the yellow peril theme, Knackfuss's allegorical painting showed:

> . . . high upon a rock in the foreground the nations of Europe, France, Germany, Russia, Austria, England and Italy, . . . depicted as mail-clad Valkyries [united] beneath a sign of a radiant cross. The Archangel . . . stood before them, sword in one hand while pointing with the other towards a horrible spectacle in the East. High in the smoke of the burning cities of Europe a Chinese dragon, symbolic of destruction, emerged bearing a seated Buddha upon its back. Beneath the picture the Kaiser placed the words, "Nations of Europe! Join in Defense of Your Faith and Your Home!"[39]

The painting evoked the need for an Occidental alliance against the threat to Christian civilization supposedly posed by the rising races of the Orient—an alliance that would unite a militarily as well as morally rearmed consortium of Western nation-states against a heathen menace. Although, with the exception of the temporary alliance of Western nations that put down the Boxer uprising (1900),[40] no such alliance was ever cobbled together—and, within less than two decades of the circulation of the Kaiser's call to arms, the nations of Europe would be embroiled in the first of the new century's two internecine global conflicts—the more or less inchoate yellow peril thesis of previous eras had been revitalized in 1895, given a sharpened focus, and introduced into the West's political, cultural, and social life and literature. In the United States it would find its expression not only in public policy but also in virtually every sociocultural venue, genre, and medium in which it could be expressed.

In point of fact, it is important to note that American apprehension over the races and peoples of Asia had arisen before the Kaiser's painting had reached the United States. It focused on both an "awakened" China and on the effects of Chinese immigration to the United States. The "peril" that the Chinese Empire and its nationals overseas allegedly posed was composed out of a collage of fear-inspiring stereotypes. These included a belief that, whether as warriors or immigrants, or, as some would have it, warriors-as-immigrants, Asiatics from the "Middle Kingdom" were "invading" America with an eye to "conquest";[41] moreover, that, as part of the invasion, Chinese arrivals would spread leprosy and other loathsome diseases;[42] induce innocent Americans to smoke opium;[43] undermine moral values through their whoremongering[44] and gambling;[45] and undercut the higher wages and much-needed benefits that, in their absence, would go to white workingmen and women.[46] Of these, only the first-named—the fear of a Sino-American war—began to fade in the decade before 1905, to be replaced by what would become a decades-long apprehension about the military danger to the United States presented by Japan. In the years preceding Japan's victories in the Sino-Japanese (1894–1895) and Russo-Japanese (1904–1905) wars, it was China, its army and its people, that constituted the focal point of America's vision of a military "yellow peril."[47]

The Yellow Peril in Fiction

From 1880 to 1907, tales imagining a Chinese invasion of the United States were a staple of the futurological fiction published in such prominent journals as the *Californian* and *Overland Monthly.* In fact, the scenario presented in the very first of these tales had so mastered the basic idea involved in this burgeoning genre that when, in 1882, Robert Wolter's novel-length work, entitled *A Short and Truthful History of the Taking of California and Oregon by the Chinese in the Year A.D. 1899*[48]—to be discussed further below—appeared, imagining the Chinese navy in control of the entire Pacific coast,[49] a reviewer for the *Californian* observed that it was a poorly written elaboration of an idea that had already been sufficiently developed in an earlier short story by a different writer.[50] Wolter's book neither began nor brought an end to what would later be called the genre of yellow peril literature; it had been preceded by such book-length fictions as H. J. West's *The Chinese Invasion* (1873), in which it was proclaimed, "The Chinese in California are the advance guard of numberless legions that will, if no check is applied, one day overthrow the present Republic of the United States";[51] Atwell Whitney's *Almond-Eyed* (1878), whose plot told how hordes of Chinese immigrants had invaded California, driven white workers and shopkeepers into ruin, and introduced a smallpox epidemic;[52] and Pierton W. Dooner's *Last Days of the Republic* (1880), purporting to describe how Chinese immigration would become the prelude to an invasion, eventually achieving imperial control over the whole of the United States and obliterating America's political, cultural, and moral institutions. But there would be more fictions to come.

And, what would result from the conquest? Dooner spoke for his fellow yellow peril writers when he ended his novel: "[I]n America, the representatives of the one race of man, which, in its relation to the family of men, had borne upon its crest the emblem of sovereign power since the dawn of history, saw now the ancestral diadem plucked from its proud repose, to shed its lustre on an alien crown."[53] Fictional variations on the twin themes of the security of the United States and the Chinese threat to Western civilization would continue through the first decade of the twentieth century, despite the passage and renewal of laws restricting Chinese immigration, a growing number of reports of Manchu military weakness, and widespread belief in the impending disintegration of the Qing empire.[54] Thus, to mention one outstanding example from the later period, Marsden Manson's *The Yellow Peril in Action* (1907),[55] treated its readers once more to a full-scale Sino-American war and to the threat of Western civilization's certain doom.

In addition to the threat of a Chinese invasion, a Chinese immigrant's socioeconomic success in America was also seen as a challenge to Western civilization. Thus, Jack London (1876–1916), whose ideology combined a form of radical socialism with a selectively racialist social Darwinism—one of his colleagues asserted that "Jack stood with one foot planted in the soil of social democracy but the other foot was . . . clogged in the morasses of the philosophical teachings from which have sprung fascism"[56]—penned a short story in which the coolie trade, merchant capitalism, and miscegenation work together to subvert the happiness of the beneficiaries of a Chinese laborer's cunning: "Chun Ah Chun," a laborer impressed into service on a Hawaiian sugar plantation, rises to become a partner in the import business, marries a woman of Polynesian, Italian, Portuguese, English, and white American descent, fathers a dozen daughters, each of whom he marries off to a wealthy white man, and then, as Clarice Stasz summarizes the *denouement* of this oddly plotted tale, Chun "flees to Macao, where he lives his final days in peace, free from the family fighting caused by the corrupting influence of the money his crafty capitalism had earned."[57] In 1904, London had written an article entitled "The Yellow Peril" in which he had wondered, "Why may not the yellow and brown [races] start out on an adventure as tremendous as our own and more strikingly unique?"[58] In a short story published in the same year, he had imagined China's "Unparalleled Invasion" of the United States, brought about, as tenBroek's, Barnhart's, and Matson's *precis* puts it, by apprehensions over "China's mounting population [and fears that it] might soon surpass that of all the rest of the world." Similar to the idea put forward a decade earlier by Kaiser Wilhelm II but more specific and deadly, London proposed not only an anti-Asian alliance by the nations of the Occident, but also a final solution to the problem created by the awakened giant of Asia, namely, that the Western nations engage in a "primitive form of bacteriological warfare against the Chinese"[59] and wipe them out.

Above all other charges heaped on the denizens of China (and of Chinatown)—for example, their alleged "immorality," "treachery," "savagery," and slavish willingness to work for low wages[60]—the "talk of 'yellow hordes' or the 'Yellow Peril' in the period 1885–1915 derived its force from the fact of 400,000,000 Chinese, just as . . . other American ideas concerning China [would, in future years, also derive their] . . . force from the size of the Chinese population."[61] Thus, in Oto Mundo's bizarre science fiction novel, *The Recovered Continent: A Tale of the Chinese Invasion* (1898),[62] in which a mentally retarded white man is restored to rationality and becomes a general leading Chinese armies against the Occident, as the nations of eastern Europe and the eastern Mediterranean succumb before China's invading troops, headlines scream "FOUR HUNDRED MILLION CHINESE ARE POURING LIKE A FLOOD OVER EUROPE!"[63] Later, during the period of post-Qing civil war in China, as well as in the years of Japan's aggressions in Manchuria, Nanjing, and Shanghai, China's millions of people would be reconceptualized in popular American literature more benignly—as "four hundred million customers."[64] Cutthroat or customer, however, the Chinese in China or America were conceived primarily as an "Other," outsiders, foreigners, aliens.

Although the imagery and the scenarios originally developed in yellow peril tales about China would be recycled later as anti-Japanese stories, after the latter nation had become Britain's and America's chief rival in the Pacific, their picture of a threatening China had been firmly established, available for a revival if foreign affairs or domestic difficulties seemed to call for them. Designated as "romances and narratives which may be called the Yellow Peril fiction" in the exhaustive but all-too-neglected investigation carried out by Limin Chu,[65] several of these fictions about China had originally appeared as short stories in the *Overland Monthly,* a journal that in the years 1868–1875 and 1883–1935, "excepting in its last few years, . . . provided month after month, almost without fail, some treatment or mention of China or the Chinese."[66] One of the most developed of these, published in 1880, was penned by an author writing under the nom de plume "Lorelle" and entitled "The Battle of Wabash." It unfolded a futuristic drama whose action took place in the year 2078, by which time the government, society, and culture of the United States, having been overwhelmed by Chinese immigrants and their unacculturated descendants, as well as by miscegenation and its supposedly subversive biocultural effects, had become irrevocably Sinicized. In 2081, seeking a last stand against total Chinese domination, the remaining elements of the white population rise in armed rebellion. Chu provides a pithy summary of the fateful outcome:

> In the fall of 2081, the resident Chinese army, after sacrificing half a million men, succeeded in joining forces with the army of expedition from China in lower Illinois. On November 3, thirteen Chinese columns, massed on a front eleven miles wide, moved against the American positions. While the U.S. troops withstood the frontal assault, their reserves in the rear were pressed back to back against the men in front by a Chinese flanking movement, so that the entire American army was surrounded. At the end of the Battle of Wabash, the Chinese left five million dead or wounded on the field, but the American forces were exterminated, the Republic fell and her people passed into slavery.[67]

"The Battle of Wabash," like the succession of yellow peril fictions about China and the overseas Chinese that preceded and followed it, linked the Qing empire's threat to America's national and cultural security to what its author derisively called "milksop philosophy," that is, the belief that Chinese immigrants to the United States ought to be regarded as "assimilable," that they be not merely tolerated, but encouraged to become U.S. citizens, admitted into the labor force on terms equal to those of whites, allowed to marry across racial and cultural lines, and permitted to procreate offspring who would be treated as full-fledged Americans. In Dooner's aforementioned *Last Days of the Republic,* a novel that appeared in the same year as Lorelle's short story, the same warnings are spelled out. China's supposedly ancient aim at global domination is credited with finding a new but ready starting point in California's gold rush "golden age"; Qing emigrants enter and subtly subvert first California's, then the South's cultural, social, agricultural, and industrial ways of life, obtaining civil rights and political influence through subterfuge and white America's greatest weakness, tolerance. When, at last, the peril is perceived and an armed uprising has begun to halt it, it is too late. "Owing in some degree to the comparatively simple wants of the Asiatic soldier, considered in connection with those of the American, but chiefly to the act of an uninterrupted communication between the army and China, and to the productiveness of the rice fields of the Southern States, the invading army suffered but little inconvenience from the lack of the usual and necessary supply food."[68] Soon, Dooner's cautionary tale concluded, the "character of the war . . . [had become] a slaughter—or more properly a war of extermination . . . The soldiers of the Republic . . . saw . . . the land that their fathers had wrested from the primeval forests and inhospitable wilderness of the New World, and erected into the most glorious, and one among the most powerful, independencies upon the globe—a land whose liberties, whose power, whose wealth, whose enlightenment, were theirs by creation, and which had known no civilization other than their own—saw all this already hurled beneath the tread of the rude conqueror . . . Their loss was irreparable . . . The destruction was complete."[69] Two years after Dooner's work was published, Wolter's *A Short and Truthful History of the Taking of California and Oregon by the Chinese in the Year A.D. 1899* appeared. This novel relocated the place and foreshortened the imminence of the danger, imagining the Chinese seizure of two of the Pacific coastal states to take place a bare seventeen years after the book was published and devoting veritably its entire first half to a one-sided but factual history of Chinese immigration and proposals on how it might be halted.[70] In that same year, Congress enacted the first of what would become six decades of legislation barring the immigration of Chinese laborers and their wives to the United States and denying all Chinese immigrants, regardless of class, the right to naturalization.[71]

Although one short story—Adele F. Battele's "The Sacking of Grubbville,"[72] published a decade after the enactment of the first Chinese Exclusion Act—would appear to have treated the belief that Chinese immigration threatened the United States as nothing more than a product of sensational rumors started or inflamed by dissolute Irish laborers, the publication of William W. Crane's "The Year 1899"[73] in the same journal seven months later not only restored the yellow peril to its older place in American thought but reinvigorated it, as Chu puts it, "with a vengeance."[74] For this tale imagined a Chinese-led Asian confederacy that not only included Japan—until the retreating Chinese army treacherously betrayed its Japanese volunteers, leaving them to die, after which Japan joined with Britain and the United States to punish China—but also recruited and allied itself with African Americans, Puerto Ricans, various Caribbean peoples, and dissident tribes of American Indians. Invaded by sea in the Southern states and by the Chinese navy in the Pacific, the defenders of a white America are able to rout the Negro and Cherokee bands hidden in the swamps. But the "white" forces are not able to defeat the Chinese invaders of the South who have joined with and led the black, brown, and red insurgents in their struggle. Eventually, America and Europe—for the Asiatic confederacy has also fallen on Europe like Genghiz Khan of old—are saved from utter annihilation and given time to regroup and invade China (with a now chastened and pro-Occidental Japan), when internecine fighting breaks out among the Hindus and Moslems, who constitute an important contingent of the allied Asian forces invading Europe, forcing China's leaders to order her troops in America and Europe home for defensive purposes.[75]

Crane's story did much to impugn the credulity of the U.S. State Department, but even more significant is the fact that his tale testified to a gnawing fear among some Americans that the "white republic" (to borrow Alexander Saxton's term for the United States)[76] could be vulnerable to assault by a joint effort mounted by all those who live on the "other" side of the "color line,"[77] and that only the divisions that currently existed among the nonwhites could keep them from forging a unity that might rise up against their Euro-American oppressors. "One of the most serious questions resulting from the Asiatic awakening," wrote Maurice Muret in 1926, "is, whether, as some people assert, there is a growing sentiment of unity and fraternity among those peoples."[78] Muret believed—and hoped—that such an alliance would not be formed, and for the same reason that had been offered in Crane's tale: He cites as a telling fact the less than friendly reception given to the Hindu philosopher, Rabindranath Tagore, by Chinese intellectuals. "No," he observed, "the great fraternity of brown and yellow people in the Orient is not yet founded, that fraternity . . . which is to be the signal for an immense insurrection of all Asia against Europe."[79] Nevertheless, Muret argued that China—then in the midst of both internecine warlord politics and the conflict between the communists and the Kuomintang[80]—needed to be watched: "China is . . . a critical spot in the danger zone of our world. The lust of which she is an object, the anarchy of which she is the example, her complacency toward Bolshevism, her hatred of the West, all constitute serious dangers."[81]

The Chinese Immigrant as a Yellow Peril

Even before his ghettoization in America's Chinatowns, the Chinese male immigrant laborer was imagined to be one more undesirable and unwanted addition to the growing multiethnic American population. His wife and children would also be proscribed after 1882. Chinese were ranked with African and Native Americans, but, with the exception of Crane's fiction,[82] rarely perceived as possible allies in a rebellion of the latter peoples. A cartoon by Thomas Nast, who expressed some sympathy for the Chinese, pictured a Native American "Red Gentleman" telling a "Yellow Gentleman," "Pale face 'fraid you crowd him out, as he did me";[83] another Nast drawing depicted "Columbia" standing guard over an abject and despairing Chinese immigrant while holding back a white mob with the admonition: "Hands off, Gentlemen! America means fair play for all men."[84] But, while Nast would depict Chinese immigrant families, Native Americans, and ex-slaves sitting around a dinner table with friendly whites while all celebrated "Uncle Sam's Thanksgiving Dinner,"[85] and would satirize the Sinophobic slogan in the West, "The Chinese Must Go," by placing it side by side with a cartoon of the Southern view, stating "The Nigger Must Go," subtitling both "The Poor Barbarians Can't Understand Our Civilized Republican Form of Government,"[86] other cartoonists would dwell on such interracial conflicts as those dividing Chinese laundrymen from African American washerwomen,[87] as well as those drawn by G. F. Keller depicting scenes from Dooner's *Last Days of the Republic.*[88] Still others would focus on the moral threat to white American women and children allegedly posed by the Chinese situation of womanlessness, opium addiction, and criminal association.[89] In the latter decades of the nineteenth century, such images were transferred to the stage in the form of minstrel shows and comic sketches that both established and reinforced hostile or humiliating stereotypes. Robert G. Lee, who has conducted an exhaustive examination of these vaudevilles, points out:

> For its audience of urban workers who were being shaped into a working class, the minstrel show constructed and displayed a line-up of racial and ethnic characters. Blacks, Jim Crow, and Zip Coon, Indians and John Chinaman were compared and contrasted with European Americans, Tommy the English sailor, Mose the Irish fireman, Siegal the German. Even as these characters interacted on the stage, the minstrel show drew sharp boundaries around racial difference and made clear the unacceptability of racial amalgamation.[90]

And John Kuo Wei Tchen has shown how these same shows assisted the Irish immigrants in their effort to become "white," while leaving their Chinese fellow immigrants to wallow in the slough of permanent alienage.[91]

Although the image of a militarized China menacing the West faded after 1905, not to be revived until the communist takeover in 1949, apprehensions about the effects of Chinese immigration on the United States would continue, a diminished yellow peril perhaps, but one that argued that the immigrants from the Middle Kingdom threatened basic American institutions and culture. Thus, even if China did not have an army and navy sufficiently well equipped to overcome the armed resistance of American soldiers and sailors, the Qing empire's emigrants might undermine the nation's moral infrastructure. Ambrose Bierce's newspaper, the *Wasp,* trumpeted this theme. In numerous of its ink sketches, the writer/artist warned:

> . . . [I]t is not alone in the field of labor that the evils of the Asiatic interloper are felt. He is the ruin of the household . . . The leering idiotic and immodest attitude of the daughter of the house shows the damning influence of the opium-pipe; the father, driven from employment, despairingly seeks relief in a suicide's death, leaving his widow destitute, famished and despondent; the son, driven to stealing bread for himself and mother, finds himself a felon . . . ; while . . . in a huge manufactory may be seen the cause of all the

> evil in the fact that Chinese are driving the white men from employment, hurling them from the windows and kicking them out of the doors. Surely such a spectacle must stir the blood in the veins of either Saxon or Celt.[92]

An undated cartoon in the *Wasp* countered Nast's image of the ethnically ecumenical Thanksgiving by imagining what a Fourth of July celebration would be like after Chinese hegemony had triumphed:

> . . . [T]he role of subserviency is reversed: one white man sells Chinese newspaper[s] while another is the laundryman; a white barber gives the Chinese a haircut; a white cabby drives for Chinese passengers; and a Chinese policeman is arresting a white pauper.[93]

Still another *Wasp* cartoon, by G. F. Keller, the illustrator of Dooner's novel, dated November 11, 1881, and entitled "A Statue for Our Harbor," was published five years before the Statue of Liberty had been put in place. It showed a "Chinaman" holding an opium pipe in his left hand while the torch in his right lights separate emanations saying "win to," "white," "labor," "diseases," "immorality," and "filth."[94]

The poem that would fasten the most infamous image onto the Chinese in America, Bret Harte's "Plain Language from Truthful James," popularly known as "The Heathen Chinee," was penned by a writer who not only served as the *Overland Monthly*'s first editor, but also supported the civil rights of Chinese immigrants and wrote scathing editorials attacking their Sinophobic enemies.[95] Nevertheless, despite Harte's persistent denials, authorship of other stories in which Chinese characters are portrayed sympathetically, and his claim that others had read much more than he intended into the poem,[96] it was quoted often, its central character "Ah Sin" became the representative figure of the Chinese immigrant, and its never-to-be-forgotten refrain—

> Which is why I remark,
>   And my language is plain,
> That for ways that are dark
>   And for tricks that are vain
> That heathen Chinee is peculiar,
>   Which the same I am free to maintain[97]

—became a standard part of popular American Sinophobic literature.

Republished in 1900, the poem failed to halt the decline of China's standing as America's yellow peril enemy in the Far East, a descent that had begun when Japan whipped China in the Sino-Japanese War (1894–1895), and would be reinforced after the combined forces of Europe and America put down the Boxer uprising. Although the militant martial artists called "Boxers" had laid siege to the foreign legations in the Chinese capital for fifty-five days, after their ignominious defeat, the popular image of the Chinese shifted downward rapidly, from a people feared and despised to one laughed at and pitied.[98] No longer would "Chang, the Chinese giant"—a victim of acromegaly, billed as "standing nearly 9 feet high . . . combin[ing] the Strength of Hercules and the beauty of an Apollo"[99]—serve as a symbolic reminder of China's monstrous strength and its people's overdeveloped virility. Although American cartoonists had once drawn "boxers as giants breaking from their chains . . . , chas[ing] westerners through the streets ready to kill them with long knives," once they had been routed by the Western forces, the Chinese masters of kung-fu no longer appeared as hulking brutes of Oriental occult strength. "The ultimate humiliation," observes Jonathan G. Utley, "is shown in a cartoon where the powers use his [i.e., the Chinese boxer's] queue as a clothesline on which they hung their flags."[100] By the time, nineteen years later, when the gentle-looking Richard Barthelmess (1895–1963) would portray "'Cheng Huan,' the 'Yellow Man'" in D. W. Griffith's film, *Broken Blossoms,* Americans had become prepared to see a Chinese man looking and acting slight and effete, and spouting a mix of Confucian and Christian philosophy, engaging in a vain attempt to rescue a young white girl (Lillian Gish) from her cruel and sadistic father (Donald Crisp). The Chinese variant of the yellow peril had become softer. Except for the global machinations of Sax Rohmer's fictional villain, Fu Manchu, whose international all-Asian force threatened to overwhelm the West,[101] America's Chinatowns, rather than the shores of the California coast, would become the dreaded place for that people's far more local crimes and community-based cunning. As Robert McClellan has pointed out, "The attitude toward China expressed at the turn of the century was formed out of the needs of American ethnocentrism rather than by the realities of the situation in the Far East."[102] Those needs had changed—and they would change again.

A New Yellow Peril: Japan

"Prejudice against the Japanese," observe Robert F. Heizer and Alan F. Almquist, "sprouted in the rich soil that had nourished anti-Chinese attitudes shortly before."[103] Like the Chinese, Japanese immigrants to America were perceived in both anthropological literature and public law as "Orientals," "Asiatics," "Mongolians," or "people of the yellow race,"[104] but, after Japan's emergence as a formidable power in Asia and the one nation threatening America's and Britain's designs on a Pacific hegemony, they appeared far more menacing.[105] *Organized Labor,* a San Francisco journal that in 1900 had argued that "the sniveling Japanese, who swarms along the streets and cringingly offers his paltry services for a suit of clothes and a front seat in our public schools, is a far greater danger to the laboring portion of society than all the opium-soaked pigtails who have ever blotted the fair name of this beautiful city,"[106] had, in effect, set forth one of the main themes that would find literary and political expression as the Japanese variant of a yellow peril threat to the United States. Five years later, however, the same journal warned its readers of a more formidable challenge:

> A characteristic among Japanese . . . is their propensity for spying . . . Put a huge roof over the Japanese Empire, and you have a national Japanese detective agency, with which there is nothing to compare in the rest of the world . . . Their spying has been done long ago about this country, and more particularly so, California, and the results are shown now. Japan intends to make California its Manchurian fields.[107]

The *San Francisco Chronicle* reiterated the accusation one year later, combining it with the charge of unassimilability: "The Japanese who come here remain Japanese . . . Every one of them, so far as his service is desired, is a Japanese spy."[108] Of course, older and in some cases less vicious images of the Japanese were available when events in the real world called for their presentation. As Earl Miner would point out in 1958, the "stock stage types of the 'Jolly Jap,' the unbelievably refined or intrepid Japanese, and the cruel Oriental have lived on in plays, motion pictures, and comic strips in spite of the more mature understanding of Japan which has been gained in recent years."[109] But, the idea that Japanese presentations of themselves to white Americans were, in fact, calculated deceptions, crafted by an aggressive people who plotted nefarious schemes behind an impenetrable facial mask,[110] seemed to predominate over all others,[111] especially as the Japanese empire competed for prestige and power in the Pacific region with Britain and the United States,[112] and as Japanese immigrants seemed to thrive in their small-scale agricultural, shopkeeping, labor-organizing, and educational pursuits in Hawaii,[113] California,[114] and other parts of the American West.[115] It would be no less than one of the foremost sociological authorities on race relations in general and Asian Americans in particular, Robert E. Park (1864–1944), who would observe in 1913, that "the Japanese . . . is condemned to remain among us an abstraction, a symbol, and a symbol not merely of his own race, but of the Orient and of that vague, ill-defined menace we sometimes refer to as the 'yellow peril.'"[116]

The Russo-Japanese War (1904–1905) seems to have been the final as well as the single most important factor in the shift of *fin de siècle* America's version of yellow peril fears from China to Japan. This is truly ironic since Japan's Cabinet Resolution of December 30, 1903, took account of such Occidental fears, imagining them to be primarily European in origin, and sought to allay them:

> The doctrine of the "yellow peril" [the official resolution stated] is not too prominent a concern among white people nowadays, but it still persists among some Europeans. There is a risk that it might readily return and induce them to rally together to this far-fetched notion. If, therefore, Japan and China were to join together in any war against Russia, the anxiety over the "yellow peril" might recur and persuade Germany, France and other countries to intervene.[117]

However, it was the American response that proved to be crucial. President Theodore Roosevelt, who brokered the Treaty of Portsmouth ending that war, seemed to have encouraged Japanese imperialism on the Asian mainland so long as China remained an object of the "Open Door" policy and Japan did not expand any further in the Pacific. However, in later years it would be the "Japanese [nation and the *Issei* in California who] bore the burden of all the conventional misconceptions about Orientals entertained by Americans." The immigrants "were criticized for likening their emperor to a god; [moreover,] there were rumors that Japanese aliens working at United States army bases were gaining knowledge of fortifications which they transferred back to Japan; [and, to make matters even worse,] the Japanese were even accused of crowding American children out of schools."[118] In the years immediately following the settlement of the Russo-Japanese War, one war-threatening crisis after another—for example, the enforced segregation of Japanese schoolchildren in San Francisco's public schools; the riots against *Issei*-owned businesses in the same city; the rumor that Japan was rebuilding its military forces in order to dislodge the United States from its holdings in Hawaii, the Philippines, and Guam; and the belief that Japanese immigrants to Mexico and Canada were a disguised military force planning the invasion of the United States[119]—arose to trouble American-Japanese relations.

In November 1906, *Harper's Weekly* editorialized:

> Japan is at this moment the strongest naval power in the Pacific . . . In a word, rich as we are, and poor as she is, we could not afford to go to war with Japan, for in the Philippines, in Hawaii, and on our Pacific Coast, we are vulnerable.[120]

That vulnerability was made even more palpable three years later with the publication of *The Valor of Ignorance* by Homer Lea (1876–1912), a self-styled military analyst, and, later, a military advisor to Sun Yat-sen.[121] Lea proclaimed a

> law that the boundaries of nations are never, other than momentarily, at rest; and [he went on to observe] that there are two phases to this state of agitation,

> expansion or shrinkage. Expansion of a nation's boundaries is indicative, not only of its external growth, but of the virility of its internal constitution; the shrinkage of its boundaries, the external exemplification of its internal decay.[122]

The "virility" of a nation's "internal constitution" turned, Lea would insist, on its maintenance of a monoracial population. "Homogeneity of race," he claimed, "has been recognized as an invariable principle in determining the stability of national institutions."[123] And from this theorem it followed that the "deterioration of a political entity subject to the diversity of its constituent elements, is slow or rapid in proportion to the fractional facets of its racial heterogeneity."[124] As Lea saw the matter, "Should Germany . . . and Japan . . . continue to adhere rigorously to these laws [and their corollaries], resisting the deteriorating influence of industrialism, feminism, and political quackery, they will, in due time, by the erosive action of these elements on other nations, divide the world between them."[125] With Japan's defeat of China in 1894–1895, of Russia a decade later, and the neutralization of England achieved by the Anglo-Japanese Pact (1902), Lea insisted that only the nation formed out of the heterogeneous population of the United States stood in the way of racially homogeneous Japan's imperial advance.[126]

Lea believed that America's multiethnic and multiracial population was a recent development, that until "the time of the Civil War the American could be considered a homogeneous people."[127] He pointed out that although at "the beginning of the Civil War the foreign non-Anglo-Saxon element was less than one-twelfth of the population, . . . [by the turn of the new century,] the Anglo-Saxon homogeneity . . . had declined to less than seven-twelfths . . . and [s]ince that time this declination . . . has gone on at even greater speed."[128] In many of the states of the former Confederacy, he noted, "the negro outnumbers the white in inhabitants, while in most of the other states in the South they exceed one-third of the population."[129] Nor were matters much better above the Mason-Dixon divide: "In the Northern States ninety-four per cent of the European immigrants become domiciled, and at the present time there are in this country over thirty million persons of foreign parentage."[130] And, if these statistics were not enough to warn white Anglo-Saxon Americans of the danger they faced, Lea added, "Should the present rate of immigration continue, it is only a question of a few years when the voting majorities in all [of America's] great cities will be foreign."[131] In those great cities, Lea warned, "are to be found, more or less entire, those human factors that determine the course of nations within whose boundaries they are placed."[132]

But nothing mattered more to Lea's estimate of America's vulnerability than the fact that Japan—to him the true representative of the yellow peril[133]—was sending more and more of its immigrants to live and work near military installations in Hawaii and along the Pacific Coast.[134] In fact, he argued, the immigrants who had settled in Hawaii since 1900—many of them alleged to be hardened veterans of Japan's recent victories over China and Russia—had already rendered "the military occupation of Hawaii tentatively accomplished."[135] Thus, with Hawaii already lost, if the United States wished to avoid the situation created by its too liberal immigration policies and its lack of preparedness for the inevitable war with Japan—to prevent, that is, the time when "this heterogeneous Republic . . . shall disintegrate, . . . [falling] into the palm of re-established monarchy . . . [and, by that fact, paying] the toll of its vanity and its scorn"[136]—it would have to recognize that the "principal consideration that now concerns this Republic is the defense of the Pacific coast."[137] Like Wolter and Dooner before him, but with Japan rather than China designated as the source of the peril from the East, Lea believed that "primarily, the defence of the Pacific coast belong[s] to a navy."[138] To this end, he laid out the strategy and tactics appropriate to holding back the onslaught from Japan that he was sure was coming.[139]

Seven years after Lea's sensational book was published, George Bronson Rea, editor of the prestigious *Far Eastern Review,* issued a pamphlet entitled "Japan's Place in the Sun—The Menace to America," a work so provocative that Toyokichi Iyenaga, professorial lecturer in political science at the University of Chicago, edited an entire volume of replies to its arguments.[140] Fortified by *feuilletons* by such white Americans of prominence as J. I. C. Clarke, Sidney Gulick, R. B. Teusler, and Russell Dilkes, and supported by two editorial letters composed by Japanese scholar C. Ohira, Iyenaga sought—in vain as it turned out—to allay the apprehensions about Japan's danger to the United States that Rea had set forth. Although he did not shrink from criticizing California's enactment in 1913 of an Alien Land Law ("We consider this as in violation of the treaty existing between us"),[141] Iyenaga denied that this would become a "cause for war."[142] Furthermore, he held that the "Pacific is broad enough to accommodate without jostling all the navies and merchant fleets of both nations on its opposite shores."[143] But, he did insist that the United States recognize and acquiesce to Japan's "most vital political interests in China,"[144] a nation, he claimed, for which Japan zealously seeks "regeneration."[145] As for Rea's charges—namely, that Japan "regards the United States as her future enemy; that she is secretly and heavily arming for the contingency; that [Japanese in America] are acting as agents to conceal with malicious intent from American eyes actual facts about Japan and thus proving, while loyal to our native country traitors to the country wherein we now reside"—Iyenaga dismissed the entire body of these charges as but the products of press-promoted propaganda about a "yellow peril." Japan, he argued, ought to be regarded as a nation that, since the turn of the century, has been rightfully "entitled . . . to rank among the first-rate Powers."[146] Iyenaga scorned the vulgar characterization of Japan that were to be found in popular journals, and retorted, "It is indeed a strange coincidence that the royal painter, [i.e., Kaiser Wilhelm II], who drew for the first time a picture of a 'yellow peril' for the edification of the Russian monarch, is the same ruler who is now deluging Europe with blood." And he pointed to the "fact that the world has not yet seen any 'yellow peril' materialize except in yellow journalism!"[147]

However, not all spokespersons for Japan were as optimistic as Iyenaga, who counted on American forbearance and Japan's "deep conviction that America's greatness rests upon her sense of justice, fairness, and humanity."[148] The views of two contemporaries of Iyenaga—Iichiro Tokutomi and K. K. Kawakami—will suffice to illustrate a less sanguine and more truculent outlook on Japanese-American relations: Tokutomi, a member of Japan's House of Peers and editor-in-chief of the *Kokumin-Shimbun,* having examined the several outstanding issues affecting relations between Japan and the United States, appraised America's attitudes toward Japan, and traced the historical relations between the two nations, turned his critical pen on such then-current sources of tension as the racially restrictive U.S. immigration policy, the recently enacted Alien Land Law, and the as-yet-unresolved disputes over the "Shantung Question," Japan's annexation of Korea, and various Russo-Japanese border disputes. Japan, Tokutomi believed, had already conceded too often and too much to the United States. "How can we be optimistic?" he inquired and answered his own question:

> We do not know what more our country can hereafter concede to America . . . When she said the Japanese immigrants were troublesome, our country put a stop to emigration by making the "Gentlemen's Agreement." When she complained about "picture marriages," our country had them discontinued. It is true that our special position in Manchuria was recognized by America, but in order to participate in the consortium initiated by America for the benefit of China, we have abandoned the greater part of our rights in Manchuria and Mongolia . . . Rarely did we make any protests . . . In short, our guiding principle has been to make concessions, whereas America's principle is "high pressure." So far, this has been the course of events between the two countries.[149]

And, Tokutomi concluded, "We must say that the outlook for the relations between Japan and America can never be so optimistic as [either] the pro-American or the pro-Japanese claim."[150]

K. K. Kawakami, a Japanese publicist residing in the United States, who wrote a number of books on aspects of the Japanese question and international relations from the 1910s through the 1930s, had begun his journalistic career as an avowed socialist (e.g., "Asia's deliverance from the Occident lies in its employment of much the same method as has been employed by labor in its deliverance from its bondage to capital").[151] By 1921, however, he had become a proponent of what would become an "island-for-peace" proposal by which one or another of the Occidental colonial powers would be encouraged to give over to Japan one of its possessions in the Pacific,[152] helping in this way to solve the excess population problem that, supposedly, was driving Japan's new aggressiveness. ("It is obvious that the great Powers of the West have accumulated more land than they should rightly own—than they can hold without doing injustice to the smaller nations, which find themselves in sad plight, due to the impossibility of finding room for their surplus population.")[153] Eleven years later, Kawakami, having become the Washington, D.C., correspondent for the *Tokyo Hochi Shimbun,* published a book-length *apologia* for what had become the new Sino-Japanese crisis. To an introduction by Tsuyoshi Inukai, prime minister of Japan ("Japan is not imperialistic. She is not activated by land lust. All that the Japanese desire in Manchuria is to live and toil peacefully and harmoniously with other peoples. Only when that privilege, to which we are fully entitled by treaty and by the great sacrifice we had made for China, was persistently denied us through thirty years' deliberate policy of obstruction and exclusion did we resort to an armed intervention which seemed the only means to cut the Gordian knot"),[154] and his *tu quoque* justification for Japan's intervention in Manchuria ("Japanese expansion in Manchuria is far more defensible than American expansion in the Caribbean and in Central America"),[155] Kawakami did add a rebuke for Japan's ill-timed move on Shanghai ("Whatever the official explanation, whatever the extenuating circumstances, Japan's single-handed intervention in the Shanghai area is a blunder of the first magnitude").[156] If Kawakami thought his reasoning would calm American anger over Japan's policies, he was sadly mistaken. One year later his *Manchouko: Child of Conflict* would be published in the United States. A sequel to the previous year's volume, this book would explain, indeed it would celebrate, what the author called "one of the most significant developments in the present century—a great experiment in the reorganization, regeneration and rejuvenation of an ancient nation long wallowing in chaos and maladministration so serious as to have become a menace to her neighbors."[157] Thus, reminiscent of, and perhaps derived from, Japan's post–Sino-Japanese War propaganda and popular anti-Chinese songs, he treated the Chinese and Manchurian peoples as backward, cowardly, contemptible or, perhaps pitiable, and as unworthy heirs of a once-great tradition that Japan could restore.[158] However, neither such apologies nor justifications would turn many Americans away from their belief that Japan as well as the Japanese immigrants in the United States[159] represented a danger to Western civilization in general and to American moral, cultural, and military security in particular.[160]

Visions like those of Lea and Rea, insisting that Japan and the overseas Japanese threatened the national security of the United States, would continue to be a feature of both policy debate and popular culture in America during the first five decades of the twentieth century. So pervasive was this outlook that Jesse Frederick Steiner's sociological study of Japanese immigration to the United States, released in 1917, was entitled *The Japanese Invasion.*[161] It included a chapter on "The Japanese 'Menace,'" whose inverted commas over the tendentious word were not matched by a thoroughgoing critique of its connotations.[162] In some ways, Steiner's book echoed but softened the anti-Asian attitude adopted by the more truculent sociologist Edward Alsworth Ross (1866–1951), who, in 1900, had ended his address to a mass meeting of white workers with the recommendation that "should the worst come to the worst, it would be better for us if we were to turn our guns upon every vessel bringing Japanese to our shore rather than permit them to land."[163] With words like these the seeds of hostility toward Japan and its emigrants would be planted so deep in America's sociopolitical soil as to assure their flowering at a later date. Although Professor Steiner acknowledged, in what must be regarded as a remarkably ambiguous manner, that the "Japanese problem was a matter of race prejudice compounded by economic as well as cultural differences"—and, in a later article, urged granting the opportunity to acquire U.S. citizenship to the *Issei*[164]—he nevertheless chastised his fellow Americans for not recognizing what he regarded as the reality of a genuine yellow peril: "We seem to lose sight of the fact that the few thousand Orientals in our country are but the vanguard of many millions in Asia who are eagerly awaiting the chance to cross the Pacific"; and he predicted, "When this oriental horde reaches America it is inevitable that the situation should be [even] further complicated by the factor of racial prejudice."[165]

Throughout the 1920s and 1930s, Lea's fears about Hawaii and the west coast's Japanese were given both widespread publicity and intensive and sometimes secret policy considerations not only in the American territory but throughout the area of the Pacific rim. John S. Chambers, writing in 1921 in his capacity as state controller in California, warned that "the Japanese in Hawaii today would hold political control if the Islands had statehood"; moreover, he asserted, in California the *Issei* and their American-born offspring had adopted a policy of "peaceful penetration" of the state's arable lands that would result "in time, . . . [in] the dispossession of the whites in such areas."[166] Royal D. Mead, former secretary of the Hawaiian Sugar Planters' Association, seeking to replace union-oriented and strike-prone Japanese field workers[167] with what he supposed would be the more tractable Chinese, testified before a congressional committee that the Japanese were not only unassimilable ("Without doubt, as a race, the absolute coherence and solidarity of the Japanese is marvelous,") but also a threat to national security, a fact with which "we have to contend . . . from a military standpoint."[168]

A few years later, the "military standpoint" was extended beyond Lea's naval perspective—despite, or perhaps because of the inadequacy of the several Anglo-American-Japanese capital-ships agreements[169]—by the recognition that a lead in air power and the island or carrier bases from which bombers and fighters could be launched might make all the difference in a war fought in the Pacific. According to Colonel Warren Jefferson Davis, by the mid-1920s Japan had become both the "Gibraltar" and the "air menace of the Pacific" because of its control over numerous strategic island bases and its coordinated build-up of its own army and navy forces.[170] However, Davis went on to warn America that not only was its military unpreparedness a veritable invitation to an air attack by Japanese planes—("Our coast defences from the Pacific to Alaska are woefully deficient, and at best would offer only a limited protection to the few fortified spots, and this protection does not extend to the air")[171]—but also that its own resident alien population constituted an equally serious threat—("We have been over-run with a great mass of immigrants, who have not desired to be assimilated, and who will not subscribe to citizenship; who live apart in our crowded centers of population, and are spreading their insidious and poisonous doctrines throughout the country, protesting against military training in our schools, and by their very action are trying to overthrow our Government").[172] Although his comments on America's immigrant population did not single out the Japanese, in other parts of his book Davis made it clear that their "racial pugnacity"[173] made them the source of the nation's peril: "The Japanese are trained from infancy to glorify war. They are peace loving in their homes but daring and desperate fighters in the field and they are not restrained by the more humanizing and benevolent emotions which often quite dominate America's policy."[174]

The combination of themes that had arisen from the writings and speeches of Lea, Rea, the Hawaiian and Californian Japanophobes, and such military experts as Davis, were given added support by the publication in 1924 of a futuristic novel, *The Great Pacific War,* by Hector C. Bywater (1884–1940),[175] a leading authority on naval warfare. Reminiscent of the early Sinophobic invasion fantasies, but containing much more strategic detail, and, later, said to have influenced both American plans for an island-hopping strategy in the Pacific and Admiral Isoroku Yamamoto's idea for the attack on Pearl Harbor on December 7, 1941,[176] Bywater set forth a tale of an American war with Japan that would break out in January 1931 and end with an American victory of sorts—(". . . the great conflict of which the salient phases are described in the foregoing paper has proved, in its material aspects at least, scarcely less disastrous to victors than to vanquished")[177]—in March 1933. In his preface, the author, apparently unaware of earlier fantasies with yellow peril invasion motifs, claims, "to the best of my knowledge, this book constitutes the first attempt that has been made to forecast the progress of a future naval war in the Pacific from a Western point of view."[178]

By 1934, Japan, as John E. Orchard pointed out, "stands isolated, condemned by world opinion, withdrawn from the League of Nations, feared as a menace to the peace of the world."[179] Carl Crow, a writer sympathetic to China, had published *Japan and America* eighteen years earlier, laying out a succinct summary of the grievances that divided Japan and America, as well as a forceful description of the many ways that Japan threatened the United States. Insisting that Japan's economic woes and the absence of a true democracy were sufficient to prevent its leaders from embarking on a war with the United States, Crow concluded, "Japan is a menace, not only to the United States but to all Western civilization, but our protection is found in the inherent weakness of the Japanese state."[180] However, by the 1930s neither American military strategists nor the purveyors of popular culture felt they could count on a weak Japan to help them. In strategy and story each took up matters of military preparedness and counterespionage, the latter directed at the Japanese in Hawaii and on the Pacific coast. America's turn-of-the-century acquisitions in the Pacific—Hawaii, American Samoa, and Guam—had, from their initial occupation by the United States, been perceived in terms of military strategy and national security. Guam remained under the control of the United States Navy from 1898 to 1941 but had not been sufficiently fortified to prevent its conquest by Japan after that year. A number of military projects were undertaken at Tutuila, American Samoa, in the 1930s.[181] Hawaii became America's naval center for any future war operations in the Pacific.[182] Fears about the Japanese living on the west coast led the FBI to conduct a clandestine "cointelpro" operation in the Little Tokyos of California, Oregon, and Washington through much of the decade of the 1930s.[183] When, on December 7, 1941, Japan's carrier-based planes bombed Pearl Harbor in Hawaii,[184] despite "the conclusion of the Army's board of inquiry that there was 'no single instance of sabotage' and 'in no case was there any instance of misbehavior' on the part of Hawaii's Japanese, Secretary of the Navy Frank Knox told the press in mid-December that Pearl Harbor resulted from 'the most effective fifth column work that's come out of this war, except in Norway.'"[185] Plans, some already made, for the surveillance of, and projects for the incarceration of Japanese Americans, were soon underway.[186] The belief that the yellow peril enemy must carry out its insidious plans in stealth—employing sneak attacks whenever possible, utilizing cleverly disguised espionage, and, at all times, exploiting both its overseas nationals and their American-born offspring as advance agents—had triumphed over what an investigation of the actual situation might have shown.[187]

On February 14, 1942, Lieutenant General John L. DeWitt, appointed military commander of the Pacific coast area of the United States, included in justification for his request for extraordinary authority over California's, Oregon's, and Washington's civilian population, what is perhaps, the most succinct summary of a racially based anti-Japanese variant of the yellow peril:

> In the war in which we are engaged racial affinities are not severed by migration. The Japanese race is an enemy race and while many second and third generation Japanese, born on United States soil, possessed of United States citizenship, have become "Americanized," the racial strains are undiluted . . . It, therefore, follows that along the vital Pacific Coast over 112,000 potential enemies, of Japanese extraction, are at large today.[188]

And, as is well known and needs little further discussion here,[189] armed with the authority of Executive Order 9066,[190] and, in 1943 and 1944, given approval by the United States Supreme Court,[191] General DeWitt saw to it that 120,000 persons of Japanese descent, residing along the Pacific coast, were not only evacuated from the Pacific coast but imprisoned, for from two to five years, without a trial, in specially constructed camps, for the most part located in remote and desolate areas of the American interior.[192] In addition, a considerable number of *Nisei* were persuaded to foreswear their United States citizenship and were deported to Japan, only regaining their lost naturalization after years of litigation.[193] Peruvian Japanese were in effect kidnapped from their South American home country, imprisoned in Texas, and, with only rare exception, deported, against their will, to Japan after the war had ended.[194]

The U.S. military's official attitude toward Japanese American men of age to serve in the armed forces indicates both race-based ambivalence and a suspicion about their loyalty. Denied enlistment in the days immediately following Japan's attack on Pearl Harbor, Japanese American men were later formed into segregated units—(the 442nd Regimental Combat Team,[195] the 100th Infantry Battalion,[196] and the 1800th Engineer General Service Battalion);[197] a few were enlisted into a special military intelligence unit (MIS);[198] a small number helped to prepare the secret but-never-put-into-operation plans for invading Taiwan;[199] several thousand served in the Pacific, many in General

Joseph W. Stilwell's nonsegregated units stationed on the China-Burma-India front;[200] and another group—called the "derelicts of Company K" by their sociologist-biographer—were so demoralized that their commander saw to it that they never left the United States.[201] When, in 1944, a military draft was instituted together with further loyalty tests for those in the so-called relocation centers, seventy-five *Nisei* in the camp at Heart Mountain, Wyoming, resisted complying with the War Relocation Authority and were imprisoned, to be pardoned by President Truman only in the war's aftermath.[202] A loyalty-security program, employing a questionnaire and arousing considerable feelings of distrust, resentment, and insecurity among the *Issei, Nisei,* and *Kibei,* was implemented in what were at first called "concentration camps," resulting in a further segregation of the "loyal" from the "disloyal."[203] In 1947, the historian Henry Steele Commager observed, "It is sobering to recall that though the Japanese relocation . . . was justified to us on the ground that the Japanese were potentially disloyal, the record does not disclose a single case of Japanese disloyalty or sabotage during the whole war."[204] The myth of Japanese American perfidy had needed no facts to buttress the draconian actions taken by the government of the United States.

Forty-six years later, in 1988, when Congress debated whether the survivors of the incarceration incident were owed both an apology and a monetary compensation, opponents of the measure—which eventually passed and was signed by the president—argued that Japan should be made to compensate the families of those killed in the bombing of Pearl Harbor, causing *Nisei* senator Spark Matsunaga to point out that the proposal "presumes that we Americans of Japanese ancestry had something to do with the bombing of Pearl Harbor. That is absolutely false . . . The amendment . . . would obscure this distinction [between Japanese and Japanese Americans] by denying compensation to Americans for what the Japanese Government did at Pearl Harbor."[205] In the course of his speech, Senator Matsunaga took note of the fact that "a stigma has haunted Japanese-Americans for the past 45 years. We are seeking Congressional action to remove that cloud over their heads."[206] But for some, the stigma had not been lifted by the passage of the redress bill. When, for example, in September 1999, a proposal was made to erect a historical marker at the place that had served as an internment camp for Japanese Americans near Santa Fe, New Mexico, a survivor of the Bataan Death March objected: "They're not showing very much respect . . . to these guys who took the brunt of it. The Japanese [American men imprisoned in Santa Fe] lived a great life . . . and I don't think they should be glorified."[207]

The Japanese Farmer as a Yellow Peril

However, as was the case with the original Sinophobic yellow peril argument, the package of Japanophobic fears and apprehensions included a domestic component—namely, white growers' opposition to the "unfair" competition posed by Japanese vegetable farmers. Major support for the evacuation of Japanese Americans residing on the Pacific coast had come from associations of white grower-shippers, especially strong in California.[208] Austin Anson, managing secretary of one of these associations, complained to a reporter for the *Saturday Evening Post* about the situation in the Salinas valley:

> We're charged with wanting to get rid of the Japs for selfish reasons. We might as well be honest. We do. It's a question of whether the white man lives on the Pacific Coast or the brown men. They came into this valley to work, and they stayed to take over. They offer higher prices and higher rents than the white man can pay for land. They undersell the white man in the markets. They can do this because they raise their own labor. They work their women and children while the white farmer has to pay wages for his help. If all the Japs were removed tomorrow, we'd never miss them in two weeks, because the white farmers can take over and produce everything the Jap grows. And we don't want them back when the war ends either.[209]

But, while Pacific coast journalists vented their anger at Japanese Americans —(e.g., "I am for the immediate removal of every Japanese on the West Coast to a point deep in the interior," thundered Henry McLemore in the *San Francisco Examiner.* "I don't mean a nice part of the interior either. Herd 'em up, pack 'em off, and give 'em the inside room in the badlands . . . Personally, I hate the Japanese. And that goes for all of them.")[210]—Herbert B. Maw, the governor of Utah, saw in their exile from California, Oregon, and Washington an opportunity to obtain a labor force at no cost to his state. However, his request that the federal government hand over 10,000 to 20,000 evacuated Japanese, and provide a subsidy to pay for the guards necessary to keep watch over them, ensure their labor, and remove them from Utah when the war was over, was rejected by officials in Washington, D.C.[211] Chase Clark, the governor of Idaho, was also worried about whether, because of the war, his state would be forced to receive a population of undesirables: The Japanese, he explained, "live like rats, breed like rats, and act like rats. We don't want them becoming permanently located in our state."[212] From 1942 until 1945, and in some cases even longer,[213] the Japanese along the Pacific coast were uprooted from their homes, jobs, and schools and impounded—a people not wanted.

All these, together with those who were not imprisoned—Japanese already settled in the midwest or eastern parts of the United States; *Nisei* and *Sansei* serving in the armed forces; and the persons recently designated as belonging to the "new categories of eligibility" for redress—(i.e., children of parents who were excluded from the Pacific coast but not incarcerated; children born to mothers who left the camps and then reentered them; children born to mothers who left the camps in order to be near their husbands in the armed forces; children of Japanese who volunteered or were ordered to teach the Japanese language in the Naval Language School at Boulder, Colorado; children of Japanese repatriated to Japan in 1942 and 1943;[214] Japanese Americans deprived of education, job, and the ordinary amenities of life by the military's drawing of the exclusion boundary down the middle of the main streets of Phoenix and Glendale, Arizona; Japanese American railroad and mining employees working outside the exclusion areas, but fired and abandoned at the sites of their jobs; Americans of Japanese ancestry residing in Hawaii who suffered racial discrimination during the war; and Latin Americans of Japanese descent who were kidnapped, impounded, and in many cases, deported to Japan.)[215]—are, in their sheer humanity and socioeconomic, cultural, and national diversity, proofs of how the racist sophistry of the yellow peril can impact destructively on the ordinary lives of disparate individuals.

The Yellow Peril after 1945: The Reemergence of China

In the course of the nearly five and one-half decades since the Second World War has ended—except for a brief period in the 1970s and early 1980s when an expanding Japanese economy and a very large U.S.-Japan trade imbalance[216] reawakened fierce Japanophobic passions that had seemed to have been repressed for good by the atomic bombs that fell on Hiroshima and Nagasaki,[217] or which only occasionally emerged from their slumberous state on annual anniversaries of the bombing of Pearl Harbor[218]—China, or, rather, the Peoples Republic thereof, has been moved into that place in the pantheon of U.S.-threatening yellow peril nations. The wars that the United States fought in Korea[219] and Vietnam[220] were in one sense surrogative conflicts, that is, aggressions and counter-aggressions pitting the evils, committed or anticipated, by the USSR—sometimes thought of as a non-European, even Oriental, empire—and Mao's China against America's emergent status not merely as the single most important world power, but also, as the global defender of Western democracy.[221]

Unlike American Japanophobia, which tended to organize itself around either fears of invasion, worries about California's farmlands and fisheries, or apprehensions about an "unfair" trade war, today's Sinophobia is caught up in the unresolved questions about U.S.-China trade—whether commerce should be linked to China's record on human rights and to suspicions about the aggressive aims of the People's Republic.[222] With China's recovery of Hong Kong from Britain,[223] Macao from Portugal,[224] and continuing pressure for the restoration of its sovereignty over Taiwan,[225] "Chinese influence," in the words of Robert D. Kaplan, "is seeping into more and more of Asia."[226] Further, both China and Taiwan have established footholds on the Panama Canal, no longer a possession of the United States, [227] and an arena long held to be of strategic importance to the West. With the firing and subsequent arrest of Wen Ho Lee, whose indictment accused him of acting "with intent to secure an advantage to a foreign nation,"[228] the elements of a revived yellow peril imagery found a point of focus. Since then, it has been reported, both scholars and students from China are finding it more difficult to obtain visas for entry into American universities and colleges. Allegedly, these intellectuals and postgraduate scholars are potential risks to America's national security,[229] while new revelations about Chinese being smuggled into the United States via Hong Kong are alleged to herald "a new and troubling trend."[230]

Missions, Markets, and Marxism: Awakening America to the Chinese Dragon

So long as China appears to beckon to America with a promise of 400,000,000 or more customers, docile but hard-working people who will also be willing converts to both free-market commerce and faith-driven Christianity,[231] the threat of its people, culture, and armaments to the security of the United States is lowered. However, since the 1920s, a falling off of missionary endeavor and the rise of both nationalism and communism have undermined the earlier sanguine outlook. Pearl S. Buck (1892–1973), born to missionary parents and a missionary herself until conditions in China led to her outspoken critique of the West's default on its humanitarian obligations,[232] had, by the early 1930s, worried over the future of Protestantism in Asia:

> How much will remain of Christianity in the future of the Far East it is impossible to tell . . . There is in the Orient as in the Occident a genuine spiritual hunger . . . In the midst of eager, experimental youth the Christian Church continues to proceed in the main with formal and uninspiring creeds and forms, and communism and People's Movements are supplying this idealism . . . [I]t may be that . . . the strength of communism will be the next chief cultural missionary movement in the world. No one can say.[233]

In the same year and published in the same volume of essays in which Ms. Buck's essay appeared, Tyler Dennet offered a stinging critique of what had been the cornerstone of American foreign and trade policy with China since 1899, that of the "Open door":

> The . . . Open Door notes of John Hay, American Secretary of State, in the last year of the last century . . . sought to secure the voluntary assent of the trading nations . . . to the principle that the trade of China should remain subject to the conditions of free competition for all nations . . . Underlying the notes was the assumption, patently correct, that the ancient Chinese empire was unable to be its own doorkeeper . . .
>
> McKinleyism, in which the Open Door and the integrity of China doctrines were the initial chapters, contemplated a political world of harmonious states held together by enlightened self-interest . . . The idea was sensible enough, but it could not be realized . . . In the world as we find it thirty years later the Open Door and the other principles . . . are seen to be not principles of cohesion but of division. They are in practice policies of intervention, essential neither to prosperity nor to peace . . . [T]he Open Door principle is likely to turn out to be little more than the old imperialism with a new name.[234]

Two decades later, John King Fairbank, perhaps America's leading authority on China, would apply a different twist to the matter in his reexamination of the sociocultural and ideological changes that had occurred in China in the one hundred years since the Qing emperor's representatives had been forced by Great Britain, France, and the United States to sign the first "unequal treaties" (1842–1844). His analysis stressed the ignorance, indifference, and confusion of the Chinese leaders who had had to deal with the incursions made by the West.[235] He concluded that "the long-term patterns of Western history as they impinged upon China contributed to the destruction more than to the creation of any observable rhythm in the Chinese social process."[236] In contrast, he asserted, the same century had witnessed an entirely different history of modernization for Japan: "Japan . . . had a patriotic and adaptable ruling class. China did not. Japan had the medieval tradition of the samurai as a basis for modern chauvinism. The early bankers of Osaka and Tokyo were forerunners of the modern Zaibatsu. By the nineteenth century, Japan . . . was a nation somewhat like Western nations, while the Middle Kingdom was a state of a different political species altogether."[237] Thus, precisely because of China's failure to fit into a pattern comparable to that of Japan, as well as its "inability to meet the West on equal terms,"[238] it had, from the time of the treaties until 1943, been a part of that "treaty system which had . . . been created to serve as a vehicle for British and other Western trade diplomacy, and evangelism in China,"[239] a system which, while it contrasted fundamentally with the "preceding millennia of the [Chinese empire's] tribute system . . . , contrasts . . . less sharply with the new international order of communism of which China has become a part."[240] The burning question of the moment, Fairbank believed, was "how to integrate into a world community one-fifth of the human race whose social heritage is essentially at variance with that of the West."[241] The issue was made more urgent, he observed, by "the fact that this effort is currently being made under the banner of communism."[242] However, even if there were to occur a respiritualized Christian missionary movement in China, or a renewed intellectual effort at understanding how China's trade and diplomatic history had gotten both it and the United States into such difficulties, neither would be sufficient to halt the revival of the once-slumbering Chinese dragon. Its awakening was once again said to be imminent.[243]

From Asiatic Coolies to Armed Enemy

Hostile anti-Chinese remarks had in fact been noticed during World War II, in those very areas where *Kuomintang* soldiers fought side by side with troops from the United States in the struggle against Japan's imperialist advance. Ordered not to use the term *Chink* to refer to America's Chinese allies, the U.S. "G.I.'s" turned to, or perhaps invented the ethnophaulism *slopey* (derived, perhaps, from "slope-eyed" or "slope-headed"), adding, after the onset of the Korean War and continuing into the Vietnam War, the term *Gook* (which at one time referred to Filipinos and would become a feature of military slang designating any nonwhite person in the Pacific area or the Far East).[244] Harold Isaacs, a searching analyst of both the Chinese revolution,[245] the nature and consequences of the Second World War in Asia,[246] and American images of ethnoracial peoples,[247] explained the wartime rise of anti-Chinese prejudices thus:

> Consider what happened: the previous direct contacts of Americans with Chinese in China were confined to a small number of missionaries, officials, businessmen, scholars, and students. These were abruptly widened to include about a quarter of a million young Americans drawn from a cross-section of the whole American population. This large and significant body of men emerges from the experience nursing violent prejudices. They return to their homes attributing to the Chinese people as a whole all the brutality and venality and ugly viciousness of China's ruling cliques, its big and small officials, its generals and many of its soldiers, its exploiters. They bring to the traditionally amorphous American feeling of sympathy for China a sharp and bitter and explicit contradiction.[248]

However, a long-lingering image of Chinese soldiers as a "human sea" of Asiatic coolies incapable of either combat artfulness or techno-military skills would begin to give way in the face of Chinese military successes in the Korean

War. "Before the Korean War ended," Isaacs observed, "the new image of the Chinese warrior and foe became something more than a vision of vast numbers of massed barbarians akin to the Mongol hordes. These were Mongol hordes with big guns and jet aircraft and a growing number among them who knew how to use these weapons with considerable precision and skill."[249] Moreover, according to a now declassified CIA memorandum dated December 29, 1950, apprehension about a Chinese military incursion into Vietnam, then in conflict with France, was a principal fear in the U.S. intelligence community: "The Chinese Communist regime is already furnishing the Viet Minh materiel, training and technical assistance . . . The intervention of Chinese Communist troops in force in support of the Viet Minh would render the military position of the French untenable . . . Direct intervention by Chinese Communist troops may occur at anytime . . . The strong probability is that the loss of Indochina to Communist control would mean the eventual loss of all mainland Southeast Asia."[250] When by 1966, the much-feared Chinese invasion of South Vietnam had not occurred, William P. Bundy provided a more nuanced variation of China's threat:

> To accept Mainland Chinese domination in Asia would be to look forward to conditions of external domination and probably totalitarian control, not merely for twenty years but quite possibly for generations . . .
>
> But essentially we are dealing here not with the power of ideas but with the power of subversive organization—perhaps the one field in which Communist China has shown real innovation and skill . . . [251]

The awakened dragon was once again, as in the days of the Boxer uprising, about to be perceived as "cruel and revengeful."[252] Suspicions about the real aims of Chinese in America had been rekindled after the outbreak of the Korean conflict and would become even sharper during and after the Vietnam War. When, during the first year of the Korean struggle, Chinese "volunteers" halted the American military advance across the thirty-eighth parallel,[253] there were roundups of alien Chinese along the east coast of the United States.[254] Although during that war both American-born and immigrant Chinese "experienced the wrath of the larger society because they were considered 'enemy-images,'" Rose Hum Lee, the first Chinese American to chair an American university sociology department, took comfort from the fact that "they were not placed in concentration camps, as the Japanese had been during World War II."[255] However, Professor Lee would point out in 1960, "most persons of Chinese ancestry, regardless of birthplace, feared the repetition of an established precedent: the deprivation of civil rights and privileges, without due process of law, confiscation of property, and imposition on them of all the onus of enemy-subversive status."[256] A few years later, in 1966, these fears were made palpable by a rumor reported in Jerome Beatty Jr.'s column in the *Saturday Review* to the effect that detention camps were being prepared to "relocate" all the Chinese in the United States in the hope of preventing them from sabotaging the U.S. war effort in Vietnam.[257]

The policies and perspectives that would culminate in the arrest and indictment of Wen Ho Lee can be traced to the return of yellow peril fears during the first years of the People's Republic. The fall of Nationalist China in 1949 had, in effect, threatened the status and the future of five thousand overseas Chinese students, professionals, trainers, government officials, and visitors to the United States with displacement and statelessness.[258] By 1951, Public Law 535, coupled with the U.S. attorney general's collateral regulation, had relieved the plight of many of the stranded students, allowing those who had entered the United States before 1950 to complete their studies, find employment, and—perhaps most important—convert their nonimmigrant student status to that of permanent residents.[259] Nevertheless, most of the members of this aggregate suffered in numerous ways from the effects of the marginality that events had thrust upon them.[260] Worse, these students and intellectuals were not infrequently regarded as security risks, with some officials holding that they should be repatriated to the People's Republic and others believing "that the Chinese Communists would give their highest medal to the immigration department for sending back these students to Peking."[261] Those Chinese students whose visas had expired were subjected to Justice Department interrogations with "Catch 22"–style queries not unlike the infamous Questions 27 and 28 given to the already incarcerated *Issei, Kibei,* and *Nisei* by the War Relocation Authority in 1943:* The Chinese students were asked which of two Chinese governments, that of Chiang Kai-shek or that of Mao Tse-tung, they supported or had some positive feelings toward. As an editorial in the April 12, 1952, issue of the *Nation* pointed out:

> The Chinese student faces a particularly difficult position. If he rejects Chiang's leadership, this does not necessarily make him a follower of Mao . . . this fact is often overlooked . . . They have to prove their innocence of any disloyalty to our government instead of being presumed innocent until proven guilty, as the American system of justice prescribes.[262]

Fears about the knowledge and skills that American-educated Chinese might give to China after they returned to their homeland eventually led the presi-

---

* The questions are reproduced in Paul R. Spickard, *Japanese Americans: The Formation and Transformation of an Ethnic Group* (New York: Twayne Publishers, 1996), p. 118.

dent of the United States to invoke a restraint on any who sought to depart. This restraining order continued in full force until 1955, when, after numerous protests, seventy-six students, among the hundreds who sought to return, were permitted to depart for China.[263] Suspicions about Chinese students in America would be renewed after China entered the "nuclear club."

Concerns about what kind of assistance Chinese scientists and technicians might be able to give to the weaponry of the People's Republic of China became even more serious when it became clear that Mao's regime had sought and received aid from the Soviet Union in its drive to join the nuclear club.[264] From 1950 to 1960, the USSR supplied China with eleven thousand "advisers,"who helped in the construction of 141 industrial projects that included building the Anshan steel complex in southern Manchuria, developing the Sinkiang oil fields, as well as advising on the construction of numerous railway networks, automotive and tractor factories, and hydroelectric power plants. In 1955, Soviet specialists set up an atomic reactor and a cyclotron inside China, while a score of Chinese nuclear physicists studied at the USSR's Joint Institute of Nuclear Research at Dubna. Although an agreement of 1957 had pledged Russian aid in supplying China with the "new technology for national defense," the developing rift in Sino-Soviet relations soon prevented further assistance. After 1960, when all Russian technicians had been withdrawn, the Chinese proceeded on their own. On October 16, 1964, claiming that it was "a major contribution made by the Chinese people to the cause of the defence of world peace," China detonated what President Lyndon Johnson called "a crude nuclear device which can only increase the sense of insecurity of the Chinese people."[265] In May 1965, China set off a second bomb; one year later, still another, ten times larger than the second and using some thermonuclear material; five months later, a bomb that could be carried on a missile; and, two months after that, a 300 kiloton device. Then, on June 17, 1967, China exploded a true hydrogen bomb of at least three megatons, a device one hundred times more powerful than the bomb that had been dropped on Hiroshima in 1945. Americans as well as the other Occidental nations had to recognize that the Chinese dragon was no longer somnolent. If aroused, it could breathe thermonuclear fire.

The Yellow Peril and the Cox Report

For a brief moment in 1900—that is, until, five years later, Japan's startling emergence as the first Asian power to defeat a European state eclipsed it—China and its "Boxers" awed and frightened Americans. "In the West," observes Paul A. Cohen, "in the early decades of the twentieth century, the Boxers were widely viewed as 'the Yellow Peril personified.'"[266] After nearly a century-long hiatus, during which Japan took its place, China's new thermonuclear "boxers" revived Occidental apprehensions of the perfidy that supposedly characterized the dreaded demons from the East. "The Boxer Uprising," recalled Jonathan G. Utley, "proved to Americans what they had already believed, that the Chinese were not a trustworthy people, that they valued duplicity and deceit rather than honesty."[267] China's people, once admired in Pearl Buck's stories about their sturdy peasantry, were transformed into a Cold War enemy after 1949. Whereas the original view of China's threat achieved its legitimation through futuristic novels and stories, occasional American military ventures in China, labor union-inspired screeds denouncing immigrant Chinese laborers, and, after the threat of invasion had receded, lurid tales of crime and vice in America's and England's Chinatowns, the current version finds its legitimation in concerns over Asiatic communism, China's military and foreign policies, and—most significantly—the possibility that Chinese scientists, technicians, and engineers, working in American laboratories, universities, and corporations on secret, arms-related, and other thermonuclear matters, might use their positions of knowledge, authority, and privilege to aid the People's Republic of China.

That this belief might be rooted in some factual matters does not remove it from the realm of racial prejudice—from which it came and to which it belongs. Herbert Blumer has pointed out how race prejudice is formulated as a "sense of group position."[268] Further, he noted, the prejudicial process takes place in public arenas, wherein representative spokespersons, for example, "leaders, prestige bearers, officials, group agents, dominant individuals, and ordinary laymen," employing "tales, stories, gossip, anecdotes, messages, pronouncements, news accounts, orations, sermons, preachments, and the like," take up a "big event," giving it a meaning that develops the particular racist image, and designating the position of the racial group with respect to it. The history presented in the body of the present essay, describing the formation, development, vicissitudes, and applications of yellow peril discourse to Asian countries and Asiatic peoples, clearly matches this pattern.

However, in the present situation, rather than popular fiction, Asiatic exoticisms, laborite hostility, and sensational stories—all of which have been stored away in the American consciousness, able to be called up for both cognitive and cathectic support whenever needed to buttress its reappearance—the onset of the still developing anti-Chinese thesis is given its impetus by breaking news reports and hastily completed government investigations. Thus, on March 6, 1999, on the front page of the usually staid and colorless *New York Times,* a "special report" broke the story that would lead not only to the dismissal and later the arrest of Dr. Wen Ho Lee, but also, and more ominously, to the lowering of a cloud of suspicion over virtually all Chinese in, or coming to, the United States, with the headline: "Breach at Los Alamos: A Special Report; China Stole Nuclear Secret for Bombs, U.S. Aides Say."[269] Within two days Dr. Lee was fired from his job and a new yellow peril campaign had begun. According to Robert Schmidt, "The *Times* onslaught continued for five months. In a series of front-page articles . . . the *Times* pressed the case against Lee, insinuating that he was guilty of various nefarious deeds."[270] When, on September 7, the *Times* saw fit to publish an article by a different journalist, complaining "that the Federal investigation [had] focused too soon on the Los Alamos National Laboratory, and . . . Wen Ho Lee,"[271] it was too late. Five days earlier, Paul D. Moore, from 1978 to 1998 the FBI's chief analyst for Chinese counterintelligence, had published an op-ed essay in the *Times* suggesting that "China may have succeeded in devising an espionage strategy that can, over time, consistently defeat our ability to investigate or prosecute spying offenses."[272] On November 19, the *San Jose Mercury News,* a local California newspaper that had been skeptical of the *Times'* reports on Wen Ho Lee from the beginning, published Vernon Loeb's and Walter Pincus's (*Washington Post*) article headlined "New spy data suggests scientist is innocent,"[273] but it had little effect. Dr. Lee was arrested three weeks later.

"Several Asian-Americans," observed *New York Times* reporter James Sterngold on December 13, "said the event merely brought to a head four years of growing anger at the way they were being treated and portrayed in the media."[274] FBI investigations of Chinese Americans who had contributed to political campaigns were intensified. Chinese Americans, beset with new revelations about a Buddhist Church's role in Vice-President Gore's fund-raising activities, and confessions by Chinese campaign workers who had collected and given improper and perhaps illegal contributions from suspicious sources to President Clinton's election,[275] began to experience what Lisa Lowe calls that feeling of being the permanent "foreigner-within," the people who, regardless of birthplace and citizenship, are forever under suspicion about their "true" loyalty.[276] Asian American civil rights groups—including the Organization of Chinese Americans, the Committee of 100, and the Steering Committee of the Wen Ho Lee Defense Fund—began to coordinate efforts to douse what they perceived as a smouldering fire of Sinophobic race hatred.[277]

The capstone thus far on the current revival of yellow peril Sinophobia is to be found in *"U.S. National Security and Military/Commercial Concerns with the People's Republic of China," The House of Representatives Report of the Select Committee on U.S. National Security an Military/Commercial Concerns with the People's Republic of China,* popularly known as the "Cox Report," after Christopher Cox, the chairman of the House Policy Committee.[278] Enjoying unanimous and bipartisan support from committee members, this report is a fine illustration of how what Richard Hofstadter calls the "paranoid style" that so often colors sudden shifts in American policy and perspective[279] can be conjoined with a yellow peril thematic. Among its accusations the report claims:

> "The PRC [People's Republic of China] has mounted a widespread effort to obtain U.S. military technologies by any means—legal or illegal . . . The . . . Intelligence Community is insufficiently focused on the threat posed by PRC intelligence and the targeted effort to obtain militarily useful technology from the United States . . . In June, 1993, . . . a former Chinese philosophy professor, Bin Wu, and two other PRC nationals were convicted . . . of smuggling third-generation night-vision equipment to the PRC . . . Wu appears to have been part of a significant PRC intelligence structure in the United States. This structure uses "sleeper"agents, who can be used at any time but may not be tasked for a decade or more . . . The [PRC's] State Science and Technology Commission was involved in efforts to elicit nuclear weapons information from a Chinese American scientist . . . Peter Lee, a Taiwanese-born naturalized U.S. citizen who formerly worked at the Los Alamos Laboratories, passed classified information to the PRC in 1977 and in 1985 . . . In 1993, PRC national, Yen Men Kao, a North Carolina restaurant owner, was arrested by the FBI and charged with conspiring to steal and export classified and export-controlled high technology items to the PRC . . . The PRC also relies heavily on the use of professional scientific visits, delegations, and exchanges to gather sensitive technology . . . Another risk in scientific exchanges is that U.S. scientists . . . are prime targets for approaches by professional and non-professional PRC organizations that would like to coopt them into providing assistance to the PRC. In many cases, they are able to identify scientists whose views might support the PRC, and whose knowledge would be of value to PRC programs. The Select Committee has received information about Chinese-American scientists from U.S. nuclear weapons design laboratories being identified in this manner . . . The People's Republic of China . . . has stolen classified information on all of the United States' most advanced nuclear warheads . . . The stolen U.S. secrets have helped the PRC fabricate and successfully test modern strategic thermonuclear weapons . . . The PRC employs various approaches to co-opt U.S. scientists to obtain classified information . . . : appealing to common ethnic heritage; arranging visits to ancestral homes and relatives; paying for trips and travel in the PRC; flattering the guest's knowledge and intelligence; holding elaborate banquets to honor guests; and doggedly peppering U.S. scientists with technical questions by experts, sometimes after a banquet at which substantial amounts of alcohol have been consumed . . . Until at least the year 2000, the Department of Energy's counterintelligence program will not be adequate.[280]

In a preface to the Cox Report, Kenneth deGraffenreid writes: "The American people should be in no doubt about this—*in important ways Communist China might pose a more dangerous threat to the United States than did the Soviet Union.*"[281] And in his "Foreword"[282] to the same report, former secretary of defense Caspar W. Weinberger reinforces deGraffenreid's point, noting, "The PRC in the past twelve to fifteen years has changed from being a friend that is anxious to have our support in its attempt to wield a strong defense against the Soviets, to being a power that has made a conscious effort to replace the former Soviet Union as a superpower rival of the United States." Moreover, he went on, "To achieve that goal, the leaders of the PRC will use—and have used—every available means to make Communist China our strategic equal." In effect, Weinberger seems to be arguing that Communist China has risen once again, as the Qing empire had over a century earlier, to be the representative yellow peril nation of the Far East. To achieve its nefarious ends, he charges, it will steal or buy U.S. technology, oppose and block U.S. foreign policy actions, and try "to displace American influence in Asia and the Pacific region." However, Weinberger goes further: In passages that do not mention but will be reminiscent to all who recall how fanciful and false tales of espionage, subversion, and fifth-column activities in the years before Japan's attack on Pearl Harbor helped fuel the justification for imprisoning without a trial the Pacific coast Japanese Americans,[283] he links the findings of the Cox Report to the 1993 People's Liberation Army publication of a textbook entitled *Can the Chinese Army Win the Next War,* a work that identified the United States as China's "principal adversary" but, he complains, one that had not aroused President Clinton's administration to undertake any significant counteraction. Weinberger then asserts that "the Clinton-Gore administration stands condemned of some of the worst and most damaging national security decisions of this century," and praises the Cox Report for uncovering "the most serious breach of national security since Julius and Ethel Rosenberg betrayed our atomic secrets to the Soviet Union and Aldrich Ames sold us out for a mess of pottage." Neither Wen Ho Lee nor any Chinese in America could take comfort from Weinberger's ominous conclusion: "For their crime, the Rosenbergs were executed. The crimes uncovered . . . by this Report have yet to be redressed."

Lest anyone might have missed the implications for Chinese Americans of the Cox Report, Lars-Erik Nelson, in one of the few critiques of this foreboding document, points out: "most irresponsibly, the Cox report suggests that every Chinese visitor to this country, every Chinese scholar, every Chinese student, every Chinese permanent resident, and even every Chinese-American citizen is a spy, potential spy, or 'sleeper agent,' merely waiting for the signal to rise up and perform some unimaginable act of treachery."[284] From all this it would appear to be the case that Charlie Chan, the unacculturated book-and-reel-life Chinese detective who used his Oriental cleverness to help Americans to be safe from domestic criminals and foreign spies during World War II, has died,[285] and been succeeded by the real-life minions of that preternaturally brilliant scientist, Dr. Fu-Manchu ("Imagine a person, tall, lean and feline, high-shouldered," Sax Rohmer, his creator, wrote, "with a brow like Shakespeare and a face like Satan, a close-shaven skull, and long, magnetic eyes of the true cat-green. Invest him with all the cruel cunning of an entire Eastern race, accumulated in one giant intellect . . . Imagine that awful being and you have a mental picture of Dr. Fu-Manchu, the yellow peril incarnate in one man")[286]—with Caspar Weinberger and the members of the committee that wrote the Cox Report self-appointed detectives who, with public support, might save America from an otherwise awful fate.

The Yellow Peril in the "Asian Century": A Clash of Civilizations?

As the twentieth century drew to a close Ian Buruma, a prominent writer on the relations of Asia to the West, pointed out how "silly" it now seems to recall the fears voiced in the 1970s and 1980s by "politicians, pundits and . . . novelists [who] rode the bandwagon, explaining how Japan, with the rest of East Asia in tow, was about to conquer the world."[287] Yet, he goes on, despite the fact that "Michael Crichton's 1992 novel, 'Rising Sun,' in which predatory Japanese conglomerates virtually take over Los Angeles, looks as quaint these days as Sax Rohmer's stories about the demonic Dr. Fu Manchu," China, "the last large Asian country still trying to combine authoritarian government with capitalist enterprise," survives. Believing that "it is hard to imagine how a nation's economy can keep on growing without freedom of information, without its citizens having the right to question their leaders and without laws that are based on popular consent and that people will obey," Buruma nevertheless cannot refrain from noting that "anyone who has recently been to Shenzen, Canton or Shanghai will have seen young Chinese, computer-literate, enterprising, free-spirited and almost frighteningly eager to take on the world." He concluded, "If only China were to follow South Korea, Taiwan, the Philippines, Thailand and, one hopes, Indonesia, then I would raise my glass and propose a toast to the coming Chinese century."

Buruma's glass is not likely to be hoisted in the near future. China's record on just those acts that arouse suspicion and fear has been enlarged: Two days after his essay appeared it was reported that on August 7 Chinese authorities in Beijing had arrested Professor Yongyi Song—an applicant for American citizenship and a research scholar from Dickinson College, Carlisle, Pennsylvania, specializing in the analysis of the Chinese Cultural Revolution (1966–1976)—charging him with making "illegal provision of intelligence to foreigners." He was released six months later and permitted to return to the United States.[288] Four months earlier, in a wide-ranging news report on undocumented Chinese in Vancouver, British Columbia, James Brooke of the *New York Times* added still another element to allegations of Chinese deceptiveness.[289] He reported, "Every year about 5,000 people flying to Canada tear up their documents on airplanes, and then apply for refugee status. An increasingly popular practice is to apply for refugee status, and then disappear during the one year review period. That abuse has increased 20-fold during the 1990s, reaching 4,203 documented cases last year . . . Most are presumed somehow to have sneaked or been smuggled across the border to the United States." Six days after Buruma's essay appeared, the *New York Times* reported on a new wrinkle in smuggling Chinese into the United States—hiding them in the containers used on cargo ships that ply the Pacific, crossing from Hong Kong to port cities in Washington and California.[290] Further, in two essays designed to lessen Sino-American tensions (e.g., "China and the United States are likely to be the two dominant world powers during the twenty-first century. It is imperative that these two continental giants learn to live and work together productively and cooperatively."),[291] David Shambough describes China's military capability (e.g., "Its current weapons inventory remains ten to twenty years or more behind the state of the art in almost all categories")[292] in a manner that, unintentionally, to be sure, could exacerbate adherents of the Cox Report to even greater heights of concern about Chinese attempts at theft and espionage. However, in two "human interest" stories about ordinary Chinese—one, a bylined item in the morning edition of the *New York Times,* January 2, 2000, reporting that cat-nabbing has become a problem in Beijing because "some Chinese pay good money to eat cat, in a Cantonese dish called Dragon and Tiger Fight, which combines the meat of snakes and cats"; the other, a report on the eighty-two thousand rural migrants in Beijing who are forced to root through the garbage to avoid starvation and who live in constant fear of apprehension by the police, harassment, and deportation to the countryside from which they have fled[293]—the "dragon" has been, for some, cowed, while the "tiger" is once again regarded as weak as its "paper" icon. Will it arise, reassert its strength, and retaliate?

In academic Western post–Cold War analyses—as well as in instances of published fiction in the United States of the 1930s* and, more recently, in *samizdat* and new fiction in both the PRC and Taiwan—there have appeared

*In two works of fiction that bridge yellow peril themes of the late nineteenth to early twentieth century with the nonfictional allegations of the present, China and the Chinese people employ chicanery and seduction to undermine Western civilization. [For a summary and commentary on Charles Finney's 1935 tale, "The Circus of Dr. Lao" and John Steinbeck's love-and-death story of 1939, "Johnny Bear," see Jonathan D. Spence, *The Chan's Great Continent: China in Western Minds* (New York: W. W. Norton, 1998), pp. 183–86.]

modern civilizational variants of a revived yellow peril discourse. In 1993, Samuel P. Huntington's "The Clash of Civilizations"[294] announced that "world politics is entering a new phase . . . [T]he fundamental source of conflict in this new world will not be primarily ideological or primarily economic. The great divisions among humankind and the dominating source of conflict will be cultural." Although he allowed that "nation states will remain the most powerful actors in world affairs," Huntington insisted that the "principal conflicts of global politics will occur between nations and groups of different civilizations." Positing the existence of "Western, Confucian, Japanese, Islamic, Hindu, Slavic-Orthodox, Latin American and possible African" civilizations, he projected a future in which the clash of these civilizations will occur at both the micro and macro levels. At the former, "adjacent groups along the fault lines between civilizations [will] struggle, often violently, over the control of territory and each other"; at the latter, "states from different civilizations compete for relative military and economic power, struggle over the control of international institutions and third parties, and competitively promote their particular political and religious values." China, Huntington argues, as a "Confucian" civilization, is already involved in a conflict with the West over cultural differences and in terms of control over "nuclear, chemical and biological weapons, ballistic missiles and other sophisticated means for delivering them, and . . . guidance, intelligence and other electronic capabilities." The greatest danger to the West—for Huntington sees the basic clash as "the West versus the rest" of the civilizations—would arise if—reminiscent of William W. Crane's short story, "The Year 1899," which, of course, Huntington does not acknowledge—a Confucian-Islamic coalition brought their combined military power to bear on the Occident. Such a coalition is already in its nascent state, he believes. Huntington does not favor intercivilizational warfare; rather he warns that the West "will increasingly have to accommodate . . . non-Western modern civilizations whose power approaches that of the West but whose values and interests differ significantly from those of the West." However, he believes that the Occident will have to "maintain the economic and military power necessary to protect its interests . . . , to develop a more profound understanding of the basic religious and philosophical assumptions underlying other civilizations . . . , [and] learn to coexist with the others." He does not say how these necessities are to be obtained.

Huntington's thesis has evoked a chorus of critiques, most of which are beyond the scope of the present essay.[295] In the PRC, however, the People's Republic has of late been novelized as, respectively, a fearsome yellow peril or as a triumphant survivor of global conflicts. Thus, in a startling response to Huntington's claims, Wang Xiaodong, an editor of the PRC journal *Strategy and Management,* writing under the pseudonym Shi Zhong, not only denied that China was a Confucian civilization, that China sought to Confucianize the world, or that the clashes between China and the United States were anything other than competitive struggles over which nation had the economic strength to dominate Asia,[296] but, also, in the process of developing his argument, quoted from an essay that had been appended to the 1991 *samizdat* three-volume novel, *Huanghuo* (Yellow Peril) by Bao Mi (pseudonym for Wang Lixiong).[297] The novel provided a new focus for a Chinese yellow peril. Banned in mainland China but published to acclaim in Taiwan, *Huanghuo,* said to have been inspired by the calamitous events in Beijing in 1989, seems to imagine a degraded and distorted Chinese communism as the real peril, for, according to Geremie R. Barmé, it is a piece of futuristic fiction that foretells "the collapse of Communism in China and the outbreak of a civil war that leads to a global conflagration." Its author's most outspoken contempt is directed at China's prosperous intellectuals:

> They might not talk like louts, but theirs is a realm of utter spiritual degradation. They are without integrity; they crave depravity; they are shameless and thick-skinned. They are always ready to sell out their principles, and they will take risks only if there's the chance of making a profit. They regard all that is sacred with disdain and despise all ideals.[298]

However, if Wang Lixiong sees a world-threatening yellow peril in the profit-seeking policies of the post-Mao intellectuals and the domestic and foreign policies that they are pursuing,[299] another futuristic novel, Qiao Liang's *Gateway to Doomsday,* published in China in 1995, envisions a more sanguine yet formidable future for a thoroughly modernized techno-military China.[300] Rather than being pictured as a corrupt and greedy nation, or one whose armies threaten the peace of the world Qiao Liang's China seems to be possessed by the Hegelian spirit of history.[301] Set as the millennium dawns, this China has become an economic giant, a veritable symbol for worldwide hope for an end to conflict. A Chinese computer genius, attached to the People's Liberation Army and aided by his half-Russian, Bloody-Mary–consuming lover—who has the power to divine the future but only when she is in the midst of coitus—develops an apocalyptic computer virus "like AIDS" that infects all the world's computers except China's. Having disabled the global network, China assumes a benevolent sovereignty over it. The conclusion to this melodramatic novel takes place at the female protagonist's funeral, where there is echoed the sign-off call of an astronaut who, like Hegel's Owl of Minerva, is circling the globe—"Good night America . . . good morning to the East. Good morning Asia." Should he read these two books from wherever his place is in the afterlife, Kaiser Wilhelm might smile in recollection of his own prescience.*

Chinese America and the Yellow Peril: What Is to Be Done?

In the last year of the nineteenth century, Theodore Roosevelt wrote to Spring Rice, a British diplomat, boasting, "Together . . . the two branches of the Anglo-Saxon race . . . can whip the world."[302] A few years later, he was not that sure. And neither were the U.S. presidents who came after him. For the next one hundred years first China, then Japan, then China again would rise up in America's public consciousness as a threat to the West in general and the United States in particular. In each era of this yellow peril mystique Americans of Asian heritage, whether immigrant aliens or native-born citizens, would suffer outrages directed against their character, culture, opportunities, and, often enough, their very lives. Whether cast as members of a "race," a "civilization," or a "culture," Asian Americans are treated as bearers of virtually ineradicable traits that are at least implicitly assumed to be "inherited." Thus, Professor Huntington asserts that civilizational "differences are the products of centuries"[303] and that cultural differences are "far more fundamental than differences among political ideologies and political regimes."[304] For Huntington, as Robert G. Lee has pointed out in his thoroughgoing critique of the "clash of civilizations" thesis,[305] Asian Americans, together with all those representatives of other non-Western civilizations residing in America, are imagined to threaten the U.S. with "de-Westernization." This is a fate so terrible, Huntington —sounding very much like Homer Lea—warns, that "if Americans cease to adhere to their liberal democratic and European-rooted political ideology, the United States as we have known it will cease to exist and will follow the

* The one British novel that addresses this newest version of the yellow peril is a throwback, sounding very much like the late-nineteenth- and early-twentieth-century fictions described in the preceding part of this chapter. Entitled *Dragon Strike: A Novel of the Coming War with China,* coauthored by the British Broadcasting Company's China bureau chief and a journalist on the *Financial Times,* this futuristic fiction presents a conflict between an aggressive China, bent on dominating Vietnam, Malaysia, and the Philippines, and a coalition that temporarily unites Great Britain, the United States, and a reluctant Japan in an attempt to forestall both Sinocentric imperialism in the South Pacific and a global threat of nuclear war. (See Humphrey Hawksley and Simon Halbertson, *Dragon Strike: A Novel of the Coming War with China* [New York: St. Martin's Press, 1999]. Charles Wilson, reviewing this book in the *New York Times* observed, "Considering the bombing of the Chinese embassy in Belgrade last year and the recent failure in the Senate of a nuclear test-ban treaty, this book seems remarkably prescient." [*New York Times Book Review,* Sec. 7., January 16, 2000, p. 21.])

other ideologically defined superpower [the Soviet Union] on the ash heap of history."[306]

However, it is the Asian American victims of individuals and groups that have been moved to murderous action who have become the real martyrs to such apprehensions. Robert G. Lee has summarized some of the most lethal of the attacks that have occurred since the reemergence of the yellow peril in the American mind-life and the imposition of what he calls the "mere gook rule," that is, the rule that any Asian American is a "gook" worthy of extermination:

> Most notorious have been the murders of Vincent Chin in Detroit; Navorze Mody, an Indian American, in New Jersey; . . . Vandy Phorng, a Cambodian American, in Massachusetts in 1987; Jim Loo a Chinese American, in North Carolina, and five Cambodian and Laotian American children in a Stockton, Calif., schoolyard, in 1989; Hung Trong, a Vietnamese American, in Los Angeles in 1996 . . . , [and] the killings of scores of Asian American shopkeepers and cabdrivers . . . [as well as] twenty-five Korean American shopkeepers . . . killed by non-Korean assailants [in the two years before the Los Angeles riot of 1992].[307]

And, what is to be done? Rose Hum Lee, writing in 1960, after the Korean conflict had ended but before the Vietnam War, the temporary competitive advantage of Japan, or the national security fears about China and America's Chinese had revived a new yellow peril, thought that "now is the most auspicious time [for Chinese residing in the United States] to strive for total and unreserved integration into the American society" and put the burden of accomplishing this on the Chinese themselves: "Regardless of where the peoples of the United States of America originated, they must strive to fit in to the new social climate which emerged in American society and the world after World War II."[308] Forty years later we can see that such a program, even if it is desirable—and some of the new multiculturalists have registered their dissent from it—has not been effected. Even after being designated as one element of the Asian American "model minority,"[309] a veritable role model for other ethnoracial groups experiencing race prejudice, discrimination, and poverty, Chinese Americans discover that in times of crisis they are thrust back into the special category reserved for internal enemies.[310]

The idea of America, or the entire Occident for that matter, being in peril from the "yellow" people has something of a "geological" character. It is deeply embedded in the Occidental consciousness of itself, a consciousness that, until recently, took "whiteness" to be a fact of nature needing neither an "archaeology" nor a sociological deconstruction,[311] and "Orientalism" to be its utter and absolute antithesis.[312] It is an all-too-neglected element in the "American dilemma" that, despite numerous efforts over the past half century, has not been resolved.[313]

Robert Park once pointed out that "a more thorough investigation of the facts would probably show that minorities, racial, cultural, and national, have always sought the freedom and protection of the more inclusive imperium."[314] No doubt this is true, but two questions arise with respect to that claim: How is that freedom and protection to be gained? What forms of social and cultural organization are most conducive to both liberty and security? None of the proposed processual and institutional answers to these questions—assimilation, acculturation, amalgamation, on the one hand; congregation, pluralism, ethnic power, and multiculturalism on the other—has as yet proved either effective or become likely to be fully realized.[315] The lair of the yellow peril's fire-breathing dragon is to be found in the winding labyrinth of the American psyche. It is one of the "idols" of the American mind in a society that, as Harold Isaacs pointed out so presciently in 1975, is "fragmenting and retribalizing . . . at a much more rapid rate, certainly, than [it is] moving toward any more humane kind of humanhood in the arrangement of [its] social and political affairs."[316]

Asian Americans, not only Wen Ho Lee, are thus waiting for an outcome still unclear and more than likely to be unsatisfying.

CHAPTER THREE

The "Chinese Question" and America's Labor Historians

A Wrong Turn in a Quest for a Usable Past

> The general public in this country, unfortunately, does not know or understand the Chinese. This is due partly to the remaining effect of the propaganda against the Chinese during the anti-Chinese agitation here, but primarily to the present prevalence of certain elements in this country, which makes this knowledge and understanding impossible.
>
> —J. S. Tow, *The Real Chinese in America*

> There must be candor in disclosure, honesty in inquiry and resolute determination in attack, or we will fail again, as we have so often failed before.
>
> —C. Eric Lincoln,
> *Race, Religion and the Continuing American Dilemma*

Introduction

A specter is haunting America's labor historians: It is the apparition of the Chinese workingman. Long gone from his once insecure place in the fields, factories, industries, mines, and railways on the western frontier, as well as from the shoe and cutlery manufactories where he once served as a short-term strikebreaking laborer in the northeast, the Asian immigrant from what was once called the Middle Kingdom is today being raised from the ignominious grave to which earlier labor historians had consigned him. But now he serves as a foil in an ongoing debate over whether organized labor's history contains a rich heritage of left-multiracial virtues or a clandestine legacy of right-racist vices. Arrayed on each side of this battlefield of words and documents, accusations and countercharges, are some of the finest minds and some of the newest Ph.D.-minted members of the historians' profession. Those who seek honor for a nonracist laborite heritage are led by the late Herbert Gutman and count among their number Eric Arnesen, Bruce Laurie, Leon Fink, Alan Dawley, Alex Lichtenstein, Daniel Letwin, and numerous other epigoni; those who examine the patterns and consequences of white working-class racism are a dissident element among labor historians, and include Herbert Hill, Alexander Saxton, David Roediger, Nick Salvatore, Noel Ignatiev, and Gwendolyn Mink, among others. To this force and counterforce must now be added works addressing the role of the Chinese workers and the anti-Chinese movement in the annals of American labor history. In support of the followers of Gutman there has recently appeared Andrew Gyory's *Closing the Gate: Race, Politics, and the Chinese Exclusion Act;*[1] while several works on labor matters within and affecting America's Chinese by Peter Kwong[2] stand in virtual but unstated opposition to the former's roseate thesis, as do portions of the researches conducted by John Kuo Wei Tchen and Herbert Hill.[3]

When it comes to bringing the Chinese back into the history of organized labor in America, followers of Gutman must fight on two fronts. For it is an undisputed fact that America's first labor historians took great pride in the role played by organized labor's exclusion of the Chinese worker not only from the United States but also and equally significantly in his (and her) exclusion from trade union membership and eviction from jobs once dearly held. E. Salyer is thus quite correct when she observes, in a blurb written on the back cover of Gyory's book, that "he challenges the standard interpretations which have stood for years and become incorporated into the 'textbook' versions of American history." Although Salyer has exaggerated the extent to which standard textbooks had adopted the outlook of the previous generation's labor annalists, she is referring to Gyory's attempted repudiation of the thesis about Chinese workers and organized labor's response, best represented in a statement made by the much-revered Selig Perlman in 1922:

> The anti-Chinese agitation in California, culminating as it did in the Exclusion Law passed by Congress in 1882, was doubtless the most important single factor in the history of American labor, for without it the entire country might have been overrun by Mongolian labor and the labor movement might have become a conflict of races instead of one of classes.[4]

Whereas Perlman and such other traditional labor historians as John R. Commons[5] and Philip Taft[6] justified the anti-Chinese actions taken by America's incipient labor union movement by treating their only slightly bowdlerized versions of the rhetoric employed by the Sinophobes as part of the *Zeitgeist,* Gyory—as the disciple who voluntarily accepted Gutman's challenge that someone accommodate the issues in the Chinese question to the theses central to the "New Labor History"[7]—insists on denying that white workingmen and their labor institutions were possessed by a vigorous and pervasive anti-Chinese animus.

To simplify his argument, Gyory lumps his opponents into a single category. He passes lightly over Perlman's statement on the matter, and is equally complacent over related comments made by Commons, Taft, and such other labor historians as Joseph G. Rayback and Gerald R. Grob. But, immediately, Gyory conflates their perspective with that of such present-day critics of the racist practices of organized labor as Herbert Hill,[8] Roger Daniels,[9] and Ronald Takaki,[10] each of whom might be said to have agreed with the traditional labor historians that the anti-Chinese attitude and actions of the formative national labor movement were central aspects of its development, but, unlike the latter, each of whom *denies* that this perspective and those actions were good, proper, ethical, or necessary. Gyory aims some of his most withering fire at Gwendolyn Mink. In 1986, Mink had argued that white workingmen's support for Chinese exclusion had become "a peculiar bridge between unionism, and national politics."[11] In Gyory's opinion, Mink has erred most egregiously by "repeatedly stressing, with virtually no original evidence, that workers in the eastern United States backed the cries of their brethren in California and that their support for Chinese exclusion thereby 'nationalized labor politics'"; however, even worse, Gyory retorts, Mink has echoed "the work of [Alexander] Saxton and [Herbert] Hill and anticipated that of [David R.] Roediger."[12] Rejecting the findings of laborite Sinophobia in studies done decades earlier by Mary Roberts Coolidge,[13] Elmer Clarence Sandmeyer,[14] and Stuart Creighton Miller[15]—each of whom Gyory criticizes for adopting and elaborating up on what he regards as a false "national racist consensus"[16] on organized labor's history—Gyory counters with a postmodernist deconstruction of the racialist process, namely, "race is . . . constructed differently at the same time by people in the *same* social class."[17] And, given his assumption that this assertion is a heretofore unrecognized truth, Gyory states, "Workers' myriad attitudes toward Chinese immigration demonstrate . . . and reveal the dangers of generalizing too broadly about the extent and uniformity of racism in any single group."[18]

But, if the workingmen and their associations are not the leading sources of America's anti-Chinese movement, then who are the culprits? Gyory's answer is, as Leon Fink[19] writes in a blurb appended to the cover of *Closing the Gate,* one that "rescues our understanding of the tragedy of Chinese exclusion (and by extension other American racial practices) from the glib generalities reliant on a resort to 'racist culture' in favor of a painstaking—if painful—account of specific political agency." That "political agency" is specified by

Gyory: "The single most important force behind the Chinese Exclusion Act was national politicians of both parties who seized, transformed, and manipulated the issue of Chinese immigration in the quest for votes."[20] And thus begins his investigation, one that seeks nothing less than a "not guilty" verdict for the now nearly century-old indictment charging that America's labor movement has been scarred by its support for Sinophobic as well as other forms of a virulent racism.[21] Should Gyory succeed in his endeavor, he will not only relieve America's labor movement of its stigmatizing anti-Chinese heritage, but also (if we read between the lines of Fink's parenthetical statement above) absolve that movement of charges that its organizational practices restricted African Americans, Hispanics, and women, reducing the benefits that might have been gained from interracial solidarity and cooperation.[22] Eliminating its racist legacy might even succeed in returning the image of America's labor movement to that presented in 1891 by Edward and Eleanor Marx-Aveling.[23] More relevantly, it would provide an enormous assist to the posthumous fulfillment of Gutman's project: treating a broadened understanding of the class struggle as the unifying feature of America's labor movement, relegating labor union racism and workingmen's gender prejudices to insignificance.[24]

Gyory has chosen to undertake a daunting task. Leaving aside debates over whether the labor movement was (and, perhaps, still is) racist, whether the exigencies of the times justify or fail to lend adequate support to the exclusionary position taken by the major unions, and whether workingmen did or did not hold to the same outlook as their own union leaders, there still remains the scholarship on these and related questions carried out by sociologists and historians of the Chinese, a body of researches to which any labor historian should attend. Of these, Gyory did pay special attention to one work: *Chinese Immigration,* a well-documented analysis of American Sinophobia, published in 1909 and written by sociologist Mary Roberts Coolidge (1860–1945).[25] A scholar-activist who launched modern sex research,[26] demonstrated in behalf of women's suffrage, authored the first major work on the domestic and marital lives of middle-class women,[27] and conducted first-hand investigations of the social and cultural life of the Native Americans of the southwest,[28] Coolidge's study of the Chinese question has long been recognized as a forerunner of critical *engagé* research on this topic. For Gyory, it is of utmost importance to restrict the findings of Coolidge's "California thesis," which, as Gyory summarizes it, "blamed workers, and particularly Irish immigrants, for fanning the flames of racial hatred." Hence, he complains about the fact that "Coolidge's thesis has remained the dominant explanation for Chinese exclusion," bemoans the fact that "[s]ucceeding generations of historians have refined but not overturned her argument," and proclaims, without presenting a scintilla of evidence in support of his statement, that Coolidge's *Chinese Immigration* is "marred by class-prejudice, numerous inaccuracies, and a polemical tone."[29]

The "succeeding generations of historians" to which he must be referring would have to include Elmer Sandmeyer, as well as such social scientists as Rose Hum Lee, Betty Lee Sung, and Peter Kwong. With the exception of his unpersuasive denunciation of Coolidge's exposé of the corrupt practices of American port officials in China,[30] and his dismissal of Sandmeyer's study as one that though "a more scholarly and balanced account" than that of Coolidge, "essentially reaffirmed Coolidge's thesis,"[31] Gyory does not address the arguments about labor and racism contained in the works by these investigators of Chinese life in America. However, their findings deserve at least a hearing, if not a central place, in studies of the Chinese workingman and workingwoman. His neglect of these works is a glaring omission; it violates what it perhaps the single most important tenet of the New Labor History—namely, the demand for a "rich and detailed study of the many varieties of past American working-class experiences."[32] Unless, that is, Gyory intends to evict the Chinese worker from the annals of American labor history! But more on this point below.

Gyory does not bother to mention, much less refute, Rose Hum Lee's statement that America's Chinese immigrants "were excluded from skilled occupations by the labour unions' concerted efforts to bar them from shoe, textile, and tobacco making, heavy machinery and other industries."[33] Nor does he acknowledge the comparative point to be made with respect to the allegation that the Chinese workingmen were a peculiar species of "cheap labor," although Betty Lee Sung had done so some thirty-one years before his book was published: "The greatest antagonism against Chinese immigration in former years was directed against the threat of cheap labor. Not that the Chinese were different from other immigrant nationalities in this respect . . . But it was felt that because of the greater endurance and efficiency of the Chinese laborer, he was a threat to the job tenure of the white laborer."[34] Moreover, Gyory fails to recognize what Peter Kwong has shown, namely, that the American Federation of Labor and its affiliated unions continued their hostility to the Chinese worker[35] well into the twentieth century. "Capital," writes Peter Kwong in his recent and devastating critique of the conditions under which undocumented workers live and labor in the United States, "counts on labor's traditional racism and exclusionary practices, for it recruits precisely those whom organized labor excludes."[36]

On December 17, 1943, Congress approved H.R. 3070, entitled "An Act to repeal the Chinese Exclusion Acts, to establish quotas, and for other purposes."

It became Public Law 199, thus ending sixty-one years of prohibited entry for Chinese.[37] Gyory, who claims his "book answers a simple question: Why did the United States pass the Chinese Exclusion Act of 1882?" insists and seeks to demonstrate that "most workers evinced little interest in Chinese exclusion," and that "organized labor nationwide played virtually no role in securing the legislation."[38] In effect, when, in the same paragraph, he quotes an otherwise unidentified midwestern congressman declaring, "To protect our laboring classes . . . the gate . . . must be closed,"[39] Gyory seems to be implying that the laboring classes were being protected from something—Chinese immigration—of which they had no fear and little concern. But not even his own distorted picture of the events leading up to the passage of the Exclusion Act will sustain this remarkable thesis. However, even if one were to accept the latter thesis for purposes of discussion, there would remain the need to account for organized labor's persistent pursuit of exclusion after the original law had been enacted, a pursuit that continued up to and including the congressional debates over H.R. 3070, during which, to give but one example, Lester M. Hunt of the Teamsters' Union argued that the repeal was being "instigated by the communists and that Congress was being coerced into passing the bill,"[40] and to which the American Federation of Labor offered "stiff opposition."[41] Gyory has not attended to this profoundly important question. His investigation ends in 1882, sixty-one years short of where it should have gone.

Gyory's Strategy: The "Culture" of the White Laborer, the Allegations of Contract Labor, and the Periodicity of the New Labor History

There is a triadic structure to Gyory's argument. Its architectonic is that of a three-legged stool upholding New Labor History's precepts as set forth by Gutman[42] and elaborated upon by David Montgomery[43] and Leon Fink.[44] One leg purports to show the white workingman's commitment to an antiracist abolitionism, an antislavery emancipatory outlook, and a position not unlike that of the postwar Reconstructionists. Because they were steadfast in these beliefs, Gyory insists that the white workingmen of the East Coast were either hostile to, indifferent toward, or only occasionally aroused to action by the anti-Chinese rhetoric and Sinophobic prejudices of both their West Coast compatriots and their labor movement's own leaders. Instead of race prejudice, Gyory insists there was manifested a vague but powerful toleration of worker solidarity amidst ethnic diversity. As he would have it, it was that sense of interracial union that was manipulated by unscrupulous politicians who turned the legitimate fears of these workingmen into support for the exclusion of Chinese from the United States. The second leg of Gyory's argument gives substance to these fears by reviving the "coolie" thesis, namely, the belief that virtually every Chinese who set foot on America's shores was an involuntary, "imported contract laborer." Denying that this epithet and allegation were products of an anti-Chinese stereotype, Gyory virtually elevates the anti-coolie hysteria of the nineteenth century to a place in the rational belief system of white workingmen as well as an appropriate rationale for public policy. The third leg consists of a subtle arrangement of the temporal aspects of labor history such that organized labor's anti-Chinese activities after the passage of the Chinese Exclusion Act are omitted altogether, in effect treating them as matters of minor significance, events outside the scope of Gyory's study, and thus outside the question of labor's responsibility for the treatment and condition of the Chinese labor force in America. Each of the legs of this three-legged thesis is dependent on the other two, and each deserves critical attention.

The Workingmen's Culture

"Contrary to Alexander Saxton's claim that 'not much of abolition rubbed off on them,'" Gyory contends, "the abolitionist movement—in which many workers had taken part—and the ideals of the Civil War had indeed affected both working-class ideology and working-class demands."[45] This statement serves a two-fold purpose in Gyory's rhetorical strategy. Simultaneously, it gives substance to the New Labor History's imperative that the culture of both immigrant and native workers be made a central feature of any investigation;[46] in addition, it puts a positive ideological spin on the white workingmen's opposition to Chinese contract labor. "In the cacophony of voices in the Reconstruction era," he writes, "workers claimed the free-labor legacy of the Civil War . . . East of the Rockies, workers clothed their protest [against Chinese immigration] not in the rhetoric of race versus race or native versus immigrant but in that of freedom versus slavery."[47] Thus does Gyory convert the coded rhetoric of latent Sinophobia into a manifest defense of workingmen's liberation.

However, as a New Labor Historian concerned not to overgeneralize a group's beliefs, Gyory might have inquired whether there in fact existed a common and uniform attitude toward abolition among the antebellum white working classes, and whether that same uniformity of thought and conduct had held during the postwar period. The evidence on this matter has long been available. It will not support such a thesis.

Abolitionists

That a persistent, pervasive pro-abolitionist stance did *not* characterize the outlook of white workingmen has been demonstrated in numerous historical investigations. Indeed, insofar as antebellum attitudes toward African Americans carried over and were projected onto Chinese workers, they were not of a kind that would likely lead to an opposition to exclusion. Paul Goodman has noted the diversity in the responses of white workingmen to abolitionism—"a small number joined the movement, others sympathized and signed anti-slavery petitions that did not commit them to immediatism, but many more remained indifferent or hostile and bitterly prejudiced toward free African Americans." Moreover, Goodman goes on to observe that "most anomalous were the radical, egalitarian workingmen who flocked to the Jacksonian Party in coalition with slaveholders and planters who held them and all free labor in contempt."[48] Nor was this much different in New York City where, even before the Draft Riots of 1863, white laborers "feared not only the competition of Negroes in the skilled trades but also the loss of social status which resulted from associating with them."[49] In nineteenth-century Chicago, as Eric L. Hirsch's investigation has emphasized, "Anglo-American workers often accepted a hegemonic ideology promoted by the largely Protestant middle and upper classes . . . Nativism and antiradicalism were part of the ideology."[50]

For Irish workers, the majority of whom would become the mainstay of the pro-exclusion forces, it is simply not true to say, as Gyory does, that later studies merely adapted Coolidge's so-called California thesis to the national scene. Rather, recent studies show that the complex civic, occupational, social, religious, and marital situation of the Irish workers is related to their decision to move against first the African Americans, then the Chinese.[51] Essentially, the Irish workers were moved by racially based status considerations. Unlike black slaves and many free Negroes, the Irish had the right to vote, to join political parties, to seek niches of influence, power, and control in urban politics—each providing a competitive advantage in the struggle to get ahead in America; each threatened by identification and association with those nonwhites who had been declared aliens ineligible to citizenship in the United States, that is, blacks in 1857,[52] Chinese in 1878.[53] What the Irish and other European immigrants sought—and gained—was not only what Roediger, inspired by W. E. B. DuBois, calls the "wages of whiteness,"[54] but something more comprehensive, the social, moral, and civic status of white men.[55] Thus, the rejection by the Irish miners of Pottsville of Daniel O'Connell's 1842 exhortation that the Irish workers "treat the colored people as your equals, as brethren";[56] thus, the antebellum Irish parade to New York City's polls shouting "Down with the Nagurs!";[57] thus the spread of anti-Negro assaults in what began as the New York City draft riots of 1863 to Albany, Troy, Yonkers, Hartford, and Boston—and, in New York City, to attacks on Chinese peddlers suspected of having liaisons with white women;[58] thus James Brewer Stewart's observation that "the unskilled Boston dock worker was always quick to repulse any challenge to his sense of fraternal 'whiteness' with the Winthrops and the Adamses";[59] thus the Catholic anathema pronounced on California's Chinese workers by the *metis* priest Father Bouchard;[60] thus Denis Kearney's vitriolic verbal volley heaping invective on Chinese domestic servants for imperiling the jobs deserved by Irish women;[61] and thus the addition of the long-queued, cunning "heathen Chinese" to the repertory of low-brow Irish vaudeville.[62] The Chinese became not merely the indispensable enemy[63] of Irish workers' opportunities, but also the morally inferior people, the men farthest down, but, more significantly, the people to be kept out of the labor movement and the country itself.

Reconstruction, Redemption, and Anti-Chinese Racism

Gyory attempts to downplay the influence of Denis Kearney's demand that "The Chinese Must Go," claiming it was given undue importance by selective and biased journalists, but he has an even bigger problem with the anti-Chinese rhetoric of an East Coast journalist, John Swinton, a Sinophobic demagogue who "would later emerge as the nation's preeminent labor editor of the 1880s, proprietor of a radical newspaper that bore his name."[64] Because, in 1870 Swinton published an editorial in the *New York Tribune,* denouncing the Chinese as "inferior," "depraved," practitioners of "indecent and obscene, foul and mortifying vices," and asked, "Can we afford to admit the transfusion into the national veins of a blood more debased than any we have known," and answered his own question, stating that it entailed but an easily understood conflict: between "the *roast rat* against the *roast beef*"[65] (an adumbration of the infamous paper by Samuel Gompers and Hermann Gudstadt, issued by the American Federation of Labor in Washington, D.C., in 1902,and entitled, "Some Reasons for Chinese Exclusion. Meat vs. Rice. American Manhood against Asiatic Coolieism. Which Shall Survive?") Gyory finds it necessary to play down the effect that Swinton's polemic would have on the rank-and-file white workingmen: "His anti-Chinese screed," he asserts, "proved an ugly and ironic segue to his brilliant career: Ugly because of its virulent racism; ironic because workers, for whom he intended it, largely dismissed his argument and disregarded his remedy."[66] However, Gyory's interpretation of this key event, offered without evidence to back it up, does not receive support from the researches of John Kuo Wei Tchen, who points out that Swinton had "articulated a pan-Euro-American nationalism that would foreshadow dominant American racial ideology for . . . years to come." Tchen calls attention to the fact that Swinton, in "contrast to the distinction . . . others made between 'coolies' and free immigration, . . . [had] emphasized unresolvable racial differences as the primary grounds for anti-Chinese protest," and he underscores Swinton's claim that "the life genius, and power of the American Republic is with the European race."[67] Tchen concludes, "I disagree with Andrew Gyory's contention that Swinton 'convinced very few if any members of the working classes,'"[68] pointing out that after Swinton, the sloppy usage of the term *coolie labor* became "a synonym for all Chinese men, eliding significant differences of contracts among Chinese laborers into a term used to refer to all Chinese laborers," and going on to observe that "hence all Chinese labor in the United States became equated with 'coolieism' which was, as [the editor of the *New York Herald*] wrote, 'but another name for African slave labor.'"[69] It is not going too far to say that Gyory carries off these same elisions in his revival of the "coolie myth" and his tendentious defense of the late nineteenth-century white workingmen.

Gyory's "politicians" thesis pales into insignificance if one compares its explanatory value with that of John Kuo Wei Tchen's briefer but all-the-more comprehensive investigation of the origins and development of exclusionism among the Irish of New York City.[70] Tchen presents a sociocultural analysis that comes closer to E. P. Thompson's demand for the inclusion of popular culture features of workingmen's lives,[71] extends the "whiteness" studies of Roediger and Ignatiev, and combines these with a showing of how ideologies supporting race and gender hierarchies were fitted together to form a Sinophobic and exclusionist orientation. "Irish competition with blacks and Chinese undoubtedly existed," he concedes, ". . . yet it is not a sufficient explanation for Irish anti-black and anti-Chinese feelings and actions."[72] Added to job competition, Tchen points out, was the rise of fears about "amalgamation," already present in the New York City riots of 1834 and 1863, but exacerbated to a much higher degree by the appearance on New York City newsstands of David Goodman Croly's and George Wakeman's pseudo-scholarly, sensation-causing pamphlet, *Miscegenation: The Theory of the Blending of the Races, Applied to the White Man and Negro.*[73] The few Irish-Chinese marriages that had occurred in the early decades of Chinese arrival in the city came thereafter to be regarded as a threat to white civilization. Further, Tchen shows, after Irish minstrels, comedians, and actors began to add scathing stereotypes of Chinese to their popular variety shows in the bowery, in the process providing Irish workers with a legitimation of their belief that there was a people further down in the social and moral scale than themselves—further down, that is, than the Anglo-American Protestants held them to be—they facilitated their own ascent into the economically and politically privileged "white" race, leaving behind both black laborers and their erstwhile fellow workers, the Chinese. "The Irish did not magically become white," Tchen points out. "Irish men were able to become Americanized by actively participating in racial masquerades of the established political culture . . . , by so doing they became increasingly viewed as 'white.'"[74] And, employing general fears of race mixing and Sinophobically stereotyped low-brow cultural displays, New York City's Irish Catholics could "defuse longstanding Anglo-American and European-Protestant hatred toward them . . . [by] symbolically displac[ing] such low valuation placed on them onto an even lower group."[75] Precisely "because they had prerequisite talents and skills for entering into New York commercial stage culture just at the point of its expansion, the Irish were in a unique position to build up their own image in mainstream society while creating new 'heathens' to displace their longstanding negative image."[76] Thus Tchen, carrying forward themes developed earlier by Ignatiev and Roediger, provides elements of "the cultural background that made possible the passage of the 1882 Chinese Exclusion Act."[77]

Gyory's assertion that white workingmen were moved in both their attitudes and their responses to former slaves and to Chinese immigrants by the ideals of abolition and Reconstruction, is further contradicted by the evidence amassed by historians. Thus, Howard Rabinowitz concludes his comprehensive empirical investigation of what happened to the freedmen and -women during the actual postwar quarter century on a doleful note: "For the majority of urban Negroes, . . . the first twenty-five years after the war were years of frustration and disappointment. The year 1890 found them at the lowest levels of the economic ladder with little prospect for improvement."[78] Organized labor, observes Eric Foner, in "its own conception of equality remained in many respects thoroughly conventional. Composed mostly of artisans and skilled industrial workers, unions proved unwilling to expand their membership beyond the ranks of white men." Moreover, he goes on, "In California, where indentured [sic!] Chinese immigrants by 1870 constituted a quarter of the wage labor force, the agitation for their exclusion, more than any other issue, shaped the labor movement's development."[79]

But were the Chinese workingmen so different from white laborers in their aims and efforts? Gyory, in effect abandoning any attempts to understand the culture of the Chinese workingman, displays no interest whatsoever in such social, economic, or community-wide institutions of the Chinatown Chinese as clans, *Landsmannschaften,* or labor guilds.[80] Nor does he give any recognition to such Chinese individuals as the crusading newspaper editor and progressive opponent of exclusionism, Ng Poon Chew,[81] or to the founder-editor-publisher, in 1883, of the first anti-exclusionist East Coast Chinese newspaper, Wong Chin Foo,[82] who appropriately entitled his short-lived but influential publication, *Chinese American (Hua Mei Xin Bao).* In any true labor history of the late nineteenth century, Wong Chin Foo should be included, for he was the principal leader of the Chinese community's attempt to overcome the citizenship provisions of the Chinese Exclusion Act, and in 1892 founder and secretary of the Chinese Equal Rights League of America, an association of English-speaking Chinese dedicated to securing the civil rights of all Chinese in the United States. According to the *New York Times,* the League's members "wore American clothes, . . . patent leather shoes and white neckties,"[83] thus displaying openly the lie of unadaptability broadcast nationwide by the spokesmen for the white labor unionists.

In contrast to the argument Gyory is advancing, the labor historian David Montgomery, in his occasional but pointed mentions of the Chinese workingman, has in effect argued that the latter showed themselves—by their willingness to labor long and hard at dangerous tasks under life-threatening conditions,[84] and, even more to the point, by their ability to organize themselves into labor guilds and proto-unions that were willing to and did in fact go on strike—to have the very characteristics that should have made them candidates for recruitment into the burgeoning labor movement. Although Professor Montgomery is not the first to take note of the fact that "when laborers unionized as laborers . . . their organizations were based on ethnic ties," he should be credited with being one of the few who observe that "the context of the exclusion movement also inspired purely Chinese unions of cigar makers, jean makers, and laundrymen."[85] Moreover, Montgomery does not treat these Chinese labor guilds as antithetical to the aims or the organizational structure of the white workingmen's associations of that era, but rather, he compares them favorably to those formed by Greek and Italian workers.[86]

But, Montgomery's studies go even further, in effect undermining much of Gyory's argument. Montgomery published his findings more than a decade before Gyory had put out his. Of great significance in this regard, is Montgomery's analysis of Chinese-initiated work stoppages and strikes, and his reports on the Chinese laborers' willingness to participate in the very unions whose white members scorned their efforts, rioted against them, and clamored for their exclusion from both the labor market and the country. "Although few in America were aware of it at the time, [the Chinese working on the Central Pacific section of the Transcontinental railway] staged, in June, 1867, one of the largest-scale strikes of the century."[87] As Montgomery goes on to observe, demanding a wage comparable to that being paid to white workers, insisting on a ten-hour day, and calling for abolition of whipping for those who quit, the Chinese refused to leave their makeshift tents for a week, won their wage demands, and returned to work. Anti-Chinese violence in Vancouver, Tacoma, Seattle, Denver, and Los Angeles, as well as the wholesale expulsion of the entire Chinese community from Humboldt County, California, nevertheless continued as one element in the white workingmen's campaign of ethnic cleansing of the labor market.[88] "White workers and farmers," Montgomery asserts, "who flocked to the Pacific Coast in search of high wages and fertile valleys quickly and virtually unanimously came to look on first the Chinese and later the Japanese as the carriers of poverty and social decay."[89] And, in direct contradiction of the thesis that Gyory is espousing, Montgomery points out, "The labor movement itself played a leading role in the struggle to exclude Chinese and Japanese from American life altogether."[90]

Contract Labor: The Chinese Workingman as a "Coolie"

A central feature of Gyory's argument distinguishes between the right of Chinese laborers to *emigrate* to America—which, he claims, white workingmen did not oppose—and the right of capitalists to *import* Chinese to America under conditions of contract—which, he insists, was the sole objection made in the white workingmen's exclusionary demands. The former was lawful under American statutes until 1882; the latter allegedly aroused the ire of white workingmen to what Gyory believes was a real socioeconomic evil, contract labor. It was this evil that provided a legitimate basis for extending a prohibition on entrance to the United States to any people who were brought into the country in that condition.[91] Thus, to buttress his claim on this crucial point (and, incidentally, to refute a charge that Herbert Hill had brought against Adolph Strasser, Cigar Makers' International Union president, namely, that this colleague of AFL leader Samuel Gompers was one of "two men, above all others . . . responsible for organized labor's crusade against Asian workers,"[92] as well as a similar accusation made by Gwendolyn Mink, namely that Strasser had "defended the anti-Chinese posture of [his] California colleagues and actively involved [himself] in the exclusion movement)[93] Gyory quotes the testimony of Adolph Douai and Adolph Strasser, two labor leaders who in 1878 testified on the Chinese immigration issue before the House of Representatives' Hewitt committee, convened to investigate the causes of the ongoing economic depression of that era. Douai, editor of the *Arbeiter-Union,* claimed, "We would not restrict anyone . . . We demand that Chinese emigration under contract ought to be stopped immediately," but "[n]ot otherwise."[94]

Strasser, pressed over and over again by Chairman Hewitt as to the precise nature of his opposition to Chinese immigration, insisted, "I am not opposed to the Chinaman, or any nationality; but I am opposed that John Chinaman or anyone else should be imported here as a coolie under contract. I don't agree that the Chinaman must go. I cannot agree with that, because you might as well say that some one else must go. That is wrong; I cannot agree to that. I am not in favor of that; but I am in favor not to tolerate the direct importation of coolies by contract." When Hewitt asked him, "You won't allow any one to be brought here under contract?" Strasser replied, "I am opposed to it."[95] However, Gyory's attempt to relieve Strasser and most of the white workingmen of the East Coast from the charge that they possessed and were possessed by a generalized Sinophobic bias will not survive closer scrutiny.

Perhaps, first, it ought to be noted that, despite all the posturing before congressional committees and in other public venues, the opponents of contract labor succeeded, as the wording of the Chinese Exclusion Act plainly shows, in prohibiting the coming to America of *all* Chinese laborers, whatever their contractual condition: "sec. 15. That the words 'Chinese laborers,' wherever used in this act, shall be construed to mean both skilled and unskilled laborers and Chinese employed in mining."[96] Indeed, subsequent renewals of the act enlarged the meaning of the term *laborer* to include salesmen, clerks, buyers, bookkeepers, accountants, managers, storekeepers, apprentices, agents, cashiers, physicians, restauranteurs, and laundry operators,[97] hardly "coolies" by any stretch of the verbal imagination, no matter how it might be attached to this kind of rhetorical imagery. Moreover, the original act and subsequent as well as earlier judicial rulings, put two additional burdens on Chinese who wished to emigrate. The first was denial of citizenship: Section 14 of the Act provided "That hereafter no State court or court of the United States shall admit Chinese to citizenship; and all laws in conflict with this act are hereby repealed."[98] Four years earlier, in the Federal District Court proceeding *In re Ah Yup,* a Chinese immigrant alien was declared to be "Mongolian," and being, therefore, neither "white" nor of "African nativity" nor "African descent," to be ineligible for citizenship in the United States.[99] The second burden took the form of an extension of legal disabilities already applicable to Chinese men to their wives: "The wife of a Chinese labourer," observed Huang Tsen-ming, associate justice of China's Judicial Yuan in 1936, "or a Chinese woman not previously a labourer, who married a Chinese labourer, was held to have or acquire the status of the husband, and was not permitted to enter the United States."[100] Just as Chief Justice Taney had in 1857 denied United States citizenship to Dred Scott and all other African Americans, foreclosing for them the possibility of being included in the Constitutional compact embracing "We, the people,"[101] so, in the court ruling of 1878, ratified by section 14 of the Exclusion Act in 1882, did the justices and legislators do the same to Chinese immigrants. While the Fourteenth and Fifteenth Amendments to the Constitution revoked the Dred Scott ruling on African Americans' citizenship, Chinese immigrants in America would not become eligible for naturalization until a provision for such was included in the repeal legislation of 1943. Organized labor from either the East or West Coasts did nothing to aid in the repeal of this law, and in fact did much to encourage its continuance. To give but one telling example: In 1924, Hugh Frayne, a New York representative of the AFL, told the congressional committee holding hearings on immigration restriction, "Labor is for the entrance of suitable immigrants from all nations except the Asiatic ones."[102]

Gyory seeks to reattach legitimacy to the fear that a "coolie trade" from China would swamp America and subvert the aims of its progressive labor movement. In this sense, his thesis seems to support the argument made by Perlman and quoted at the beginning of this chapter. However, he doesn't want to attribute this apprehension to white workingmen if it is considered a racially prejudiced stereotype; rather, he wishes to assign it to the white workers as a prescient perspective if it is based in fact. Thus, although in his text and in a footnote citation[103] he indicates that he must know about Persia Crawford Campbell's distinction between the "credit-ticket" system, by which a great many Chinese came to America,[104] and the coolie trade proper, outlawed by poorly enforced American laws of 1862 and later years,[105] by which Chinese were brought to Peru,[106] Cuba,[107] the British West Indies,[108] and other areas where exploitation of Asian laborers was the order of the day,[109] he purposefully allows this distinction to be obscured and glossed over, making nineteenth-century Chinese immigration to the United States appear to be but one more instance of the nefarious and multifaceted coolie trade. Hence, Gyory places a greater emphasis on the "Koopmanschap affair"[110]—an ultimately abortive scheme hatched at a convention of planters meeting in Memphis (1869), whereby about two hundred Chinese were inveigled, shanghaied, or kidnapped from the interior of Guangdong province and brought to New Orleans by Cornelius Koopmanschap in order to supply the South with agricultural laborers[111]—than on the more common means by which Chinese came to this country. For example, when Gyory recounts that in the three years before the Chinese exclusion law was passed, fears were noised in the press and by white labor agitators, warning that the Chinese were moving eastward into the workplaces of white laborers, he opines that "the ghost of Koopmanschap hovered ominously," and that in effect the white workingman was being told, "You are replaceable, and your replacements are ready."[112] Just as, earlier, Gyory, having discussed the meaning of the word *coolie,* had posed a series of rhetorical questions:—

> "But were all Chinese who signed contracts 'coolies' and 'almost slaves'? Could an impoverished Chinese man sign a contract and not be a 'coolie'?

And then answered them:

> Possibly, probably, but no one knew for sure."[113]

—so, in his discussion of the fears attending the rumors of a "Chinese labor invasion" of the East, rumors spread by Sam Quong, a recent immigrant, Mrs. Timothy Sargent, a promoter of Chinese domestic services, Gifford Parker, a merchant in the China trade, and planter Henry Scharett, he concedes, "There may have been little truth to their statements, but no one could be sure, and in the end it really didn't matter."[114] But, of course, it was possible to ascertain the truth *then,*[115] and it did matter *then*—to the Chinese who were to become the victims of these base canards, and to the white workingmen who should have been able to figure out for themselves, since they were not told by their leaders, that dividing the working class into excludable and eligible workmates on the basis of race would do untold damage to labor solidarity and the need for workingmen to speak to capital in a multiethnic but single voice.[116] And it should matter *now* to Gyory in particular and to labor annalists in general. For the unrepentant mendacity of the charges hurled at the Chinese by both the rank and file and the leaders of the American labor movement continue not only to dirty labor's escutcheon but also to falsify labor history itself. What the white workingmen of yesterday need is not a new form of historiographical exoneration for their racist misdeeds, but rather an acknowledgment of the role they played in the anti-Chinese movement and a recognition of the proactive effects their involvement in the "Chinese Question" had on both Chinese life chances in the United States and the labor movement itself. These desiderata, sad to say, Gyory does not provide.

Although contract labor was by no means unknown in other sectors of the labor market in the United States,[117] it was alleged to be a peculiar feature of Chinese immigration. To be sure, from time to time, the importation of Chinese under fixed contracts was proposed in order to supply certain regions with low-paid agricultural workers—the three outstanding instances being the abortive "Coolie Bill" proposed in California in 1862,[118] the antebellum proslavery "fire-eaters'" attempts to seize Cuba, make it a slave state, and, as an added bonus, import portions of that Spanish colony's small Chinese population as "warrantee" workers on Mississippi's plantations,[119] and the aforementioned Koopmanschap affair,[120] which in fact was the final and failed large-scale attempt to substitute Chinese for Freedmen on the South's plantations.[121] However, much like the Chinese indentured in the Caribbean in the same era,[122] the few Chinese who were brought to the South in the post–Civil War era resisted confinement to their proposed serfdom on plantations, settled as shopkeepers in such small towns as Greenville, Mississippi, and served for decades as middlemen proprietors selling goods to blacks, brokering commercial and occasionally local political relations between blacks and whites and, in the Delta region, intermarrying with African American women and parenting what would become biracial families.[123] These Chinese were hardly a threat to the white workingmen who organized against them. Moreover, some went to court demanding their civil rights under the Fourteenth Amendment of the United States Constitution.[124] In 1927, to take one example, one Chinese family, with the support of the community, brought an unsuccessful suit to the United States Supreme Court seeking desegregation of Mississippi's white/colored school system.[125] The Chinese coolie, as envisioned in the paranoia of the Sinophobes, and in the portrait of him provided by Gyory, was for the most part, a figment of the white racist's fertile and fetid imagination, an element in the propaganda taken up not only by politicians—as Gyory would have us believe—but also by organized and organizing labor's leaders regardless of party affiliation—as a reading of the *Proceedings of the Asiatic Exclusion League* would reveal.[126]

The actual means by which most Chinese immigrated to the United States was by incurring a debt, that is, by purchasing a "credit-ticket" in order to pay for their transoceanic passage, and, perhaps, provide for their basic needs when they first arrived. "Two middlemen systems evolved," write leading Chinese American historians Him Mark Lai, Joe Huang, and Don Wong in their careful analysis of the means by which Chinese peasants and workers could depart from China and journey overseas, in order "to facilitate emigration." In one, the credit-ticket system, "passage money was advanced to the emigrant who then repaid his debt after arrival in the new land"; the other—the coolie system proper, it might be called—"involved emigrants signing term contracts of service in foreign lands in return for their passage." The distinction in practice was familiar to the peoples of southeastern China, whose husbands and sons made up the bulk of Chinese going overseas. In the latter system, "Chinese were frequently tricked or coerced into going abroad. Cantonese called these dealings *maaijeutzai,* meaning 'selling pigs.'"[127] In the former, although abuses were not unknown,[128] there was more than a semblance of free and voluntary migration. "During the nineteenth century," writes Liping Zhu, "the majority of Chinese immigrants came to the United States by means of the credit-ticket system . . . , [But] other poor peasants simply signed a contract with either the

Chinese merchants or foreign agents, who paid all expenses for transit to the United States in exchange for their labor for a certain period, which varied from two to ten years. These people were the so-called contract laborers."[129] However, Zhu goes on to emphasize, "From the beginning, the majority of Chinese pioneers to the American West were free."[130] And, unlike Gyory, who, in his attempt to denigrate Coolidge's comments on the consular service's corrupt practices, appears to be willing to accept the consular service's analogy of contract labor to slavery,[131] Zhu points out, "Unlike African slaves, the Chinese migrated to the United States voluntarily."[132]

Indeed, Chinese migrated to the United States in several different ways. Not only were there a small number of attempts to recruit contract labor from China, but also there was a more widely used debt-based approach to immigrating, not unlike the "padrone" system used by European workers who journeyed to America.[133] In the Chinese case, Chinatown associations rooted in clanship or district of origin acted as both labor brokers and debt collectors.[134] But, in addition, there was a certain amount of utterly free and individualized migration, as has been emphasized in Tchen's path-breaking study of New York City's pioneer Chinese.[135] Thus, the coming of Chinese to the United States should be contrasted from, say, that of those who went to Cuba in the early period, where, in the 1850s and for two decades thereafter, "From an economical point of view, the Chinese became the first viable alternative to the African slaves . . . , [until, that is,] the Chinese empire's cancellation in 1873 of the agreement that had authorized the traffic in coolies." Moreover, in later years, "Spaniards, Chinese, and white and black Cubans served as [railroad] stokers, brakemen, and day laborers . . . [such that the Cuban labor-force's ethnic heterogeneity] at first [held] back the creation of a homogeneous class awareness."[136] Denise Holly, who carefully reexamined the Chinese Yamen's *Cuba Commission Report* of 1876, concluded:

> It is estimated that one million Cantonese left the two provinces of South China between 1840 and 1875, the majority coming from Kwantung . . . *The majority departed as free workers for the mines of California, Canada, or Australian Queensland,* and for the French, Dutch, and English plantations of Southeast Asia. Some Cantonese were recruited by Surinam and other Dutch possessions, and the English and French islands such as Mauritius and Réunion. Of the total number of emigrants, roughly 100,000 persons signed contracts to work in Peru, and 142,000 went to Cuba.[137]

And two more points are worth mentioning in order to lay to rest—hopefully once and for all—Gyory's raising of the coolie charge against the Chinese who came to the United States. Contrary to his claim that a great many Chinese were "imported" under contract into the United States, especially during and after the years when the Transcontinental Railway[138] was being constructed, it is to Robert G. Lee's discerning investigation into the origins and discontinuities of Chinese immigration to the United States that Gyory should have turned—for Lee shows, *inter alia*:

> While the Central Pacific did recruit laborers beginning in 1867, it had already hired many of its workers from among the Chinese already in California. After the completion of the trans-continental line in 1869 the Chinese still remained active in rail construction throughout the West, but there is little evidence to suggest that the other lines recruited fresh labor from China but rather used the massive work force laid off by the Central Pacific.[139]

Gyory also makes much of the fact that Calvin T. Sampson—the owner of the ladies boot and shoe factory in North Adams, Massachusetts, in behalf of which he sought to break a strike by white workingmen belonging to the Knights of St. Crispin—negotiated a three-year contract with Kwong, Chong, Wing and Co., a San Francisco–based enterprise, that Gyory calls "a Chinese emigrant agency." Kwong, Chong, Wing and Co. supplied "75 steady, active, and intelligent Chinamen" to act as strikebreakers.[140] But were the Chinese shoemakers of San Francisco "coolies" in the pejorative sense of that word that the white workingmen and Gyory favor? Rather than acquiescing to the white workingmen's protest—and praising those among the latter who differentiated between favoring the coming of individual Chinese workmen and opposing Chinese contractees,[141] a distinction that was not made by the National Labor Union in its resolution of 1869[142]—Gyory might have inquired into the nature and workings of the Chinese boot and shoe industry in San Francisco, from which the strikebreakers were drawn. Had he done so, he would have discovered, as Joel Franks's well-researched history of that city's nineteenth-century Chinese shoemakers shows, that "neither a trade union tradition nor labor militancy were foreign to their experiences."[143] In fact, before the 1870s Chinese shoemakers had formed their own labor guild, the *Li-Sheng Tang*. In 1876 Chinese shoemakers engaged in a violent job action, demanding, among other things, a return of the money given to a contractor who had placed 750 of their fellow workers with two Euro-American firms. In this action the Chinese strikers not only went out in open defiance of Yee Chung and Co., the contractors, but also directly opposed the actions taken by the "Chinese Six Companies," that is, the community-wide confederation of traditional associations that held sway over Chinatown's denizens for decades and that supposedly kept all Chinese in supine thralldom.[144] During the 1880s there was more strike activity by Chinese shoemakers. "In the summer of 1887, 300 Chinese initiated a work stoppage in many Chinese run firms . . . [seeking a daily] pay raise of $1.15 to $1.40, . . . full wages without being compelled to pay board to their employers," and, in some cases, cessation of the practice of fining workers for failing to meet the daily production quota, an end to night work, and the right to work in production groups composed of fellows from their own clan, village, or region. Of these demands, the compromise eventually reached allowed the workers to board themselves, but neither a wage increase nor the end of "mixed" work crews, nor any of the other demands were granted. To put down the strike, it should be noted, one of the Chinese firms brought in white strikebreakers. Franks likens these Chinese shoemakers to the more poverty-stricken members of the English working classes celebrated by E. P. Thompson;[145] Gyory, who as a disciple of Gutman is supposedly inspired by Thompson's path-breaking work, makes no mention of them.[146]

If Gyory would have followed Gutman's precept, which the latter borrowed from Sartre and associated with a similar statement by Thompson, namely, that "the essential question . . . is not what has been done to men and women but what men and women do with what is done to them,"[147] he, that is, Gyory, might have looked much more closely into Paul C. P. Siu's magnificent, posthumously published monograph, *The Chinese Laundryman: A Study in Social Isolation,*[148] wherein he would have discovered the deeper meaning and the long-lasting effects of the Chinese Exclusion Act on those Chinese classified as excludable aliens and declared ineligible for U.S. citizenship, that is, those who had to make a life in the face of organized white labor's extraordinary hostility to them. In confining his effective establishment of the boundary of the working class to white laborers, Gyory has moved labor history retrogressively to what David Roediger calls the "unexamined and indefensible proposition that the white males under consideration were somehow the 'American working class.'"[149] He thus has imposed one more exclusion on the Chinese in addition to that inflicted by the Exclusion Act—ejection from membership in, as well as the history of, the American working class.

Periodicity: Montgomery versus Gutman and Gyory

In Gyory's investigation, the New Labor History's peculiar periodization becomes a way to avoid discussing labor's role in the anti-Chinese movement in the years following Congress's adoption of Chinese exclusion. Herbert Hill[150] has taken notice of Gutman's and other New Labor Historians' peculiar approach to historical periodization, for example, that Gutman "never explains . . . why he chose to limit the scope of his inquiry [into the situation characterizing the relationship of African American workers to the United

Mine Workers of America] to the years between 1890 and 1900, why that period in the UMW's history was especially significant, and why it deserves the special attention he gives it," or why Nelson Lichtenstein, in his biography of Walter Reuther, gives great emphasis to Reuther's support for "fair employment" legislation but says not a word about the union's response after the enactment of Title VII of the Civil Rights Act of 1964. Although Hill has noted how the "significance of historical events may be distorted if they are extracted from their temporal sequence without reason or explanation," a similar practice is to be found in Gyory's work. Thus Gyory's account of the Chinese Exclusion Act ends with the statute's enactment into law and says virtually nothing about how organized labor fought for another sixty years to maintain and enlarge Asiatic exclusion from both the country and the labor sector; how Chinese, Japanese, Koreans, East Indians, and other peoples declared to be aliens ineligible to citizenship in the United States—because they were neither white nor persons of African nativity or African descent—petitioned the courts either for reclassification as whites or for the exclusion law and the naturalization statute to be declared unconstitutional;[151] or how those laws made it a virtual impossibility for Chinese laborers in the United States to live a normal family life, leading an unknown number to rectify matters through smuggling, through the documentary creation of "paper sons," and through resort to the subterfuge that the Immigration and Naturalization Service came to call the "slot racket."[152] For Gyory, however, having freed the white workingman from the charge of anti-Chinese prejudice and discrimination, his work is finished. The Chinese are left to their limbo-like fate—silenced, marginalized, evicted, not even a segment of the American working class nor a part of the *history* of the American working class.

It is David Montgomery, contrary to the arguments advanced by Gyory, who takes notice of the fact that "the unions and the Knights of Labor in the Far West not only lobbied for legal prohibition of Chinese immigration but also, after passage of the Exclusion Act of 1882 unleashed an 'abatement' campaign to drive Chinese by force away from mines, ships and lumber camps and formed a League of Deliverance, which attempted to compel all San Francisco employers to replace Chinese workers with white union members."[153] White workingmen's hostility to Chinese workers continued even after the latter had conducted such strikes and threatened work stoppages as a successful cigar makers' job action in 1884 and an unsuccessful drive for a closed shop in 1885.[154] Indeed, the Chinese successes in these struggles may have increased white workingmen's hostility toward them.[155] And this hostility extended well into the twentieth century and into other areas of work, including the kinds that seemed ripe for radical multiracial class actions.

Thus, Calvin Winslow writes: "[O]n the Pacific Coast, waterfront workers were mostly white. Chinese were excluded, and African Americans were relatively scarce until World War II."[156] Labor's support for racism was ubiquitous.

The Rock Springs Riot: A Moment in Exclusion's Proactive History

Montgomery seems to qualify his virtual indictment of white workingmen's continuing anti-Asian racism when he observes, apropos of the race-and-labor situation in Wyoming two decades after one of the worst outbreaks of labor-inspired violence against the Chinese, "By 1908, in Rock Springs, Wyoming, scene of the bloody massacre of Chinese miners by white Knights of Labor in 1885, Chinese members attended UMWA meetings, according to one reporter, together with 'nearly every nation of Europe.'"[157] Gyory, it is important to notice, plays down white workingmen's anti-Chinese violence in the 1870s and 1880s, mentioning briefly the "Chico massacre" in 1877[158] but confining his discussion of the riots in Denver (1880), Los Angeles (1881), Rock Springs (1885), and Snake River, Oregon (1887), as well as the fifty-five such riots reported in the researches of Shih-shan Henry Tsai[159] to a footnote—to which he adds, citing a *New York Times* report of December 13, 1995, apparently unaware of what it means to his general thesis, this enigmatic statement: "Violence against Chinese Americans continued throughout the twentieth century."[160] To Gyory's East Coast white workingmen of the late nineteenth century, the Chinese Exclusion Act was merely an "indirect result of the labor uprising of 1877." For, although "workers would continue to express only minimal interest in immigration restriction, other groups would begin to see it as a solution for the nation's industrial problems." These "other groups" apparently are the politicians and the forces of monopoly capitalism; for Gyory concludes, "This atmosphere of violence and uncertainty breathed new life into the anti-Chinese movement among those seeking to eliminate or defuse class tensions[!]"[161]

However, both Gyory's dismissal of the massacre at Rock Springs in 1885, as well as Montgomery's sanguine statement about labor conditions there two decades later, deserve further attention. In fact, shortly after the white laborers' violent uprising that left over forty Chinese dead, drove the rest out of their homes, and torched the town's Chinese quarters,[162] the officers of the Union Pacific Coal Department that had first introduced Chinese workingmen into the Wyoming mines, determined to rid themselves of all of the latter and as many as possible of the unionized white workers as well, replacing both with nonunion Mormon miners and, more significantly, with new labor-saving machinery. A good number of the Chinese had already fled or would soon flee to China, while others moved to what they hoped would be a safer haven in San Francisco. Nevertheless, a few Chinese remained in the area, for thirteen years protected from continuing white workingmen's depredations by federal troops.[163] The reports of the Dillingham Commission on immigrants in industries in the western states of the United States, published in 1911, pointed out that in Wyoming in 1908 there were but 23 Chinese miners at one mine and that this group was "practically all that are employed in the [entire] State."[164] On August 30, 1885, two days before the riot, there had been 331 Chinese and 150 whites in the Rock Springs coalfield, and two months later—before the Union Pacific commenced in earnest its fifteen-year program of ethnic cleansing against the Chinese—the number of Chinese coal miners had actually risen to 532 while the number of white workers had dropped to 85.[165]

The Dillingham Commission went on to observe that the "race present in largest numbers among the foreign-born was the Japanese," numbering 512.[166] When the commission took note of the fact that the "mining communities in Wyoming present a somewhat unique situation with regard to the relations between the various races," it evidenced this anomaly with the statement that "*even* orientals are eligible to union memberships, and the relations engendered by the association which such membership entails are *almost* fraternal." The commission reported that "Japanese and Chinese wear their union buttons with pride and are given the same treatment as other races."[167] However, this portrait of workingmen's racial harmony and equality is undercut by the fact the "Chinese and Japanese . . . races live apart from the others in 'bunk houses' provided for them," by the commission's notice that "natives and north Europeans are preferred in all cases by the operators for supervisory and other positions of responsibility," and by the fact that in contrast with European miners, the number of Japanese so employed was "decreasing."[168] Indeed, as Herbert Hill had documented, the coal mine operators were not the only ones unhappy with the dearth of whites and the presence of numerous Asian mine workers in the region; in 1902 the United Mine Workers had unleashed a vituperative campaign in behalf of extending Chinese exclusion and followed that with a program of opposition to Japanese immigration.[169] The comity that both the commission and Professor Montgomery say prevailed in Wyoming in 1908 was indeed an exception to labor's usual anti-Asian stance. But, as Yuji Ichioka's well-informed study of the labor-and-race issue at Rock Springs shows, the exception was the product of unique circumstances and did not set a precedent for labor-race relations in other venues: "Local conditions dictated the policy of admission [of Asian workers] in spite of . . . the union's antipathy to Japanese labor . . . Thus this notable exception to organized labor's exclusion of Japanese [and other Asian] labor was not the result of labor solidarity."[170]

Of course, adherents of Gyory's thesis are likely to dismiss this discussion of the Rock Springs riot and its aftermath by pointing out that he is for the most part willing to concede the racism of the white workingmen of the West, while insisting on the nonracist perspective of the latter's compatriots on the East Coast. But, even here, he is on shaky ground. Frederick Rudolph, a historian of the incident in North Adams, Massachusetts, whereby seventy-five Chinese shoemakers were brought to break a strike at the Calvin T. Sampson Shoe Company (the incident that is the starting point for Gyory's investigation), on the basis of his painstaking analysis of what actually happened and what the consequences were, concluded: "Sampson . . . had provided the Eastern workingmen with a laboratory from which came an indoctrination in opposition to Chinese labor and an unstinted support to all efforts at Chinese exclusion."[171] And one more point: Whereas Gyory insists it is the politicians who took the lead and the unions who lagged behind in the opposition to Chinese immigration during the pre-exclusion years, Montgomery offers an important instance in New York City when that order was reversed: "Sensing that its opposition to black enfranchisement was . . . costing more votes than it was winning, especially among German workers, . . . the Tweed Ring switched its target to the Chinese. In 1870 it *joined the unions* in a huge rally against the immigration of 'coolie labor' to the United States."[172] And, finally with respect to this aspect of Gyory's thesis, it might well be remembered that no less a figure than Selig Perlman had pointed out that "the National Labor Union came out against Chinese immigration in 1869, when the issue was brought home to the Eastern wage earners following the importation by a shoe manufacturer in North Adams, Massachusetts, of Chinese strike breakers,"[173] and that, writing to the same point, John R. Commons and his colleagues observed, "The general agitation which this action [i.e., the bringing of the Chinese shoemakers to Massachusetts] provoked among all classes of labour served to bring the national labour movement into closer sympathy with the California point of view." Commons et al., went on to note, "At the next convention of the National Labour Union in 1870 the general labour movement was ready to take the step from merely advocating the prohibition of Chinese importation to demanding total exclusion."[174] Gyory's Eastern workers had not been then, and are not now, above reproach.

The Leaders and the Led: Who, in Fact, Influenced Public Policy?

Throughout his book Gyory is at pains to distinguish the attitude of the rank and file of the white workingmen from the organizational and administrative leaders of the union movement. To be sure, Gyory in the end is forced to admit that in the spring of 1882, organized labor rallied behind the bill to ban Chinese immigrants.[175] But, he insists that at that moment the workingman's support was new, that they were "[r]ecent converts to exclusion," and that they had come to endorse that approach to resolving the debate over Chinese immigration "wholeheartedly when passage in Congress became a foregone conclusion." Before that time, his study wishes to suggest, they had been supporters only half-heartedly, that is, they had, in the words of the labor paper *Carpenter,* which Gyory quotes approvingly, regarded the Chinese as "dangerous to public health and human decency," but not opposed their immigration—provided, that is, that it could be proven to be voluntary. Indeed, they only railed against "their importation in hordes, under slavish contracts made in their native country, and held sacred by their religious fears." However, since every praiseworthy white workingman—and, it would seem, since he steadfastly eschews a critique of their views, Gyory himself—believed that virtually all Chinese immigration was involuntary, in almost every instance contracted in and from China, and but a part of the ubiquitous "coolie trade," this supposedly moderating dichotomy would appear to be the making of a distinction without a difference.

To Gyory the passage of the exclusion act was "a cheap panacea" for politicians, but for the white workers of 1882, "it was plainly the best they were going to get . . . Half a loaf—even not of their own choosing—was better than none."[176] The loaf they wanted, he argues, was an enforceable law prohibiting the importation of contract labor from anywhere in the world. However, when, in 1885, as Gyory points out in a footnote, "Congress finally acceded to workers' demands and passed the Foran Act, outlawing contract labor, . . . the law proved difficult to enforce and [was] largely ineffective."[177] But, since neither the white workingmen nor Gyory in his role as spokesperson for their instant mind-set could know that the Foran Act would be so deficient, why didn't the white workingmen clamor immediately for repeal of the Chinese Exclusion Act, in effect trading in the half a loaf that they had only grudgingly accepted in return for the whole? Of course, nothing of the sort happened, and claims that neither law was accomplishing what it was supposed to led Congress, with labor's unstinting support, to revise and extend the Chinese Exclusion Act over and over again, making it one of what Lucy E. Salyer calls the "laws harsh as tigers."[178]

In point of fact, labor's leaders became so influential in the administration of the exclusion laws that, except for the appeals granted to Chinese by the Constitution-conscious judges of the federal courts in California and the Pacific Northwest,[179] and the Chinese workers' protests and boycotts of

American goods in both China and America's Chinatowns,[180] they might have succeeded in driving the Chinese out altogether: From 1897 to 1902, Terence Powderly, former head of the Knights of Labor and an outspoken Sinophobe, served as Commissioner General of Immigration and in 1900 was placed in charge of appeals arising out of the enforcement of the Chinese Exclusion Act and its subsequent modifications; two years later, he was replaced by Frank P. Sargent, grand master of the Brotherhood of Locomotive Firemen and a friend of Samuel Gompers, the notoriously anti-Chinese leader of the American Federation of Labor, who served until 1908, and he in turn was succeeded for the next five years by Daniel Joseph Keefe, president of the longshoreman's union and a former vice-president of the AFL.[181] The alleged and much-vaunted independence of the white workingmen from their own leadership in fact came to nothing. Except for its possible influence on labor history, much the same might be said of Gyory's opus.

By and large, the men who founded, administered, lobbied, and conducted the meetings and conventions of America's labor unions favored the elimination of the Chinese worker from the labor market as well as the exclusion of the Chinese people from the United States. Gyory does not engage in a sustained analysis of these leaders and of their system of controls over the rank and file, and such omissions as these give implicit support to his belief in the class-oriented—rather than race-oriented—populist consciousness of the latter. However, he does mention such leaders as Samuel Gompers, Terence Powderly, and Adolph Strasser, carefully downplaying or avoiding altogether their Sinophobic statements, writings, and programs. There is no shortage of material on these matters, so what follows can only be illustrative and will be presented in relation to Gyory's thesis.

Samuel Gompers (1850–1924)

Gompers appears briefly in Gyory's book on three occasions: during a strike by New York City cigar makers in 1877;[182] as a supporter for the Greenback Party in the same period;[183] and as a contributor to the debates over the organizational structure of the newly formed Federation of Organized Trades and Labor Union (that was to become the American Federation of Labor in 1886) at its Pittsburgh convention in 1881.[184] Although the Chinese question figures in each of these events, a reader of Gyory's book would never learn from reading it that Gompers was perhaps the most important of the advocates of Chinese exclusion and author of some of the most racist demagoguery presented during the anti-Chinese movement. One need but turn to Gompers's autobiography and to his earlier public writings to learn that he made no apology for his Sinophobic outlook or for the labor practices he instituted in its behalf. In addition, perusing these, one might uncover evidence and argument that works against the class-oriented workingmen's thesis advanced by Gyory. For instance, in his *Seventy Years of Life and Labor,* published in 1925, Gompers claimed:

> . . . [W]e were contending against a menace to our trade [that] federal legislation alone could remedy. In 1878, of forty thousand cigar-makers in the entire country at least ten thousand were Chinamen employed in the cigar industry . . . California did not have authority to exclude Chinese workmen and Federal law was needed. Our International recognized that though competition with Chinese cigar-makers was then confined to the [Pacific] coast, the cigar industry of the East had to compete with the industry of the West in all markets, but alone it was not strong enough to secure protective legislation. During several strikes in the East, we had to meet the threats of employers to import Chinese strike breakers. This was an element in deciding the cigar-makers to give early and hearty endorsement to the movement for a national organization of labor unions, for the help of all wage-earners was needed in support of Chinese exclusion.[185]

That Gompers perceived the labor problem as a race problem is made clear not only in the words used to refer to nonwhite, non-Anglo workers in his autobiography, but also, and more viciously, in the pamphlets he wrote on the Chinese question and in his efforts to eliminate the Chinese presence from the American labor market both *before* and *after the passage of the exclusion act.*

From the mid-1870s Gompers would make opposition to Chinese immigration a central plank of his labor union platforms. He admired the adoption in 1875 of the "white label" by San Francisco's white cigar makers. When, on November 8, 1877, the *New York World* reported, falsely as it turned out, that three hundred Chinese cigar makers would be brought to New York City as strikebreakers, Gompers addressed a meeting of the Cigar Makers' International Union, saying "he desired that a warning should be given that if the manufacturers imported any large number to New York they would be responsible for any violent action that might be taken to protect their wives and children, and provide them with bread."[186] In November 1881, Gompers and his fellow unionists lent their support to a resolution reported one month later: "declaring the presence and competition of Chinese [laborers] with free white labor as extremely dangerous and demanding the passage of laws entirely prohibiting their *importation.*"[187] But, less than a year later, the Chinese Exclusion Act prohibited their *immigration.*

Gompers's fulminations against the Chinese, together with demands for stricter prohibitions on their immigration, did not cease after the Chinese Exclusion Act had been adopted. Fearful that the law would not be administered with appropriate acuity, Gompers presided over a meeting of the Federation of Trades and Labor Unions at which the organization's committee on legislation suggested that "a supplementary act" would be needed in order to ensure "the strictest enforcement of the present Anti-Chinese law."[188] On August 17, 1893, Gompers wrote to John O'Brien, an AFL organizer, applauding the latter's petition urging a more vigorous enforcement of the Geary Act of 1892, the law which had extended for another decade, and made more stringent, the provisions of the original Chinese Exclusion Act.[189] Six months earlier, Gompers had written to Hermann J. Schulteis, one of the clerks who had served on the U.S. Immigration Commission and who had authored the commission's *Report on European Immigration to the United States,* suggesting that because the "Immigration, the Alien Contract Labor and several other laws which were enacted through the efforts of our organizations should at least have men to execute them who are known to be in sympathy with those laws . . . [that] in the appointment of men to fill those positions it certainly seems reasonable that the views of the Executive Officers [of the AFL] should be consulted and met."[190] These wishes would be granted later with the successive appointments of Powderly, Sargent, and Keefe to head the agency. On April 4, 1894, in a letter to U.S. vice-president and former Democratic congressman from Illinois, Adlai Stevenson, Gompers suspended the subterfuge that Gyory would have his readers take to be both valid and reasonable, namely that organized labor opposed the immigration of Chinese labor solely on the ground that the latter came involuntarily as imported contract workers. Hoping to prevent ratification of the proposed China-U.S. treaty of 1894, Gompers observed:

> The Scott Exclusion Act [1888] and the Geary Law [1892, upheld by the United States Supreme Court in 1893, by a vote of 5 to 3, with Justice Harlan absent] were not passed in response to maudlin sentiment nor a national antipathy . . . They became laws . . . at the earnest demand of the toiling masses of our country . . . It is needless here to discuss the impossibility of the amalgamation or assimilation of the Chinese in America with our people. That has been so clearly demonstrated as to need no elucidation at my hands . . . In the name of more than half a million of organized working men and women of America, I enter my most solemn protest against the ratification of the Treaty by your Honorable Body, and earnestly hope it will be rejected.[191]

The treaty was ratified, however. In subsequent years, Gompers would not only oppose American expansion into the Pacific because more Chinese would become part of the labor force, but also attempt to evict from their jobs

Chinese already at work in America. When, in 1898, the House of Representatives was considering a bill authorizing the annexation of the Hawaiian Islands, Gompers protested to Thomas B. Reed, Speaker of the House, reminding him that "it [had] required more than twenty years of constant organization, agitation, and education to legislatively close the gates of our country to the Chinese"; claiming, beyond all considerations of fact, that of the 100,000 inhabitants of those islands there were 50,000 contract laborers of whom approximately 80 percent were Chinese and Japanese; and predicting that the "annexation of Hawaii would . . . obliterate that beneficent legislation and open wide our gates, . . . [threatening] an inundation of Mongolians to overwhelm the free laborers of our country."[192]

Although—because he favored Chinese exclusion over both imperialism and the "open door" policies enunciated during the McKinley and Theodore Roosevelt presidencies[193]—Gompers failed in his attempts to thwart the ratification of the China Treaty of 1894, halt the takeover of the Philippines in the aftermath of the Spanish-American War, and prevent the annexation of Hawaii, he was more successful in forcing union-sponsored cooperative industries to fire their Chinese workers. Thus, in one instance from 1897, Gompers chastised the Columbia River Fishermens Protective Union No. 6321, chartered by the AFL in 1894, for allegedly reneging on its promise to "have your work done exclusively by white labor . . . [and for having] entered into a contract with a Chinese boss to furnish the labor . . . [such] that now they are all Chinamen who are working there, . . . [as well as for posting a notice] that 'no white labor need apply.'" The union quickly surrendered: Sofus Jensen, an AFL organizer and the union secretary with whom Gompers had lodged his complaint, wrote back that while the story of the posted notice was false, the union had replaced "Chinese and coolie labor" with "American workmen."[194] The eviction of the Chinese worker from nearly every industry to which he and, in lesser numbers because of the restriction on the coming of Chinese women to America, she, had contributed would continue apace, abetted and coerced by white workingmen's strikes, until by 1911, there were few if any Chinese to be found in any of them, as the Dillingham Commission's statistics would show.[195]

As the twentieth century dawned and with it the possibility that the already once-renewed Chinese Exclusion Act would expire, Gompers put forth efforts to secure permanent exclusion. In February 1902, he testified before the Senate Committee on Immigration, insisting that "the exclusion of Chinese laborers from the United States is asked for by all of the wage workers of our country, particularly all the organized wage earners, regardless of any section of the country from which they hail and in which they are located."[196] And once again, but even more vehemently, he buttressed his argument with an attack on the social, moral, and civic aspects of Chinese society and culture:

> The presence in our country of a people entirely out of harmony and training with American comprehension of liberty and citizenship, who are alien to our customs and habits, as different from us in political and moral ideas as it is possible for two peoples to be, who are so thoroughly grounded in race characteristics that even the generations born and reared among us still retain them, can not but exercise a most demoralizing effect upon the body politic, the social life, and the civilization of the people of our nation.[197]

And, lest the senators not be informed about the unsalubrious effects that Chinese immigration had already inflicted and would continue to inflict on America unless their coming was halted altogether, Gompers set forth a parade of horribles drawn, he claimed, from facts about the Chinese situation of the state of California:

> All impartial observers agree, and official reports confirm it, that the condition of affairs in the State of California, the people of which had and still have to bear the brunt of this Asiatic contamination almost incredible to our people, in which gambling hells, opium joints, dens of iniquity and vice [abound,] are but superficial evidences of a moral standard as degrading in its exhibition as it is demoralizing by its contact.[198]

A number of exclusionist measures were laid before the Congress in 1902, but Gompers found most of them wanting in severity and scope, including the one that eventually secured passage and the signature of President Theodore Roosevelt. In 1902, together with Hermann Gudstadt, Gompers coauthored the most infamous of his screeds on the matter, *Some Reasons for Chinese Exclusion. Meat vs. Rice. American Manhood against Asiatic Coolieism. Which Shall Survive?*[199] (Perhaps it is needless to say, given his ideological stance, that this farrago of lies and tendentiousness is not mentioned in Gyory's text, notes, or bibliography.) Setting all claims of racial tolerance, ethnic empathy, or labor solidarity aside, the two veteran Chinese exclusionists reiterated and embellished with purple prose every accusation that had been made against Chinese immigrants, insisting on their mendacity, their womanless and hence immoral lifestyle, their willing submission to cheap labor contracts made in China, their murderous intra-communal conflicts, and, lest these not be sufficient to undermine any notion of their worthiness to come to the United States, Gompers and Gudstadt added a new charge, namely, that Chinese male immigrants seduced chaste, prepubescent white girls and boys into drug addiction and prostitution:

> Passing through the upper end of Kearney street, in the vicinity of [San Francisco's] Chinatown, after nightfall one may see a number of what were

> once men and women, but are now but mental and physical wrecks of humanity. . . . Who and what are these beings, and why are they seen only in San Francisco, one of nature's most favored cities? . . . Some time in the past these poor, miserable, and degraded wrecks were the beloved children of fond parents . . . They have become what is known in the parlance of the street as "dope heads"—opium fiends in the ordinary language. In some manner, by some wily method they have been induced to use the drug. Time was when little girls no older than 12 years were found in Chinese laundries under the influence of opium. What other crimes were committed in those dark and fetid places when these little innocent victims of the Chinamen's wiles were under the influence of the drug are almost too horrible to imagine . . . [T]here are hundreds, aye thousands, of our American boys and girls who have acquired this deadly habit and are doomed, hopelessly doomed, beyond a shadow of redemption. Better death a hundred times than to have become a victim of this worst of all oriental opium habit.[200]

Gyory, who denies that Sinophobia infected much of the white working class and seeks to separate the thoughts and deeds of the rank and file from those of the trade union leadership, omits the latter from his investigation. In so doing, he does a disservice to the candidly stated beliefs of the white workingmen. To take one example from many that might be noted, the *Report of Proceedings of the Twenty-fifth Annual Convention of the American Federation of Labor, 1905*, includes the following:

> [We make] no pretense that the exclusion of Chinese can be defended upon a high ideal, ethical ground . . . Surely, America's workmen have enough to contend with, have sufficient obstacles confronting them in their struggle to maintain themselves in their humanizing movement for a higher and better life, without being required to meet the enervating, killing, underselling, and under-living competition of that nerveless, wantless people, the Chinese.[201]

The effectiveness of Chinese exclusion, coupled with the latter's forced expulsion from the agricultural and urban labor markets, led Gompers to turn his exclusionist/evictionist attention to another Asian people, the Japanese, and to nip in the bud a possibility that they might form a labor alliance with working-class Mexicans. In 1886, it had been estimated that seven-eighths of the work being done in California's vineyards and orchards was being carried out by Chinese.[202] However, a series of race-baiting strikes by rural and urban white workingmen, beginning in 1893, had driven most of the Chinese from the fields.[203] By 1911, twenty-nine years after the Chinese Exclusion Act had been passed, Japanese, Korean, Mexican, and a few southern and eastern European workers had replaced the once-thriving rural Chinese labor force in California. "The Japanese," the Dillingham Commission reported, "are at present the predominant race of hand workers in most districts, because they are present in large numbers and migrate most easily having few family ties and little property to keep them in one community."[204] Their family ties, however, would soon be strengthened by *shashin kekkon* ("picture marriage") and their settlement on the land as small holders hastened as they sought to overcome the obstacles created by California's and ten other states' Alien Land Laws.[205] However, the outcome of the Oxnard strike of 1903 and the hostile stance toward Japanese and Mexican agricultural laborers taken by Gompers and the AFL surely did much to convince the nonwhite, non-Anglo workers that labor solidarity meant little when race matters loomed in the minds of the union's leadership.

To put the matter briefly:[206] Rural Japanese and Mexican agricultural laborers had organized a union, the Japanese-Mexican Protective Association (JMPA), in the early months of 1903. On March 18 of that year, the union, composed of eight hundred Japanese and four hundred Mexicans, struck the Western Agricultural Contracting Company (WACC), protesting WACC's hiring through contractors (a common practice over which Gompers supposedly justified his opposition to Chinese immigration), payment in goods rather than money, and threats of a wage cut. The strike turned violent and eventually ended with a compromise agreement. When JMPA and another Japanese union applied for charters from the AFL, Gompers wrote the secretary of the local labor council: "If you think it wise that the Japanese be organized, you may do so, but no charter will be issued to them by the American Federation of Labor nor can they be accorded representation in an affiliated Central Labor Union." The local organizer protested this action as well as an earlier letter from Gompers that had insisted "that this charter is issued to you [Mexicans] with the express understanding that under no circumstances shall you take into your union any Chinese or Japanese." Gompers would not be moved however; not even when F. C. Wheeler, an AFL district organizer, angrily wrote the union's national secretary, quoting the Mexican workers' statement that "we had a hard bitter fight and now when our victory is absolute and complete you ask us to deny our Japanese brothers the same right we ask for ourselves. We will not do it. We will stand by the men who stood by us." Gompers would later assure the secretary of the Honolulu Trades and Labor Council that the AFL had "steadfastly refused to issue charters to organizations composed of Japanese laborers." Lest anyone suppose that Gompers was pursuing some working-class ideal in jettisoning the JMPA from the AFL, note his remark, reported in the September 1905 edition of the *American Federationist:* "The caucasians are not going to let their standard of living be destroyed by negroes, Chinamen, Japs, or any other."[207]

Gompers's hostility to Asian workers would continue throughout his life. In his autobiography, Gompers recalls an unforgettable if hasty trip he made into San Francisco's Chinatown. In that memoir, Gompers's remarks indicate the prejudicial source of his opposition to Chinese immigration. Class was not the issue.

> I made a trip through Chinatown—not the especially prepared route for tourists. It was an awful experience with all its hideousness. I had read Dante's *Inferno,* but Chinatown seemed to me a greater horror with its reeking smells, the human wrecks, gambling and mad licentiousness. The picture burned into my mind that night came to me vividly throughout future years when Chinese immigration was under consideration.[208]

So sure was Gompers that Asiatic immigration constituted a major threat not only to American labor but also to American society that, from 1905 until his death two decades later, he entertained dark suspicions about some kind of evil force at work to thwart his exclusionist efforts.[209] Thus it was that in his autobiography he recalled meeting a man—never named—who informed him of a vast conspiracy whereby unknown numbers of Chinese were being smuggled illegally into the United States with the connivance and collusion of a clandestine network of district attorneys and court interpreters. Moreover, after his chosen enforcer, immigration commissioner Terence Powderly, told him that he had been ordered to "cease his activity" with respect to exclusionary enforcement, and Frank Sargent, Powderly's successor, had become so disenchanted with his inability to bring a halt to the illegal entry of Chinese that he gave up governmental service and returned to his presidency of the Brotherhood of Locomotive Firemen, Gompers became convinced that there were "some . . . Federal officials . . . responsible for this smuggling [who] were so high up in administrative circles that they were able to prevent enforcement of the Chinese Exclusion Law."[210] Moreover, these officials, he claimed, were not only exercising control over the Immigration and Naturalization Service, but also operating out of the Department of Commerce and Labor.[211] A few years later, when Woodrow Wilson had become president of the United States—and, as Gwendolyn Mink shows, the AFL had begun to conduct a "politics of union preeminence," entering into a relationship with the Congress and the Executive Office that, on the one hand, "regarded social insurance and wages and hours laws for men . . . as hostile incursions by government," while, on the other, sought "policies that would promote its own autonomy"[212]—Gompers shifted the focus of his heated exaggerations, suspiciousness, and conspiratorial fantasy (i.e., the very trio of qualities that Richard Hofstadter calls the "paranoid style" that has so often modified American public policy debates)[213] to a recently formed opponent of exclusionism, the National Liberal Immigration League, which, he insisted, was being financed by "the Hamburg-American Steamship Company, the Campagnie Générale Transatlantique, and the Steamship Companies and industries generally that found a financial profit in employing cheap immigrant workers."[214] Members of Congress were sufficiently impressed by Gompers's argument, made in behalf of the Burnett Immigration bill, already vetoed by President Wilson, to reintroduce the measure in both houses and overturn the president's second veto by a two-thirds majority.[215] On the Chinese question Gompers never repudiated his statement of 1894 in which he declared his opposition to the "evil effect of [the] Chinese invasion: [a] people . . . who allow themselves to be barbarously tyrannized over in their own country, and who menace the progress, the economic and social standing of the workers of other countries, cannot be fraternized with."[216]

Lest one take up Philip Taft's position that Gompers's Sinophobia was merely a representation of the attitude of the day, one might contrast Gompers's statement above with that of Jacob A. Riis, who traversed New York City's Chinatown at about the same time. Riis took note of the poverty, "dismal dreariness," "forbidding partitions," opium parlors, gambling dens, overworked peddlers, "teeming tenements," and womanless condition of the Chinese immigrant laborers. But, where these would lead Gompers to call for exclusion of the Chinese, the same conditions inspired Riis to call for more not less immigration from China:

> This is a time for very plain speaking on this subject. Rather than banish the Chinaman, I would have the door opened wider—for his wife; make it a condition of his coming or staying that he bring his wife with him. Then, at least, he might not be what he now is and remains, a homeless stranger among us. Upon this hinges the real Chinese question, in our city, at all events, as I see it.[217]

It is a true tragedy of scholarship that Gyory failed to consider this argument, failed, that is, to see that Chinese workers were as integral a part of the labor force as the Irish workers he lauds.

Adolph Strasser (1843–1939)

This Hungarian-born founder of the Amalgamated Trades and Labor Union of New York City and Vicinity and Gompers's hand-picked nominee as president of the Cigar Makers International Union (1877–1891) appears more often than any other union leader in Gyory's book.[218] And well he might, for throughout much of his long life[219]—he ceased his union activities as auditor, organizer, legislative representative, arbitrator, and troubleshooter, in 1914, turning for the final twenty-five years of his life to real estate in New York and Florida—Strasser served as Gompers's close colleague, coordinator, fellow union officer, and strategist for the AFL executive, as he had for its predecessors. Together with Gompers, Strasser developed his perspective out of a peculiarly American reformulation of the ideas of Marx's American correspondent, Friedrich Sorge, leader of Section One of the International Workingmen's Association, the latter having been founded by Karl Marx in 1864. If there is need for further evidence in support of one strand of the theory of "American exceptionalism"[220]—here referring to the manner in which European conceptions of class were transmogrified to become the thesis that a workingman's wages ought to be calibrated on the basis of his biosocial proximity to "whiteness"[221]—it will be found in Strasser's (and Gompers's) adaptation of German Marxism: "If there was anything exceptional about the American labor movement compared to its counterparts in other industrial countries," writes Timothy Messer-Kruse, "it was the unique way in which the teleological underpinnings and revolutionary fervor of Marxism were deracinated and engrafted upon an essentially inward-looking and racially exclusive trade union movement."[222] For, as Messer-Kruse goes on to show, Strasser and Gompers, although each had independently "absorbed the passion, commitment, and historical materialism of their German American Marxist teachers, [together they created out of these one of] the most politically conservative working-class movements of the nineteenth and twentieth centuries."[223]

A central plank of what would become the Sinophobic and racialist ideology of the burgeoning AFL was put together by Gompers and Strasser, the latter of whom adopted the insidious "white label" as a national tool,[224] analogizing the fight carried on by white California cigar makers against their Chinese fellow workers to his own ultimately successful effort to expel from that line of work the "tenement scum,"[225] that is, rival socialist cigar makers who had broken with the Gompers-Strasser faction and formed the Progressive Cigar Makers' Union. Gyory wishes his readers to believe that Strasser's testimony before the Hewitt Committee favoring the exclusion of all contract laborers from the United States regardless of race—which he reprints[226]—refutes the charges made by both Herbert Hill and Gwendolyn Mink that Strasser, together with Gompers, to use Mink's way of wording the issue, "defended the anti-Chinese posture of their California colleagues and actively involved themselves in the exclusion movement."[227] But, Mink's statement is in accord with the facts on this issue. Strasser took a major part in bringing California workingmen's anti-Chinese prejudices to the East Coast locals and to the national executive council of what would become the AFL. On October 27, 1878, addressing a mass meeting of New York City's tobacco workers engaged in the struggle to end tenement house production of cigars, Strasser, according to a news report in the November 5 issue of the *New York Tribune,*

> made a speech in which he said that when the Chinese cigar makers in California began to crowd the whites out of the work, the latter succeeded in passing a State law requiring every cigar factory to affix on each box a union stamp, by which cigars made by white men could be distinguished from those made by Chinese; and the public showed their condemnation of Chinese work by refusing to smoke cigars made by Chinamen.[228]

The *Cigar Makers' Official Journal,* a monthly publication of the CMIU, established in November 1875, began to editorialize against Chinese cigar makers on a regular basis after November 8, 1877, when, in the midst of the tenement house work stoppage, the *New York World* printed the aforementioned false rumor that cigar manufacturers had requested that three hundred Chinese cigar makers be sent to New York City to replace the whites on strike.[229] According to the notes supplied by the editor of Volume I of the *Gompers Papers,* "The journal subscribed to the view generally expressed in the American press of the time that *Chinese workers unlike other immigrant groups,* could not be assimilated into American culture."[230] Thus, the CMIU, over which Strasser presided for fourteen years, took a position based not on the generality of working conditions or the universality of class consciousness, but rather one rooted in the assessment of each ethnic group's assimilability. Largely composed of German and Bohemian immigrants—whose separate language-based locals Strasser managed to merge—the CMIU, whose rallies Strasser often addressed in German, had no doubts about the Americanization capabilities of these European workers but no sympathetic concern for the working and living situations of the Chinese laborers in the same industry.

Had Gyory consulted articles on the labor question that appeared in *Die Gewerkschafts-Zeitung,* a German-language publication that was published for only a few years in New York City and edited and contributed to by Adolph Strasser, Carl Speyer, and Hugo Müller, he would have discovered more evidence of Strasser's support for Chinese exclusion. In the formative years of America's trade union movement, this journal had a significant influence not only on its German-reading subscribers, but also on August Sartorius von Waltershausen (1852–1938), a German economist who visited the United States in the 1880s, carefully consulted its pages, and wrote comprehensively and critically about many aspects of the labor movement.[231] In 1883, Sartorius published a lengthy essay entitled "Die Chinesen in den Vereinigten Staaten von America,"[232] which, while it concluded with support for exclusion, offered what David Montgomery calls "both a thorough account of the harassment and exclusion of Chinese by state and federal legislation, labor movement boycotts, and mob action between 1844 and 1882 and a serious informative effort to analyze the economic and institutional framework of the Chinese immigrant community itself."[233] Sartorius had met and talked with Strasser, among others, and adapted his own, already established racist outlook on the allegedly inferior races—(influenced, as Montgomery reminds us, by the writings of a German social geographer, Friedrich Ratzel [1844–1904], a right-wing National Liberal, imperialist and Social Darwinist, who had also visited the United States and written on the Chinese question)[234]—to the Sinophobia of the white trade unionists.[235] Moreover, Sartorius praised the use of the boycott and the white label,[236] tactics championed and introduced to the East Coast white workingmen by Strasser, describing with obvious approval how the boycott and the label were combined in a two-fold attack on Chinese cigar makers:

> In the last three years during which the labor movement has made such extraordinary strides in terms of organization, the label system has been more successful than ever, particularly since it has been linked to boycotts. In saloons and shops union members demand label cigars. If the owner or the manager does not supply them, the establishment is boycotted. When he accepts the workers' demands, they make further demands, for instance that he stock *only* label cigars (i.e., for all smokers). If he does not accede, the workers will again boycott his goods. In the smaller cities, where unionization is strong, this approach has been successful on many occasions.[237]

To understand Strasser's role in the anti-Chinese movement one must examine what he (and Gompers) learned from watching the fractious divisions within two American sections of the International Workingman's Association. Strasser and Gompers were at first sympathetic to socialism and to much of the efforts of IWA Section One, Sorge's largely German group. Sorge perceived as his greatest rival the leaders of the mostly American-born Section Twelve, headed by feminist, spiritualist, and candidate for the presidency of the United States, Victoria Woodhull (1838–1927), and by the utopian socialist sociologist who had translated and published in *Woodhull's and Claflin's Weekly* the first English language version of Marx's and Engel's *Communist Manifesto,* Stephen Pearl Andrews (1812–1886).[238] Strasser and Gompers carefully noted how Sorge utilized expulsion and the boycott to rid the American branch of the IWA of its left-wing deviationists.[239] Thus, in 1872, when, Woodhull and Andrews formed the Equal Rights Party with Woodhull self-nominated for the U.S. presidency and African American ex-slave Frederick Douglass as her vice-presidential running mate,[240] Sorge appealed to Marx for assistance in ridding the IWA of this wholly unprecedented move. Marx complied, denouncing Section Twelve members as "bogus reformers, middle class quacks, and trading politicians" and Andrews and Woodhull and their followers as "middle-class humbugs and worn out Yankee swindlers in the reform business."[241] Section Twelve was suspended and then expelled from the International, the electoral campaign failed, and Sorge and Section One emerged the victors.[242] What Strasser and Gompers learned from this incident was that their enemies might also be boycotted and if necessary expelled from the trade union movement. Whereas the Woodhull-Andrews group thereafter "rejected the trade union tactic of winning a larger share of the capitalist pie by controlling access to labor markets and rejecting women and racial minorities from their membership rolls," moving toward "egalitarian and inclusive unionism," Adolph Strasser and Samuel Gompers became two "of the most famous architects of the skill-, race-, and sex-defined trade union model,"[243] rejecting their older adherence to socialism in favor of "trade unionism, pure and simple."[244] The Chinese worker—and later other Asian, nonwhite, and non-Anglo workers—became the permanent, indeed the ideal enemy, a functional equivalent of the Woodhull-Andrews Equal Rights Party, toward which their Sorgean-derived expulsion strategy was irrevocably directed.[245]

Terence V. Powderly (1849–1924)

Grand Master (after 1883, General Master) Workman of the Knights of Labor (KOL), (1879–1893); elected mayor of Scranton, Pennsylvania, three times on the Greenback-Labor ticket (1878–1884); opponent of workingmen's strikes; active participant in the struggles between the KOL and the CMIU; for many years rivalrous enemy of Gompers and the latter's approach to trade unionism; advocate of political rather than economic action with respect to the Haymarket affair (1886); clandestine member of the secret Irish nationalist society *Clan na Gael;* appointed U.S. Commissioner-General of Immigration (1897–1902) by President McKinley; and Chief of the Division of Information in the Bureau of Immigration and Naturalization (1907–1924),[246] Terence Vincent Powderly is mentioned but three times in Gyory's book.[247] However, a reader would not learn from these brief entries that Powderly was one of the most vitriolic and vituperative of the labor movement's Sinophobes. Powderly's role in the alliance of the KOL with the Greenback-Labor Party is mentioned in the context of the latter's program opposing "imported," that is, contracted, Chinese labor and favoring voluntary immigration; his statement, "I am disgusted with Kearney" is presented as evidence of the KOL leader's anger over the San Francisco's sandlot salesman of Sinophobia's attempt to win over Scranton's workingmen to his extraordinarily vilifying approach to Chinese exclusion. His receipt of KOL founder Uriah Stephens's request that Kearney "be favorably launched as an element in the Labor Movement on the Atlantic Slope" is presented without any report of Powderly's reply.

However, Powderly's own adamant hostility to Chinese immigration is not difficult to document. In part, in his case, it is related to a larger religious division—the jurisdictional dispute between the Catholic church and various Protestant denominations over the appropriate trade union gospel, ultimately over the salvation of the workingman's soul.[248] In California, the Catholic church had chosen to serve its new-immigrant Irish and Italian constituencies and turned its back on Chinese immigrants, its leading local priest becoming a well-known speaker favoring exclusion.[249] In the same state—until the few conversions they were able to effect dampened their ardor[250]—Protestant missionaries, called back from China, took up the cause of the Chinese and also sought to cure their souls.[251] With the spread of the anti-Chinese movement to the East, coupled with the migration of Irish Catholics to the Pacific coast, the religio-ethnoracial conflict that threatened to divide Irish Catholic workingmen from their white Protestant fellow workers was heightened but also deflected in great part by the Chinese question.[252]

Powderly took a leading position on the latter issue when he evicted Chinese workers from his own laborite organization. When, in 1887, Chinese assemblies of the Knights of Labor were organized by District 49, Powderly ordered that they be disbanded forthwith, he having already "gone on record as not only opposing Chinese labor but also declaring that Chinese and Japanese were unfit to reside in the United States."[253]

Powderly's popularity with white workingmen—and, later, his coming to agreeable terms with Gompers—arose in great measure from the rhetoric with which he peppered his anti-Chinese diatribes. Like Kearney—whom he may have seen as more a disturbing Orangeman than a disgusting rabble-rouser—Powderly's speeches and articles were filled with Sinophobic vitriol. However, to influence his Irish Catholic followers and alleviate the worries of those papacy-fearing Protestant workingmen who on most secular matters supported his position, he linked his advocacy of stronger anti-Chinese legislation to the protection and preservation of a generalized Occidental Christian civilization in America. Thus, on January 8, 1892, an article in the *San Francisco Chronicle* quoted him censuring employers who opposed exclusion: "Standing behind them [i.e., the Chinese] are Christian employers of this land, who would rather import heathen willing to work for barely enough to sustain life than retain a brother Christian at a wage sufficient to live as becomes a Christian. We do not want opium or the Chinese who grow it."[254] In the same article, Powderly also aligned his concerns about Chinese immigration with those said to be worrying white laboring men, and, warming to his subject, to those frightened by the prospect of the destruction of the American polity itself. Thus, he warned his readers that "the substitution of the Mongolian slave for the American freeman, the abandonment of home for the street and slum and the final overthrow of the republic," were likely consequences of a weakened exclusion law.[255] A decade later, Powderly, having become Commissioner-General of Immigration, and after 1900 in sole charge of enforcing Chinese exclusion,[256] was still unsatisfied: "No graver danger has ever menaced the workingmen of America," he thundered, "than that which faces them when the possibility of lowering the bars at our seaports and border-lines to the Chinese is presented."[257] Again seeking strengthening of the exclusion law, Powderly laid out his own version of a parade of horribles, a comprehensive and irrevocable indictment of the Chinese whether considered as a people, a sociological entity, or a civilization:

> BAR JOHN CHINAMAN TO ETERNITY!
> The opposition to the Chinese coolie is not alone because of his race or his religion, but because of the economic position he occupies in this country . . . They do not assimilate with our people, do not wear our clothing, do not adopt our customs, language, religion or sentiments. It is said that the Chinese, if given an opportunity, will become Americanized. The Chinese coolie will no more become Americanized than an American can take on the habits, customs, garb and religion of the Mongolian . . . American and Chinese civilizations are antagonistic; they cannot live and thrive and both survive on the same soil.[258]

Powderly closed this peroration with a dire prophecy: "One or the other must perish."[259]

Powderly served not only a five-year term (1897–1902) as U.S. Commissioner-General of Immigration and a one-year term as special representative of the Department of Labor and Commerce to study European immigration problems, but also accepted appointment as chief of the Division of Information in the Bureau of Immigration and Naturalization, a position he held from 1907 until his death in 1924. In each of these offices he (and his successor Commissioners-General: Frank P. Sargent [1902–1908], grand master of the Brotherhood of Locomotive Firemen, and Daniel Joseph Keefe [1908–1913], a sometime vice-president of the AFL)[260] came into regular contact with and pressure from Samuel Gompers for whom the relentless pursuit of ever-stricter enforcement of Asiatic exclusion had, as we have seen, become a veritable obsession.[261]

Gyory, of course, makes no mention of any of this. Having ended his investigation with the passage of the Chinese Exclusion Act in 1882, he does not report on how Powderly, Gompers, and the other exclusionists were challenged by Rev. Wu P'an-chao (1866–1931), known in America as Dr. Ng Poon Chew, founder and editor of *Chung Sai Yat Po,* the first Chinese-language newspaper in the United States.[262] Ng, who succeeded in obtaining a reclassification of newspaper editors as educators rather than laborers, toured the United States in behalf of a repeal of the law,[263] published an eloquent refutation of the exclusionist position in the *New York Times,*[264] and debated both Powderly and Gompers when, in 1905, they sought an even harsher measure prohibiting the coming of Asians to America.[265] Nor does Gyory take account of the study published in 1916, by Tien-Lu Li, professor of English at Peking University, who, having not only examined the facts and forces associated with the Burlingame Treaty of 1868, the modification of the latter in 1880, the treaty of 1894, the Exclusion Acts of 1882, 1884, 1888, 1892, 1893, 1902, and 1904, the extension of the exclusion laws to Hawaii and the Philippine Islands after 1898, and also critically appraised both the pro- and the anti-exclusionist positions, concluded, "It is no solution of the problem that omits the main . . . question . . . , the exclusion of Chinese laborers . . . If the present policy is sound, wise, and in accordance with eternal truth and justice, then let it be pursued and maintained, cost what it may. But it would do no harm to pause and think whether it is."[266] A singular shortcoming of Gyory's investigation is that he did not take up the kind of challenge that Professor Li had thrown down more than eight decades before his book was published.

Conclusion

A Heritage of Anti-Asian Hostility

In a statement directed at British subscribers to the internet bookseller Amazon.com U.K., Gyory wrote, "At the dawn of a new century, the Chinese Exclusion Act still casts a long, dark shadow over American society and our nation's treatment of immigrants."[267] True enough, but the argument of his book, especially his revival of the coolie mystique, darkens that shadow. Suspicions about the character, intentions, and loyalty of the Chinese in the United States, whether recently arrived or American-born, did not disappear after the repeal of the exclusion laws in 1943. "Without a doubt," historians Philip P. Choy, Lorraine Dong, and Marlon K. Hom write, "Chinese exclusion . . . left a legacy of racism."[268] Some examples: When, in the midst of the Korean War, troops from the People's Republic of China hurled back the American advance, there were roundups of alien Chinese on the East Coast of the United States.[269] In 1966, with the war in Vietnam raging and threatening to engulf the great powers in a wider conflict, Jerome Beatty Jr., a *Saturday Review* columnist, hinted that America's Chinese could face the same fate as that which befell the Japanese Americans on the West Coast in 1942:

> An unconfirmed rumor has come to my attention that our FBI is well prepared for a World War III in which our major enemy will be China. Detention camps have been secretly prepared in which will be "relocated" all the Chinese in the United States so that they may be screened, and prevented from sabotaging the war effort and signaling Peking with short-wave radios.[270]

Twelve years later, Ming Hai Loo, a twenty-four-year-old Chinese American, residing in Raleigh, North Carolina, was gunned down by two white men who insisted he was Vietnamese and held him responsible for the deaths of American soldiers in Vietnam.[271] In 1983, Loren W. Fessler, a journalist who had served as an adviser with Chinese airborne troops during the Second World War, pointed out that "the legacy of anti-Chinese feeling built up in the nineteenth century remained strong all through the first four decades of the twentieth century."[272] But, ironically, his statement offered a premature closure to this mode of Sinophobia. To take but what is, arguably, the most egregious example: When, after two unemployed Detroit auto workers, on June 19, 1982, beat Vincent Chin, a Chinese American engineer, to death with a baseball bat, calling him a "Jap" and screaming, "It's because of you motherfuckers that we're out of work," and a local judge sentenced Chin's killers to probation and a fine of three thousand dollars each, a federal attempt to charge Chin's murderers with violating his civil rights failed.[273] "[H]ate crimes against Asians still . . . [occur]," Choy, Dong, and Hom point out, "testifying to the continued scapegoating of Asians in America during times of economic decline and unemployment."[274]

Nor is the current version of apprehensions about a "yellow peril"—the term authoritatively introduced into the racist rhetoric of the Occident by Germany's Kaiser Wilhelm II around the turn of the nineteenth century[275]—limited to fears about job loss to Asian immigrants or to "outsourcing" of American manufactures to countries where a supply of cheap labor is available. By 1990 the Chinese had become the largest of more than twenty Asian peoples living and working in the United States. Their numbers had grown and the shortage of women among them had been relieved because of such post-repeal laws as the War Brides Act (1945), Displaced Persons Act (1948), McCarran-Walters Immigration Act (1952), Refugee Relief Act (1953), and two of the post-repeal Immigration Acts (1968, 1981).[276] One aspect of these changes has been a peculiar distribution of occupations. Foreign-born Chinese are to be found at both ends of the occupational scale: some in well-paying, professional, technical, scientific, and high-tech positions; while others are at the low end, working as waiters, dishwashers, hotel and restaurant workers, and in the garment industry. American-born Chinese college and university graduates are more likely to be found in the white-collar professions or in business.[277] Having avoided the blue-collar sector where a lingering Sinophobic animus discouraged when it did not absolutely prohibit their entry, however, neither the foreign- nor the American-born Chinese professionals have been able to put off the badge of suspicion and distrust the earlier exclusion had done so much to spawn: Thus, the recent allegations of espionage against government-employed Chinese scientists, engineers, and technicians employed at Los Alamos National Laboratory and the corrupt practices admitted by two Chinese political fund-raisers working in the arena of national politics[278] have sent a chill into the ranks of this most successful part of the Chinese American community. "Because of the incidents at Los Alamos," Raymond Ng, a Chinese American engineer employed at the Sandia National Laboratories at Livermore, California, pointed out, ". . . a cloud of suspicion appears to hang over all Asian Pacific Americans."[279] One can almost hear echoes of Gompers's and Powderly's warnings about the threat that Chinese civilization poses for America when one reads Caspar W. Weinberger's "Foreword" to the House of Representatives *Report of the Select Committee on U.S. National. Security and Military/Commercial Concerns with the People's Republic of China* ("the Cox Report"), which stated, "Communist China's long march against the United States is as tenacious as it is diverse—from campaign contributions used to buy influence in the White House, to purchasing an interest in American corporations, to hi-tech spying, [and] to a plain old-fashioned military buildup and threats."[280] Further, when it is reported that 450 of the employees at Los Alamos are "foreign citizens," and that this number includes "more than 30 from Russia, China, North Korea, and seven other 'sensitive' countries,"[281] one senses that Chinese scientists, whether "imported" or American-born, alien or citizen, have become the era's current version of the "coolie menace." Unlike the Irish and other Euro-American workingmen, whose grandparents sought and achieved the perquisites of "whiteness" by excluding them and scorning their ancestral culture, Chinese Americans of whatever socioeconomic class are transformed into "honorary whites" when denied a place in affirmative action programs, but otherwise and all too often regarded as permanent "immigrants."[282] The deeper and more pervasive legacy of the Chinese Exclusion era has been captured by Lisa Lowe when she writes:

> A national memory haunts the conceptions of the Asian-American, persisting beyond the repeal of actual laws prohibiting Asians from citizenship and

> sustained by the wars in Asia, in which the Asian is always seen as . . . the "foreigner-within," even when born in the United States and the descendant of generations born here before.[283]

Gyory's book does nothing to dispel this national memory.

Chinese Exclusion and Labor History

Despite his claim that Herbert Gutman's "spirit and vision infuses every page of this book,"[284] a closer reading of both mentor and disciple would suggest that Gyory has not been faithful to what might be called the nonmaterialist elements of his teacher's perspective. Of the shifts that occurred in Gutman's thought, the one most relevant to Gyory's study is the former's growing interest in the spiritual side of the white workingman's mind.[285] Although most of the current New Labor Historians claim their patrimony from Gutman and E. P. Thompson—and, in one study, acknowledge the role of Christianity in inspiring urban black labor activism[286]—their general tendency is to broaden the term *class* so that it encompasses religion, race, and culture but does not give up its primacy as the essential element in the struggle between labor and capital.[287] Gutman, however, although he did not openly acknowledge a diminution in his faith in class and class struggle—as E. P. Thompson did in 1993[288]—could not deny the instances in which his historical investigations opened up features of labor activism that were not comprehendible by traditional class analysis. Of these, his study of Gilded Age Protestantism and its role in structuring the consciousness of white workingmen is crucial.[289]

David Roediger has noted that "when [Gutman] attempted to discuss race relations within the working class, a desire to recover antiracist traditions led to a straining of the evidence and an unwillingness to probe the extent of white working class racism."[290] However, although his faults in that regard are clear,[291] his commitment to factual-based study caused him to uncover evidence that tended to undermine his unfailing conviction that class solidarity and class consciousness characterized the working class.[292] For example, his startling observation—that in Protestantism there "was a religious faith that justified labor organization and agitation, encouraged workers to challenge industrial power, and compelled criticism of 'natural' economic laws, the crude optimism of social Darwinism, and even the conformist Christianity of most respectable clergymen"[293]—not only introduced a significant role for Protestant ideology in the make-up of the working-class *mentalite,* but also, if only implicitly, raised the question of the role that Catholic ideas might have played in the minds of white laborers adhering to that religion. Gutman did not explore the implications of Catholic thought for working-class consciousness, although he claimed to have collected data on the subject.[294] Had he done so, he might have uncovered how religious tensions within the working class were reduced by fomenting a campaign against Asiatic heathenism.

When Gutman flung down the challenge—as quoted by Gyory, who accepted it—"This event in North Adams needs to be looked at in a fresh light. Who wants to tackle it?"[295]—he might have been posing precisely the kind of research problem that Gyory *did not* choose to solve. That would have been—indeed, should have been—an investigation that, taking Gutman's favorite aphorism, Sartre's statement that "the essential is not what 'one' has done to him,"[296] would have pursued the largely Catholic Irish workingmen's story in terms of their anomalous status as objects of both religious and racial bigotry—and how they sought to overcome their situation by seizing upon the "Chinese Question" and turning their own and other workingmen's attention to the "threat" presented by a "Chinese invasion."[297] Putting together their refusal to associate with black and Chinese workers, their boasted identification with a generalized Occidental Christian civilization that would exclude Asiatics, and their adaptation of Sinophobic stereotopy to both their labor actions and their low-brow culture—that is, the kinds of facts uncovered in the researches carried out by Tchen, Roediger, Ignatiev, and Hill—these workers trod the path to "whiteness" and full-fledged Americanization. Gyory has not told this story. In his eagerness to exonerate the white working class from their blameworthy participation in the movement for Chinese exclusion, he has given new life to the lie that the Chinese immigrant posed a real threat to white workers' economic, social, and moral well-being.

"All too frequently, and for too long," observes historian and Sinologist Franklin Ng, "the separation of Chinese American history, like that of black history, from immigrant and ethnic history has worked to the detriment of both."[298]

And, I would add, to the detriment of labor history as well.

PART III

The "Jewish Question" and the Lost Tribes of Israel

CHAPTER FOUR

The Lost Tribes of Israel as a Problem in History and Sociology

> During a four-thousand-year history the Jewish people have survived Egyptian slavery, Babylonian captivity, Roman dispersion, the Crusades, the Inquisition, the Holocaust, and more. Jews adapted to the realities of their times and the places where they were permitted to exist, sometimes with only bare-bones knowledge of their covenant with God that determined their identity and their fate.
>
> —MARVIN D. SCHWARTZ, "Afterword," *Middletown Jews*

Ten of the original twelve tribes that comprised the ancient Hebrew people disappeared from conventional history and other secular annals sometime immediately before and shortly after 721 B.C.E., when the Northern Kingdom of Israel was overrun by the Assyrians and its people were sent into exile. Sacred histories and biblical prophecies hold that the ten lost tribes will be reunited with their tribal brethren descended from the Southern Kingdom of Judea just before, or as a signal of, the coming messianic age. A quest for the descendants of the lost tribes has been begun many times, usually associated with the resolution of immediate, local, secular, or sacred issues that emerged in a particular era and at a particular place. Various peoples (e.g., the Falasha of Ethiopia, the Lemba of Zimbabwe, the Pachucans of Mexico, various tribes of the American Indians, the imperial family of Japan, and the British Israelites) have proclaimed themselves to be, or have been designated as, the saving remnants of the lost tribes. This investigation of an allegedly scattered peoplehood has been carried out within aspects of the emerging but still inchoate tradition of postmodernist social science.[1]

Every aspect of the history—and the very existence—of the ten tribes of Israel is fraught with existential controversy and epistemological conundrums. The fatefulness of the original tribal monarchical confederation—the society of ancient Hebrews inhabiting the Northern Kingdom of Israel—is largely dependent on religious sources and a few other ancient documents whose accuracy is disputed and whose usefulness for social scientific research remains a topic of intense debate.[2] As J. Maxwell Miller observes, "Given the uncertainties that arise from the biblical story, the paucity of references to Israel or Israelites in extrabiblical documents, and the very generalized nature of evidence from artifacts, it is not surprising that present-day scholars hold widely divergent views concerning Israel's history."[3] For the purposes and epistemological approach of my own investigation, however, these uncertainties, lacunae, overextended generalities, and puzzling ambiguities constitute the very data on the basis of which quondam designations of disparate peoples as descendants of "the lost tribes of Israel," or, more generally, as Jews living outside the purview of Occidental Jewry, have been made. It is these designations—their bases, acceptance, or rejection, and the consequences that have flowed and continue to flow therefrom—that form the heart and objective of a work for which this essay can serve as only an introduction.

The histories, prophecies, myths, and sightings of the Hebrew tribes of Reuben, Simeon, Dan, Naphtali, Gad, Asher, Issachar, Zebulon, Ephraim, and one-half of the tribe of Manasseh—the so-called ten lost tribes, distinguishable from the Judean tribes of Judah and Benjamin, and those in turn from the landless temple service tribe of Levites—originated in the aftermath of the catastrophe that befell the Northern Kingdom of Israel as a result of expansionist wars conducted from 733 to 721 B.C.E. by a resurgent Assyria. Using for the most part nonbiblical sources, historian William Foxwell Albright provides a pithy precis of the fateful events:

> Damascus was stormed by the Assyrians in 732, after a bloody war, and Aram was converted into four Assyrian provinces. Even before the fall of Damascus the Assyrian armies swept over Israel, devastating Galilee, and annexing all of Israel except Ephraim and western Manasseh (733 B.C.E.). In 732 the Assyrians appointed Hoshea as the last king of Samaria, but the Assyrian exactions were too much for him, and he rebelled about 724, relying on the very dubious promise of Egyptian assistance . . . Hoshea was immediately taken prisoner, but the capital held out against a besieging army for over two years, falling at last in the first three months of 721. In his inscriptions Sargon II of Assyria repeatedly boasts of his conquest of Samaria and the "wide land of Beth-Omri" (official Israelite name of Samaria). He claims to have taken 27,290 Israelites into captivity. North Israel had ceased to be a political entity.[4]

The 27,290 taken captive, following upon the deportation of the Hebrews inhabiting Galilee and the parts of the Northern Kingdom conquered earlier, constitute the nucleus of the ten tribes whose forced dispersion over the next two millennia is considered a loss and whose eventual rediscovery and redemption are promised by God. They and their descendants have become "the lost tribes of Israel."

The legend of the lost tribes is not dependent on—but does occasionally touch on—the long and torturous history of Judeophobia. "Jews," writes the contemporary sociologist David Norman Smith in a controversial essay on the nature of anti-Semitism, ". . . will never be safe as long as they personify principles hateful to authoritarians. And that, unhappily, is something wholly beyond their control."[5] But the safety and survival of the lost tribes transcends this formulation of the "Jewish problem." It is not necessary here to enter into the debates that have arisen over the etiology of anti-Semitism[6] to recognize that the several sociocultural constructions of various human beings as Jews are not confined exclusively to the maddening architectonics of what Smith calls "chimerias," that is, "an obsessional exaggeration so extreme that [Jews] are transfigured, in thought, into literally transcendental, Luciferian figures of bestiality and danger."[7] However, the various constructions put upon those peoples designated as lost tribe descendants do share one characteristic of chimerias—namely, they are, "now and in historical memory, . . . so qualitatively contrary to any conventional conception of reality that they negate it, utterly and abstractly."[8] Thus, their special place in postmodern conceptions of historical, sacred, and secular reality. Moreover, the attitudes toward peoples said to be descendants of the ten tribes of Israel run a gamut—from philo-Semitic concerns to promptings for Christian evangelization; from justifications for rescuing Occidental Jews from the Holocaust to assertions of the right to settle in Israel; from denials of their claim to Jewish identity to murderous assaults on Jews because they are not true Israelites.

The Biblical Promise

Just as the postmodern *nouvelle vague*[9] in sociology has called into question the older divide between the science of "nature" and the science of "society,"[10] so the discovery and disputes over the lost tribes of Israel—as well as other issues facing contemporary Jews[11]—have not only had effects on governmental policies and practices, but also threatened to undermine the boundary separating "sacred" from "secular" approaches to history. But, it must be noted—and as both the recent eruption of Judaic thought and practice in Poland, a post–Cold War nation that, since the time of the *Shoah,* has been characterized as "a country of anti-Semites without Jews,"[12] as well as the rediscovery of Jewish culture and an attendant rise of religious conversions in communist Cuba,[13] illustrate—the revived interest in, and quest for, lost Jews is part of a contemporary search for a spiritually fulfilling personal and sociocultural identity.

Tamar Garb has recently pointed out that the "transition from the theological paradigm of pre-modern times to the scienticist paradigm of modernity was negotiated via the Enlightenment."[14] The Enlightenment philosophy gave privileged epistemological status to the Rule of Reason. However, today's seekers after a lost heritage of the Jewish experience, the deeply sedimented hope for an end to *Galut* (exile)[15] and for a reunification of all strands of the Jewish people, are inspired by a metarational outlook. They look on every instantiation of those who might be hitherto undiscovered bearers of the ancient tradition with a hopeful eye. Each is nothing less than a possible sign of the fulfillment of prophecy, a vindication of the theodicy of Jewish identity and its place in the world. Hence, in an extension of the studies of Garb and her colleagues, who confined their investigations to representations of the Jew in modern Western civilization, the present investigation focuses on exotic and heterodoxical peoples—African, Asian, pre-Columbian Native American, British Israelite, and, though not regarded as of Lost Tribe descent, Hispanic peoples of the Southwest—that is, on those whom, to borrow Garb's phrase, "a complex, sometimes contradictory construction of Jewishness, Jewish history, or Jewish memory"[16] has been externally projected or group-consciously adopted.

Whether there still exist descendants of the tribalized Hebrews who once comprised the majority population of the Northern Kingdom of Israel has been a matter of dispute for centuries. As the sacred book of Jewish scriptures, the *Tanakh,* explains the matter, King "Jeroboam caused Israel to stray from the Lord and to commit great sin, and the Israelites persisted in all the sins which Jeroboam had committed; they did not depart from them. In the end, the Lord removed Israel from His presence, as He had warned them through all His servants the prophets. So the Israelites were deported from their land to Assyria, as is still the case."[17] However, despite secular and some religious claims that the dispersal ended their group identity, in the prophetic tradition, the forced exile of the ten tribes—that, in fact, seems to have taken place over several centuries following the Assyrian conquest of Israel in 721 B.C.E.[18]—was not to be permanent. As noted above, Assyrian records indicate that in the first year of the conquest,[19] 27,290 people were, to use a more recent phrase, "ethnically cleansed" from their kingdom homeland.[20] But, it would seem that a deportation policy lasting as long as Assyria's did entailed an involuntary removal of many more of the Hebrew tribespeople. Their descendants, so the prophets said, would be returned to their homeland, redeemed, and reunited with their tribal siblings.

Whatever the actual number, and wherever they had gone during their exile, the biblical sages assured their hearers of an eventual redemption, return, and reunification of the two kingdoms and the twelve tribes. Said by Talmudic interpreters to be residing somewhere beyond the River Sambatyon,[21] the lost tribes, so both prophets and later rabbis insisted, would not only be found but uplifted from darkness and obscurity. Thus, Isaiah (XI:11–12): "My Lord will apply His hand again to redeeming the other part of His people from Assyria—as also from Egypt, Pathros, Nubia, Elam, Shinar, Hamath, and the coastlands." Moreover,

> He will hold up a signal to the nations
> And assemble the banished of Israel,
> And gather the dispersed of Judah
> From the four corners of the earth[22]

Similarly, Hosea, an eighth-century B.C.E. prophet, although he predicted that the Lord would surely "punish Israel for its transgressions":[23]

> —For I will give the order
> And shake the House of Israel—
> Through all the nations—
> As one shakes [sand] in a sieve,
> And not a pebble falls to the ground.[24]—

nevertheless offered a hopeful outcome to the matter—an outcome that would come to pass at a later unspecified date:

> I will restore My people Israel.
> They shall rebuild ruined cities and inhabit them;
> They shall plant vineyards and drink their wine;
> They shall till gardens and eat their fruits.
> And I will plant them upon their soil,
> Nevermore to be uprooted
> From the soil I have given them.[25]

Ultimately, however, although such minor prophets as Obadaiah (1:15–21, 16–21), Micah (4–6), Zephanaiah (3:11–20), and Zechariah (8:7–8, 11–13), also predicted a reunification of the surviving House of Judah with that of Israel, it is in the words of Ezekiel that we find a thoroughgoing statement of God's promise of that return—a redemption of peoples who, by that time, will have lost both faith and culture, that is, peoples to whom He will have become "a diminished sanctity":

> Thus said the Lord God: I have indeed removed them far among the nations and have scattered them among the countries, and I have become to them a diminished sanctity in the countries whither they have gone . . . I will give you the Land of Israel. And they shall return there, and do away with all its

> abominations . . . These shall be the boundaries of the land that you shall allot to the twelve tribes of Israel.[26]

Moreover, Ezekiel's prophecy for the new commonwealth included a naturalization policy and property rights for those whom he called "strangers":

> This land you shall divide for yourselves among the tribes of Israel. You shall allot it as a heritage for yourselves and for the strangers who reside among you, who have begotten children among you. You shall treat them as Israelite citizens; they shall receive allotments along with you among the tribes of Israel. You shall give the stranger an allotment within the tribe where he resides . . . declares the Lord.[27]

Thus does a future Israel betoken a multicultural society.

The Prophetic Tradition and Its Opponents

Over the centuries, however, believers in the biblical promise have had to contend with three perspectives that, respectively: (1) denied the possibility that the lost tribes of Israel could have survived the exile; (2) proclaimed that the ten tribes of Israel had already been reunited with their Judean brethren; or, (3) announced that the biblical prophecy enjoys neither culturological likelihood nor historical verification.

The Sages

Despite the words of the prophets, one Talmudist, Rabbi Aqiva ben Yosef (ca. 40–135 C.E.), considered the father of diasporic *halakhot* and a Jewish martyr,[28] insisted that the biblical prediction about how God would punish those who persistently disobey Him and continue to flout His laws—namely, Leviticus 26:37–38: "You shall not be able to stand your ground before your enemies, but shall perish among the nations; and the land of your enemies shall consume you"—would hold for the fate vouchsafed for "the Ten Tribes which were exiled to Media."[29] In fact, R. Aqiva believed that the dispossessed tribes of Israel had been completely annihilated.[30] Aqiva's assertion has proved to be most disconcerting to believers in the promise of an eventual ingathering of the descendants of all of the original twelve tribes. However, the great Talmudist's interpretation was disputed at the very time he uttered it, as well as in the centuries thereafter. His contemporary and subsequent disputants, relying on the words of Ezekiel, contended that the ten tribes were not dead but in long-term exile only; that already some had been returned to Judea by Jeremiah; and, as the kabbalistically inclined "Ramban," that is, Moshe ben Nahman, or Nahmanides (1194–1270 C.E.),[31] had put it, that the ten tribes would certainly have survived but been driven to "an out of the way place, so that none will remain among the [conventionally known] nations, and their location will not be known."[32]

The conception of an "out of the way place" has often been combined with God's alleged placing of the ten tribes on the far side of the Sambatyon River—as in the *Targum pseudo-Jonathan,*[33] wherein it is written, "when they will be captives on the rivers of Babylon, . . . I will remove them from there and place them within the boundary of the Sambatyon river, and these [here quoting Exodus 34:10] are the 'marvels such as have not been done in all the earth.'"[34] The peculiar characteristics of the Sambatyon—that is, that on weekdays it is impassable because of the unceasingly violent flow of rocks, stones, and debris; while on the Sabbath, when it rested shielded by a wall of fire, to cross it would violate Jewish law[35]—also made the ten tribes both more difficult to find and virtually impossible to rescue.[36] One sage, R. Samuel bar Nahman, sought to resolve the matter by urging that there had been three successive banishments of the people of Israel of which only the first deportation consisted of a removal beyond the Sambatyon, the second having been to Daphne of Antioch, and the third, even more mysterious, had entailed a divine camouflage, for "a cloud came down upon them and concealed them."[37] Still another Talmudist, R. Judah bar Simon, concentrated on differentiating the exile of Judea from that of Israel, hinting that only the latter was divinely hidden: "The tribes of Judah and Benjamin were not banished to the place where the ten tribes had been banished. The ten tribes were banished beyond the river Sambatyon, while the tribes of Judah and Benjamin are dispersed in all lands."[38] No doubt the Judahites and Benjaminites would be easier to find. Centuries later, Gaon Rabbeni Zemoch, disputing the claims then being put forth in behalf of Dan as one of the lost tribes—a claim made by Eldad the Danite (of whom more *infra*)—offered even a greater number of exiles: "And our sages have taught that there were ten captivities in which Israel went captive, through Sennacherib four, through Nebuchadnezzar four, through Vespasian one, and one through Hadrian. But the tribe of Dan is not mentioned in any of the exiles because it went of its own accord to Ethiopia 135 years before the destruction of the Temple."[39] The tribe of Dan might be in Ethiopia—as the so-called Falasha would claim successfully in the twentieth century—but it was not in holy exile. Presumably, the other nine were.

The location of a portion of the ten tribes beyond the Sambatyon River was given an epistolary form in circa 883 C.E. by Eldad ben Bahli Ha-Dani, known as Eldad the Danite. Possibly an inhabitant of Somaliland, Eldad's account of his genealogy—he traced his ancestry through thirty-seven generations to Dan, the son of the patriarch Jacob[40]—and his self-reported adventures as a traveler in Egypt, Mesopotamia, Yemen, and Ethiopia, included a claim to have found all of the lost ten tribes. According to his letter to the Jews of Spain (a text of which was published in Italy in 1480 and a commentary on which was printed in Constantinople in 1519),[41] he had come across the tribe of Issachar in a mountainous area north of the Persian Gulf, Zebulon in the hills of Paron, Reuben behind that mountain region, Ephraim and one-half of the tribe of Manasseh near Mecca, Simeon and the other half of the tribe of Manasseh in "the country of the Babylonians," and Dan, Naphtali, Gad, and Asher isolated beyond the reach of the other six; and even some remnants of the Judahites and Benjaminites in a remote part of Ethiopia:[42]

> Moreover, they [i.e., the tribespeople of Dan, Naphtali, Gad, and Asher] see no man and no men see them except these four tribes who dwell on the other side of the rivers of Ethiopia. There is a place where these can see each other and speak if they cry out, but the River Sambation is between them . . . When they want anything important, they have a kind of pigeon known among them and they write their letters and fasten them to the wings or to the feet of the pigeon, and these cross the River Sambation and the pigeons come to their Kings and Their Princes . . . The breadth of that river is 200 cubits bowshot, and the river is full of large and small stones and the sound of them rumbles like a great storm, like a tempest at sea and, in the night, the sound of it is heard a day's journey [away,] . . . The river runs and the stones and sand rumble during the six working days, but on the seventh day it rests and is tranquil until the end of Sabbath. And on the other side of the river, on the side where the four tribes dwell, is a fire which flames on Sabbath and no man can approach within a mile.[43]

With the acceptance of this passage, the River Sambatyon would thereafter become a part of the lost tribes' saga.

The Jeremiah Problem

Another biblically-based objection to any special quest for the allegedly lost ten tribes arises out of a Talmudic interpretation of a passage in II Kings 22:14–20, purporting to explain the absence of the prophet Jeremiah during a critical moment in the kingdom of Judah's history. Jeremiah had prophesied the return of the Israelites to a reunited kingdom on many occasions—for example, Jeremiah 30:3: "For the days are coming—declares the Lord—when I will restore the fortunes of My people Israel and Judah, . . . and I will bring them back to the land that I gave their fathers, and they shall possess it." According to *Tanakh,* II Kings 22:14–20, King Josiah, who had ascended the Judean throne in 639 B.C.E., that is, eighty-three years after the fall of the northern kingdom and the expulsion of some or all of its ten tribes, ordered his high priest, Hilkiah, to consult an inspired representative of the Lord about an ancient but recently discovered scroll, possibly written under divine guidance by Moses: "Hilkiah and those whom the king [had ordered] went to the prophetess Huldah . . . who was living in Jerusalem" for an authentication and interpretation of the mysterious scroll.*

The puzzling issue here is that Hilkiah did not go to inquire about such a serious matter—the scroll was interpreted to predict the fall of the kingdom—with Jeremiah, clearly the superior prophet-in-residence during Josiah's reign and a favorite of the king. The commentaries on this matter by R. Azaria Min Ha Adumim, R. Abraham Yagel, and R. Shmuel Halevi Edelsh sought to lay to rest the thesis put forth by an earlier sage, R. Yochanon bar Nappaha (c. 240–279 C.E.), to the effect that Jeremiah's absence is explained by the prophet's having undertaken a journey "to fetch the Ten Tribes,"[48] and, by implication, that he had succeeded in his efforts, thus ending the latter's exile.[49] To this assertion, R. Edelsh replied that although pious King Josiah had gone to the lands from which the tribes had been banished and destroyed the pagan idols that they had left behind, the ten tribes had not returned in the days during which he had reigned and during which Jeremiah had prophesied about them. R. Yagel and R. Adumim drew on an earlier interpretation of R. Yochanan's hermeneutic, one given by one of the greatest of the commentators, R. Shlomo Yitzhaki, or "Rashi" (1040–1105), who had modified R. Yochanan's argument to say that, although Jeremiah had gone to bring back the ten tribes, only a few members of these tribes had returned with him. The rest, he continued, though not yet ingathered with their brethren, had not become so lost that they would never again be found. They are scattered among the nations awaiting their divine deliverance. To this, R. Adumim added that to grant credence to R. Yochanan's statement would not only falsify Ezra's belief that the end of the Babylonian exile, begun with King Cyrus of Persia's decree permitting a return to Jerusalem and the reconstruction of the temple, had largely been effected by the Judean tribes of Benjamin and Judah without much participation by the Israelites, but also would discredit the prophet Ezekiel's promise that the reunification of the tribes was yet to occur. Thus did prophecy hold out promise of their discovery.

---

* Huldah is one of only four prophetesses mentioned in the *Tanakh*—the other three being Miriam (Exodus 15:20–21), the judge Deborah (Judges 4:1–10), and Noadiah (Nehemiah 6:10–14)[44]—and she does have a semblance of status as "the keeper of the [royal?] wardrobe."[45] One modern Bible scholar, Adrien Janis Bledstein, has nominated Huldah as the probable author of the entire Book of Deuteronomy,[46] traditionally attributed to the prophet Samuel and thought by another Bible scholar, Richard Elliott Friedman, to have been written by Jeremiah.[47]

Secular Doubts

The foregoing disputes and their resolutions have been carried out within the epistemological frame of Talmudic hermeneutics and by believers in the historical truth of the biblical texts. However most nonreligious authorities—including some who are Jewish—discount an inner-worldly telos for the prophetic tradition and treat the fate of the ten tribes in terms of secular culturological theories and nonsacred sociocultural processes, each and all of which, taken jointly or separately, over a long period of time, are said to have resulted in their permanent disappearance. Essentially, these modernists presuppose that such well-recognized processes as acculturation, assimilation, and amalgamation, occurring over the centuries after the Assyrian conquest, would have worked to obviate any possibility that the ten tribes could survive as a self-identified, significant, Israelitish remnant that still had a role to play in future historical developments. The banished people of the ten tribes and their descendants, they asserted, had for the most part been absorbed into the later Judean exiles or into the cultures and societies of the non-Hebrew nations into whose lands they had been exiled or to which they had migrated. Thus, Erich Kahler (1885–1970) observed: "The Assyrians, who . . . destroyed the North Kingdom, . . . carried . . . the vanquished into exile. The majority of them . . . dispersed and . . . merged with other populations, sharing the fate of many peoples and realms which perished in the turmoil of human history."[50] The unsigned entry on the lost ten tribes in *The New Standard Jewish Encyclopedia,* after summarizing beliefs about their survival, argues: "In historic fact, some members of the Ten Tribes remained in Palestine, where apart from the Samaritans some of their descendants long preserved their identity among the Jewish population, others were assimilated, while others were presumably absorbed by the last Judean exiles who in 597–586 [B.C.E.] were deported to areas adjacent to the place of exile of the Ten Tribes (Media, Assyria, and Mesopotamia)."[51] According to Shmuel Ahituv and Shalom Paul, "The northern kingdom lasted approximately two hundred years; it fell to the Assyrians in 721 B.C.E., when the majority of the Israelites were deported to Assyria . . . Unlike the Judeans of the southern kingdom, who survived a similar fate 135 years later, they soon assimilated . . . [However, they add,] the loss of the ten tribes was never accepted as final by the Jews."[52]

A Christian biblical scholar, Rev. R. J. Coggins,[53] insists—and on this point he appears to have the same position as Kahler[54]—on dating the beginnings of the Jewish diaspora not from the time of the Assyrian conquest of the northern kingdom of Israel, but rather from the time of the kingdom of Judah's loss of independence and the onset of its people's Babylonian exile. He makes this claim not only because, "Much that has been written about the supposed 'ten lost tribes' can be dismissed to the realm of fantasy," but also because "we may certainly suppose that in both Israel and Judah the majority of the inhabitants continued to lead their lives in their native places; the means for mass deportation which have formed an appalling part of the technical apparatus of twentieth-century dictatorships were not available in the ancient world." Moreover, Coggins suggests that the contrasting policies pursued by successive Assyrian and Babylonian rulers might have led to a greater emphasis on the preservation of the Judean community in Babylonia and on a much more severe program of coercive acculturation for the banished Israelites in Assyrian lands. And he also notes that the theme of exile had been interpreted differently in the two kingdoms: "For [the post-exilic Judean] community exile was an important purifying experience; for the northerners, by contrast, it was the final indication of divine displeasure." The ten tribes had succumbed from their belief in God's displeasure with them.

Still another historian of antiquity, Michael Grant, concurs with respect to the sociocultural processes at work in the face of the respectively different Assyrian and Babylonian conquered peoples' policies: "When portions of the Ten Tribes had been deported to Assyria, they got 'Lost': in other words, they gradually abandoned their Yahwist faith and adopted local beliefs instead. Yet in Babylonia, although once again there were foreign cults all around, no such process of assimilation occurred, at least not on any substantial scale."[55] Grant goes on to observe that in Babylonia, after thirty-seven years of exile and imprisonment, the Judean king Jehoiachin was released from confinement, given a pension, restored to his royal title, and permitted to preside over his people's affairs.[56] Judeans, according to Grant, were permitted to own both property and slaves and also to maintain their genealogical records. Moreover, without having to give up their faith, "Some of the men became mercenary soldiers and officers in the Babylonian service, others held royal administrative posts; many became agricultural tenants of the king."[57] And, under these circumstances, he asserts, they were able to maintain their worship of Yahweh. "Strangely enough," Grant concludes, ". . . Yahweh's power to command submission became most apparent after his people had been defeated. For it was he who was now their only *real* king."[58]

At the time when Cyrus II of Persia and his successors permitted those exiles who wished to go in advance of, or, later, to follow Ezra and Nehemiah to Jerusalem in order to rebuild the temple,[59] a seemingly permanent dispersion of the Jews had already been long in progress.[60] By the time of the Maccabean revolt (167–142 B.C.E.), Jewish communities had been well established in Egypt, Syria, Pergamum, Parthia, Cappadocia, and other places where Hellenism flourished.[61] Although Simon, the Hasmonean ethnarch, as well as his successors, John Hyrcanus, Judah Aristobolus, and Alexander Jannai, wrested and ritually restored some of the provinces once held by the Israelite monarchy, and carried out population transfers of their own devising against the peoples inhabiting these lands since the time of the Assyrian conquest,[62] there seems to have been no substantial repatriation of the ten lost tribes to their partially recovered homeland. The latter, according to the diaspora historian Werner Keller, "were never heard from again."[63] However, "Large numbers of these Israelites," writes Irving M. Zeitlin, "later fused with the Judean exiles to form the Babylonian Jewish community of second temple times."[64] Zeitlin goes on to point out that Judeans were also scattered among the inhabitants of Egypt, Moab, Ammon, and Edom; that the prophet Obadiah spoke of a Jewish settlement in Asia Minor; that the Book of Esther tells of Jews in all the provinces of the Persian empire at the time of Xerxes; and that Deutero-Isaiah laments the dispersal of the Jews east, west, north, and south.[65] To these scholars, it may be concluded, the once-dispossessed Israelites are "lost" for all time and to all intents and purposes. To give one example: the Jewish historian Hayim Tadmor, buttressed in part by Assyrian documents, sums up the case for holding that the ten tribes of the northern kingdom of Israel are unlikely to have survived for very long as a distinctive ethnoreligious entity:

> Little information is preserved about the ten tribes that were exiled to Assyria, whose fate was to serve later generations as a subject of legendary speculation and messianic hopes. What transpired was that most of those exiled were settled in the vicinity of Gozan on the Habor River . . . Others were settled in Media, where they apparently served as garrison troops in units organized within the Assyrian Army. This method of annexing into the Assyrian Army complete units from the armies of conquered peoples was widespread . . . This practice may help to explain the presence in the Assyrian Army of an officer named Hilkiyau, i.e., Hilkiah, who is mentioned in a document from the time of Sargon recently discovered at Calah. Assyrian documents from Gozan itself also contain a few names that testify to the fact that an Israelite community still existed there in the seventh century. One document mentions two Gozan officials named Paltiyau and Niriyau. These, however, are scraps of information. It may be assumed that a part of the exiled tribes that still existed as a separate and conscious group in the days of Jeremiah and Ezekiel . . . subsequently joined the exiles from Judah upon their return. The majority, however, were assimilated into the surrounding Aramean population thus sharing the fate of every ethnic community displaced by the Assyrians and subjected to their policy of enforced Assyrianization.[66]

Thus does secular history dispose once and for all time of the "ten lost tribes" of Israel.

The Samaritans: An Anomalous Peoplehood

There remains, however, one additional problem, extant from the time of the Assyrian conquest to the present, namely, the survival and contested identity of the people called Samaritans. A quasi-autonomous people who in the 1990s numbered about 530, dwelling in Nablus and Holon in the state of Israel, the Samaritans are unsuccessful claimants to an Israelite descent, more specifically to descent from two of the lost tribes, Ephraim and Manasseh.[67] Rabbinical authorities for the most part subscribe to the belief that the Samaritans are descended from those peoples whom the Assyrians transplanted onto the northern kingdom's soil after the ten tribes had been moved out. But, it is at least possible that they are descendants of the original Israelites or of the unexiled Judeans, or a mixture of these.[68] But, the writer of II Kings 17:24 put it another way, the Samaritans are neither Israelites nor Judeans, but foreigners: "The king of Assyria brought [people] from Babylon, Cuthah, Avva, Hamath, and Sepharvaim, and he settled them in the towns of Samaria in place of the Israelites; they took possession of Samaria and dwelt in the towns."[69] The newly resettled peoples, as the Book of Kings tells it,[70] had difficulties adjusting to their new life in what was once the kingdom of Israel. Troubled by the murderous attacks of lions and by plagues sent by Yahweh to chasten them, they successfully appealed to the Assyrian court to send them someone who could instruct them in a Yahwistic religious ritual that would propitiate and placate the deity of the former inhabitants of the land. And, one of the exiled priests from the northern kingdom was sent to teach them. However, each of the peoples responded to the teaching by adding a syncretistic element to its own religious praxes:

> . . . each nation continued to make its own gods and to set them up in the cult places which had been made by the people of Samaria; each nation [set them up] in the towns in which it lived. The Babylonians made Succoth-benoth, and the men of Cuth made Nergal, and the men of Hamath made Ashima, and the Avvites made Nibhaz and Tartak; and the Sepharvites burned their children [as offerings] to Adrammelech and Anamelech, the gods of Sepharvaim. They worshipped the Lord, . . . while serving their own gods according to the practices of the nations from which they had been deported.[71]

As foreigners,[72] or as a group practicing a dissident sectarian and syncretistic variant of Judaism, the Samaritans are not yet counted among the lost Hebrews awaiting discovery.

Another less than friendly account of the Samaritans—one reflecting the religio-cultural interests of the Judaic community reestablished by the three migratory returns from Babylonia permitted by the Persian successors to the Babylonian empire: the first in 538 B.C.E., under former king Jehoiachin's son; the second, in 520 B.C.E., under the Davidic descendant, Zerubabel, numbering 42,360 persons; and the third, in 458 B.C.E., led by Ezra, soon to be followed by Nehemiah in 445 B.C.E.[73]—is to be found in the writings of Yoseph ben Mattiyahu ha-Cohen (ca. 38–100 C.E.), better known by his Latin *nom de plume,* Flavius Josephus.[74] Josephus's history elaborates on the version found in the *Tanakh.* Moreover, because it distinguishes the Samaritans from the Israelites, in effect lending support to the discriminations against the former by, first, the Judeans returning from the Babylonian exile, later, the Hasmonean ethnarchs, and in more recent times, the harsh judgments on them by such secular scholars as Max Weber, Josephus's observations deserve to be quoted at length:

> . . . Shalmaneser, the king of Assyria, . . . besieged Samaria [for] three years, and took it by force in the ninth year of the reign of Hoshea, . . . and [he] quite demolished the government of the Israelites, and transplanted all the people into Media and Persia . . . ; and when he had removed these people out of their land, he transplanted other nations out of Cuthah . . . into Samaria, and into the country of the Israelites . . .
>
> But now the Cutheans, who removed into Samaria . . . [from] Persia, . . . each of them, according to their nations, which were in number five, brought their own gods into Samaria, and by worshipping them, . . . provoked Almighty God to be angry and displeased at them, for a plague seized upon them, by which they were destroyed; and when they found no cure for their miseries, they learned by the oracle that they ought to worship Almighty God, as the method for their deliverance. So they sent ambassadors to the King of Assyria, and desired him to send them some of those priests of the Israelites whom he had taken captive. And when he thereupon sent them, and the people were by them taught the laws, and the holy worship of God, they worshipped him in a respectful manner, and the plague ceased immediately; and indeed they continue to make use of the very same customs to this very time, and are called in the Hebrew tongue *Cutheans;* but in the Greek *Samaritans.*[75]

Moreover, in Josephus's account of the restoration of Jerusalem, the rebuilding of the temple, and the reconstruction of the walls around the city—events that transpired after political control over the exiled Judeans had passed from the Babylonian to the Persian empire (538 B.C.E.), and that had taken place under the successive kingships of Cyrus II (d. 529 B.C.E.), Cambyses (d. 522 B.C.E.), Darius I (d. 486 B.C.E.), and Artaxerxes (465–421 B.C.E.)—much is made of the corruption, treachery, and anti-Judaic obstructionism carried on by the Samaritans. Despite Josephus's claim that, unlike the Assyrians, the conquering Babylonians had not undertaken a policy of population transfer—and, as a result "all Judea and Jerusalem, and the temple, continued to be a desert for seventy years,"[76] that is, remained virtually uninhabited until Cyrus II permitted the Jews under Persian control to return to their homeland—some Samaritans, Ammonites, and other peoples apparently had settled in or near the land of Judea and intermarried with those Hebrews who had not been carried into captivity. As Josephus tells the story:

> When the foundations of the temple were laying, and when the Jews were very zealous about building it, the neighboring nations, and especially the Cutheans, . . . besought the governors, and those that had the care of such affairs, that they would interrupt the Jews, both in the rebuilding of their city, and in the building of their temple.[77]

And, apparently, the Cutheans and their anti-Judean allies were at first successful in their endeavors. For, as Josephus goes on to relate, "these men were corrupted by them with money, [and] they sold the Cutheans their interest for rendering this building a slow and a careless work."[78] But the Cutheans did more—and worse. During the brief reign of Cyrus's successor, Cambyses, they were able to use their influence to bring Jerusalem's civic and temple reconstruction to a complete halt, work not begun again until Darius I had succeeded to the Persian throne.[79]

It is the Samaritan's opposition to a restoration of the Davidic monarchy—a possibility that Darius I seemed to have toyed with briefly when he appointed Zerubabel, a grandson of King Jehoiachin and, by this fact of genealogy, a descendant of the house of David, to the position of satrap over the returned Jews[80]—and their refusal to accept the temple in Jerusalem and its priestly code of rites and rituals as the sole source of religious belief and praxis for all Jews in diaspora that form the basis for the charge of heterodoxy against them.[81] It stands in sharp contrast to later designations of various peoples as "lost" but redeemable bodies of dispersed Jewry—groups, that is, however much they have ceased to practice the orthodoxy of Hebraic prayer and Halakhic rules, that are nevertheless said to deserve recognition, redemption, and full-fledged incorporation into either diasporic or the Israel-settled body of Jewry, or both.

During the era of Ezra and Nehemiah, both of whom worked during the reign of Artaxerxes I (465–421 B.C.E.), the Samaritans, together with Ammonites, Philistines, and Edomites, were ethically as well as ethnically distinguished from the "posterity of Jeshua the high priest, and . . . the priests and Levites, and the Israelites, who had a greater regard to the observation of the law than to their natural affection."[82] The latter of whom were quite willing to obey Ezra's and Nehemiah's command that they renounce their marriages to "foreign" women and disavow their paternal responsibilities to their offspring therefrom.[83] Even earlier, Zerubabel—because "the Samaritans, being evil and enviously disposed to the Jews, wrought them many mischiefs, by reliance on their riches, and by their pretense that they were allied to the Persians, . . . and [in addition, because] whatsoever it was that they were enjoined to pay the Jews by the king's order out of their tributes for the sacrifices, they would not pay it"[84]—had been forced to petition Darius about the matter, and, to his profound relief, the Persian monarch sided with him and with the returned Judeans and ordered the Samaritans to pay the tithe and cease their obstructionist tactics.[85] But the Samaritans did not end their attempts to undermine the redeemed Jerusalem. Nehemiah felt compelled not only to repulse the Samaritan governor Sanballat's attempts to exert political and religious influence over Judah, finally expelling from Jerusalem the latter's son-in-law, a grandson of the high priest Eliashib,[86] but also to arm the workmen rebuilding the wall around the city against Samaritan assaults.[87] To the more secularized members of the Samaritan group, as well as to the Ammonites, Moabites, and Coelesyrians, Nehemiah's wall seemed to augur the burgeoning presence of a fortified Judean citadel,[88] threatening the precarious balance of power in the region.

After Ezra and Nehemiah had at last prevailed in their purifying redemption and military reconstruction of Jerusalem, the Samaritans retreated, but they made a new demand: that they be given the right to build a temple of their own on Mount Gerizim, with the added right to worship there in terms of their own version of the rituals and requirements of Judaism. Their proposal challenged the central authority over the Jews in diaspora then held by the post-exilic theocrats in Jerusalem.[89] Josephus insists that, when Alexander of Macedon had overwhelmed the Persian empire, replacing it with his own, and, in the process, shown kindness to and respect for the petitions of the Jerusalem priesthood, the Samaritans attempted to trick him into recognizing their separate religio-cultural autonomy, granting them the right to a seventh year tribute of the kind given to the Judean temple keepers. They did this, Josephus says, by masquerading as "Hebrews" known as "Sidonians":

> . . . the Samaritans, who had then Shechem for their metropolis (a city situated at Mount Gerizzim, and inhabited by apostates of the Jewish nation), seeing that Alexander had so greatly honored the Jews, determined to profess themselves as Jews; for such is the disposition of the Samaritans, . . . that when the Jews are in adversity they deny that they are of kin to them, and then they confess the truth; but when they perceive that some good fortune hath befallen them, they imme-

> diately pretend to have communion with them, saying, that they belong to them, and derive their genealogy from the posterity of Joseph, Ephraim, and Manasseh. Accordingly, . . . the Shechemites approached . . . [Alexander] and desired that he would come to their city, and do honour to their temple also; to whom he promised, that when he returned he would come to them; and when they petitioned that he would remit the tribute of the seventh year to them, because they did not now sow thereon, he asked who they were that made such a petition; and when they said that they were Hebrews, but had the name of Sidonians, living at Shechem, he asked them again whether they were Jews; and when they said they were not Jews, "It was to the Jews," said he, "that I granted that privilege; however, when I return, and am thoroughly informed by you of this matter, I will do what I shall think proper."[90]

As Josephus seems to suggest, the Samaritans did not entirely succeed in their ethnoreligious ruse, but during the era of the internecine warfare among Alexander's successors, they continued to maintain their temple on Mount Gerizim, using it, among other things, not only as a rival to the Jerusalem temple but also as a place of sanctuary for Judean apostates: "and if any one were accused by those of Jerusalem of having eaten things common [Gr. *koinophagia,* referring to eating "unclean" foods], or of having broken the Sabbath, or of any other crime of the like nature, he fled away to the Shechemites, and said that he was accused unjustly."[91] Later, Ptolemy, one of Alexander's successors, carried away and settled in Egypt "a great many captives, both from the mountainous parts of Judea and from the places about Jerusalem and Samaria, and the places near mount Gerizzim." Subsequently, these involuntary settlers were followed by "not a few other Jews who, of their own accord, went into Egypt, as invited by the goodness of the soil, and by the liberality of Ptolemy."[92] Violent confrontations arose in Egypt over the Judean-Samaritan issue, more specifically over whether sacrificial offerings and tithes from Jews resettled there were to be sent to the temple at Jerusalem or to the holy edifices on Mount Gerizim. Among the denominations making up the Hebraic and Aramaic settlers in Egypt and their descendants, this rivalry and dissension would continue for centuries.[93]

Josephus goes on to document what he regards as the threefold proofs of the hypocrisy of the Samaritans by (1) uncovering and holding up to scorn their petition to Antiochus IV Epiphanes, Seleucid king of Assyria from c. 175–164 B.C.E., whose draconian measures against the religious practices of the Jews had evoked the Maccabean revolt, that denied that they are or ever had been Jews; held themselves to be blameless with respect to any accusations made against the Jews; insisted that they were "Sidonians," descended from a colony of Medes and Persians, and thus "aliens from their [i.e., the Jewish] nation and from their customs"; and that requested that their temple on Mount Gerizim be redesignated as the "Temple of Jupiter Hellenius";[94] 2) scoffing at their credulity in believing a religious charlatan's assertion that Moses—who had not been permitted to cross over the Jordan river—had secreted some sacred vessels on Mount Gerizim, a claim that had aroused a riotous crowd, the members of which were thought to be revolting against Rome and were scattered and killed by governor Pilate's soldiers;[95] and (3) reporting enthusiastically on the military successes of the Hasmonean ethnarch, John Hyrcanus I, who had succeeded in 135 B.C.E. to the high priesthood earlier inaugurated by the Maccabean family; taking especial note of both Hyrcanus's conquest of "Shechem and Gerizzim; and besides these . . . the nation of the Cutheans, who dwelt round about that temple which was built in imitation of the temple at Jerusalem . . ."; and of Hyrcanus's sons' fearsome siege of the Samarian city Sebaste, foisting on its denizens a famine so complete "that they were forced to eat what never was esteemed food;" and eventually demolishing the city altogether, enslaving its surviving inhabitants.[96]

However, the Samaritans neither disappeared nor died out as a people. Nor did their strained relations with the Jews decline over the centuries of diaspora. Menahem Mansoor emphasizes their syncretistic religious practices as the Yahwistic priesthood's principal objection to their incorporation within the society of returned Judeans. It is an objection that still prevails at the present time. Mansoor observes: "The religious beliefs and practices of the Samaritans came to differ widely from those of normative Judaism. The Samaritan Scriptures contain only the Pentateuch (first five books of the Hebrew Bible). Its text, written in old Hebrew script, is at variance with that of the Hebrew Bible. [Moreover, the Samaritans built a] rival Temple to that of Jerusalem . . . on Mount Gerizim. The liturgical calendar, feasts, and practices of the Samaritans differ from those of standard Judaism . . . The Jews refused [joint worship with the Samaritans] because they viewed the Samaritans as . . . incorporating other religious practices into the true faith of Israel."[97] In his masterful reexamination of the relations among Jews and Gentiles in the ancient world, Louis H. Feldman points out that the Judean priesthood was not alone in distinguishing the Samaritans from the Jews; indeed, such Roman annalists as Quintus Curtius Rufus, Tacitus, and Damascius regarded the Samaritans as members of "a religious movement totally separate from the Jews."[98]

The New Testament accounts of the Samaritans also suggest their continuing conflict with the Jerusalem temple theocracy. Thus, there is a hint of Jewish disapproval in the story of Jesus' cure of a Samaritan leper (Luke 17:11–19); an accusation that Jesus is a Samaritan and possessed by a devil thereby (John 8:48); a more telling critique of the Judean position on the matter in Jesus' parable of the good Samaritan (Luke 10:29–37); a direct reference to the rival temples at Jerusalem and Mount Gerizim in Jesus's encounter with the Samarian woman at the well (John 4:9,20); and, in contrast to what might appear as the New Testament writers' empathy for the Samaritans, there are Jesus's instructions (Matthew 10:5–6) to the twelve apostles: "These twelve Jesus sent forth, and commanded them, saying, Go not into the way of the Gentiles, and into any city of the Samaritans enter ye not: But go rather to the lost sheep of the house of Israel"—an instruction revoked, it would appear (Acts 1:8), when Jesus gives a new order to the apostles: ". . . and ye shall be witnesses unto me both in Jerusalem, and in all Judaea, and in Samaria, and unto the uttermost part of the earth." Finally, it is worthy of note that the author of the Apocryphal work entitled *Ecclesiasticus, or the Wisdom of Jesus Son of Sirach,* believed to have been written sometime before 180 B.C.E. and included in the Christian but not the Jewish canon of sacred writings, issued a veritable anathema not only on the Edomites dwelling in Seir, and on the Philistines, but also on "the foolish people that live in Shechem," [i.e., the Samaritans], who, despite the foregoing, are said to be "not even a people."[99] Commenting on this and other anti-Samaritan writings, Alfred Edersheim, a Jewish convert to Anglicanism and sometime missionary to the Jews of Romania, observes, "At every period of sore national trial, the Jews had no more determined or relentless enemies than those who claimed to be the only true representatives of Israel's worship and hopes."[100] He, of course, is speaking of the Samaritans. Yet, as Menahem Stern points out, at the time of the Maccabean revolt, the "Samaritan population was like a wedge driven between two of the centres of Jewish settlement, Judea and Galilee, and its very existence was a thorn in the side of the Jews, although the Jews and Samaritans occasionally found themselves in the same camp in the struggle against Roman rule."[101]

The Samaritan thorn in the side of Judea was only partly drawn out during the first ten centuries of the common era, when some Samaritans, as well as other peoples dwelling in the erstwhile northern kingdom of Israel, migrated into Central Asia. It is in this period, or, perhaps, even earlier, that there is heard a claim that sounds to the present day, namely, that some of the inhabitants of Samarkand are descendants of one or more of the lost tribes of Israel.[102] The Samarian-Samarkand-lost tribes connection has been much criticized, but its leading current advocate, David A. Law, believes that the original body of Israelite exiles, those whose descendants would eventually find their way to Samarkand, were forced out of Israel by the Assyrian monarch,

Tiglath-Pileser III[103] and that these comprised members of the ten tribes who were already in diaspora when the kingdom of Israel fell in 721 B.C.E. Centuries later, when the Persian king Cyrus mounted a great caravan for an expedition into central Asia, and ultimately to Samarkand, he recruited his forces from Ecbatana, the capital of Medea, and the Nisaea region, also in Medea, each places of tribal Israelite exile settlement; so that the caravan "must have consisted of the descendants of the Ten Lost Tribes of Israel or the Samarians."[104] Professor Law apparently uses the term *Samarian* as synonymous with *Israelite* and does not seem to be discussing the *Samaritans.* A historian of the peoples called "Oriental Jews," Chaim Raphael, distinguishes "the anti-Jewish Samaritan people"[105] from the ten lost tribes, pointing out that the "long-existing eastward migration [of Jews] towards the neighboring regions of Afghanistan, Turkestan, Samarkand, Bukhara and India, and in other directions to Kurdistan, the Caucasus and even Egypt [made] Persia . . . the base historically for a continuous diffusion of Jews into 'eastern communities' . . . ,[but that the latter] all claimed to be descended from the Lost Ten Tribes . . . and spoke Persian-Jewish vernaculars, written in Hebrew script."[106] More recently, Rabbi Adin Steinsaltz, a specialist in the study of Central Asian Jews and the leader of a mission to bring the Torah, "the inheritance (*morasha*) of the Jewish people," to those Jews who have lost touch with their sacred legacy through their "wanderings in the exiles, in the 'desert of the nations,' [and] even in our own land," found no difficulty in separating these deserving Jews from the Samaritans:

> Many of us believe that despite the horrifying assimilation rate [,] the maternity wards can make up for the absence of study halls. Nevertheless, if we do continue along this path, we are moving toward a non-luminous future, in which we are destined to become like the Samaritans, a small, detached, insignificant sect.[107]

The Samaritans, as distinct from David Law's "Samarians" have not yet become candidates for lost-ten-tribalhood.

How the once-proud, once-defiant Samaritans were reduced to the ignominious status of "a small, detached, insignificant sect" was one of the central problems investigated by Max Weber (1864–1920) in *Ancient Judaism,*[108] a volume in his quartet of works on the comparative sociology of world religions.[109] "In religious history," Weber wrote, the Samaritans "are . . . quite interesting in that one may study their fate in comparison with that of the Jews in order to establish negatively what the exclusively Torah oriented religion of the Israelite priests lacked for becoming a 'world religion.'"[110] As Weber saw the matter, the Samaritans, unlike the Jerusalem-bound returnees from Babylonian exile and their descendants, failed to develop a linkage to the "pathos" of the Judaic "prophetic theodicy and social-revolutionary hope for the future."[111] Moreover, they also

> failed to develop Pharisaism which gave birth to the Talmud. They rejected the hope for resurrection. . . . [T]hey lacked the confessional development which was anchored to the content of prophetic and rabbinical soteriology and the particular Pharisee rationalism. [And, ultimately, they] failed to develop a national religious ethic which could have won the Occident.[112]

Weber sums up his seemingly neutral analysis of Samaritan failures with a caustic remark that suggests his own lingering prejudices on this and related matters affecting the "Jewish Question."[113] Acknowledging that there were Samaritan revivals during the Middle Ages and that Samaritan colonies had been planted in India in the seventeenth century, Weber apparently could not resist pointing out that "They exist to this day, as but a tiny sect (and notoriously as the sharpest cheats of the Orient, whose falsifications have even victimized serious scholars)."[114]

The reputation of the Samaritans as an anti-Jewish people, although it dates at least from the time of their status as an autonomous religious community inhabiting the environs of Shechem circa 332 B.C.E.,[115] did not prevent their acceptance within the modern state of Israel. At present, they are not regarded as a lost tribe returned to the fold, but tolerated along with such other heterodoxical adamantly non-Talmudic sects as the Karaites. By contrast, the rabbinically declared lost tribe of Dan, that is, the Ethiopian Jews, whose religion is said to be involuntarily pre-Talmudic because of their long isolation from Occidental diasporic Jewry, have been allowed to resettle in Israel. The latter regard their current difficulties in the modern State of Israel as arising out of an unacknowledged but virulent racism.[116] Neither the Samaritans nor the Karaites are perceived as black.

The Lost Tribes: Inner-Worldly and Eschatological Polities

It is a contention of Max Weber that the Hebrew deity Yahwe was "the federal deity of the conquering oath-bound confederacy which had been placed under his protection by means of a covenant mediated by priests," and, as such, that "foreign affairs permanently remained his demesne and the concern of the greatest among his prophets."[117] Yet, Yahwe was less and less able to assure a Hebrew victory in every international conflict into which the two post-Solomonic kingdoms had plunged.[118] Although Yahwe "was and remained first of all a God of the extraordinary, that is, of the destiny of his people in war, . . . his people could not create a world empire of their own."[119] Surrounded over the centuries of their land-and-state-based life by such powerful empires as those of Egypt, Assyria, Babylonia, Persia, Greece, and Rome—and, after Solomon's death, divided into two kingdoms, often hostile to each other—the Hebrews succumbed, serially, to each of their enemies. Yet, Yahwe and his followers did not die out altogether. Indeed, Yahwe rose in stature as the Hebrews were defeated: they turned to an eschatological redemption. "Jehovah," Weber concludes, "could only become a 'world god' as a supramundane ruler of destiny."[120] A great part of that destiny concerned the ultimate fate of the ten tribes of Israel.

The internecine disputes among the tribes and their eventual dissolution as territorialized units of a federated monarchical political entity warn of an irresolution in Hebrew political formations. The intertribal conflicts are virtually foreordained by Jacob's dying testament to his once-lost, now-returned son, Joseph. Summoning the latter to his death bed, Jacob (now renamed Israel as a result of his wrestling match with a messenger of God, or, perhaps God Himself),[121] announces first, a political restructuring of the tribes, and, then, a new distribution of his estate:

> El Shaddai appeared to me at Luz in the land of Canaan, and He blessed me, and said to me "I will make you fertile and numerous, making of you a community of peoples; and I will assign this land to your offspring to come for an everlasting possession." Now, your two sons, who were born to you in the land of Egypt, shall be mine. Ephraim and Manasseh shall be mine no less than Reuben and Simeon. But progeny born to you after them shall be yours; they shall be recorded instead of their brothers in their inheritance.[122]

Not only did Jacob's blessing of Joseph's sons repeat the violation of the birthright—that is, Jacob's and his mother's earlier deception of Isaac[123]—deposing Manasseh, who was Joseph's first born, in favor of the latter's younger brother, Ephraim[124]—but also, when read in conjunction with Jacob's subsequent blessings to his other sons, it disinherited Reuben, his and Leah's own first born. Reuben is replaced by Rachel's first-born son, Joseph, whose sons would receive the double portion ordinarily reserved for the oldest male heir; while Judah, the fourth son of Leah, will have authority over both his younger and older brothers and, more significantly, his tribe will be paramount in the future polity: "The scepter shall not depart from Judah, nor the ruler's staff from between his feet, until he comes to Shiloh."[125] Judah's preferment is purchased not only at Reuben's degradation (for defiling the bed of Rachel's surrogate and Jacob's concubine, Bilhah, the biological mother of his half-brothers Dan and Naphtali)[126] but also in foreordainment of the Davidic dynasty which, once the Benjaminite Saul has been deposed and killed, will descend in a single line from Judah's clan.

Jacob's blessing laid a foundation for the twelve-tribe patriarchy that, under the renewed covenant with Yahwe,[127] would confederate, so Jacob both insisted and prophesied, as a *kehal amim* (community of peoples). Later, in the post-Exodus period, his confederation would become a loosely integrated polity, first ruled over by judges,[128] and, then, a theocratic hereditary kingdom over which the descendants of Judah would reign.[129] However, this divinely blessed, inner-worldly kingdom did not seem to fulfill Jacob's promise, or Yahwe's requirements. Nehemiah's and Ezra's post-exilic restoration of Jerusalem did not include a reinstatement of the Davidic dynasty. Instead, Jacob's promise that Judah's descendants would ever remain as rulers was consigned to the eschatological future, to the messianic age. As Cyrus Gordon and Gary A. Rendsburg have pointed out, "The Messiah or king who will inaugurate the golden age at the end of days, must be of the Davidic Line."[130] Thus is Jacob to be vindicated.

Buttressed by recent archaeological evidence—as well as the biblical version —it appears that the *kehal amim* uniting the twelve patriarchal tribes into a polity, perhaps like other tribal groupings of its era, passed through several different forms before becoming the short-lived but eschatologically hoped-for Davidic monarchy. Once the early post-Exodus governance of the Hebrew tribes by "judges" had proved to be both ineffective and unwieldy, the Hebrews turned to a proto-monarchical chiefdom under Saul.[131] "At the end of the premonarchic period of Israelite history," observes archaeologist Larry G. Herr, in a lengthy essay appraising the periodization of "Iron IIA (Tenth Century BCE)" and analyzing the politics, international relations, sociocultural lives, and demographic structures of biblical-era tribal monarchies, "the Bible tells of a leader (chief—the biblical term is usually *magid,* not 'king') named Saul leading Israelite tribes and mentions what appears to be a similar ruler among Ammonite groups named Nahash (I Samuel 10:27)," adding that "Other tribal entities were probably also coalescing into supra-tribal chiefdoms."[132] Later, David, a scion of the tribe of Judah, having succeeded in his revolt against the Benjaminite Saul's leadership,[133] established a hereditary monarchy so powerful that "the 'House of David' . . . became the strongest political force in the southern Levant early in the tenth century."[134] From its beginnings however, the Davidic Monarchy was beset with problems of uxoric competition for patrilineal succession[135] and a plethora of foreign wars, while its internal unity was threatened by divisive tribal conflicts.[136] The very biblical writings of the period speak to what Professor Kiyoshi K. Sacon of the Tokyo Union Theological Seminary calls "a contradictory process in full tension between the external national expansion . . . and the internal insecurity . . . [that began] shortly after Solomon's succession."[137]

"The breakup of the small empire controlled by the House of David and the resulting centrifugal forces," observes Herr, "brought about rapid and profound political and social changes"[138]—changes that would affect the survival of the divinely anointed Judahic tribal leadership and adumbrate the fate of the ten tribes that had drawn away from it. Of the two Hebrew kingdoms that arose when Jeroboam and his followers proclaimed—

> We have no portion in David,
> No share in Jesse's son!
> To your tents, O Israel!
> Now look to your own House, O David[139]

—the northern kingdom, inhabited by ten of the twelve tribes, was not only larger than the southern kingdom, the latter being composed only of the tribes of Judah and Benjamin, but also "the largest and most prosperous of the small nations of the southern Levant . . . , [with its] fruitful hills and valleys around Samaria, Shechem, and Far'ah as well as the hills of Galilee . . . [and,] especially important, . . . the Jezreel valley where the Bible says the [ninth-century] Omride dynasty had a winter capital."[140] The institutions of hereditary monarchy of the northern kingdom, however, despite or perhaps, because of, the new nation's size, population, and early prosperity, proved to be unstable. They undermined the very idea that a single non-Judahic dynasty could survive. As Herr points out, "Whereas the House of David ruled in Judah with only minor threats to its stability (most notably the massacre inflicted on the royal family by Ahab and Jezebel's daughter Athaliah), for over 400 years, the Bible records eight *coups d'etat* during Israel's history of about 210 years (Baasha, Zimri, Omri, Jehu, Shallum, Menahem, Pekah, and Hoshea) . . . [with the few] successful dynasties [continuing under] Omri (Ahab) and Jehu (Jeroboam II)."[141] The forced dispersal of the ten tribes after Assyria's conquest of the Northern Kingdom also left them without a secular ruler—unless they would return their allegiance to the House of David, that is, to the descendants of Judah.

However, the dynastic status of the less-threatened Judahite lineage did not receive complete restoration either during or after the Babylonian exile. Although the kingdom of Judah would outlast that of Israel by 135 years, the return to Jerusalem permitted by the founder of the Achaemenid dynasty, Cyrus II, who ruled over Babylonia from 539 to 530 B.C.E., did not result in an immediate reestablishment of the Davidic monarchy. Later, as mentioned earlier, although Darius I (522–486 B.C.E.) appointed Zerubbabel, the grandson of the Davidic monarch, Jehoiachin, governor of Jerusalem, also permitting him to take charge of the rebuilding of the temple, to the consternation of the prophet Haggai, Zerubbabel is neither crowned nor anointed "king."[142] Instead, he is only referred to as a "servant" and designated as the wearer of the "signet ring." The prophet Zechariah seems to consign the future of the Davidic dynasty with respect to all the tribes to the eschatological future: "And just as you were a curse among the nations, O House of Judah and House of Israel, so, when I vindicate you, you shall become a blessing."[143]

The Persian Empire had become a world empire; it would be succeeded by Alexander's, then by the Seleucid, and finally by the Roman, the empire that would initiate the final global diaspora of the Jews.[144] Amidst these successive empires, as Gordon and Rendsburg observe, "The gentile World Empire was more firmly established than ever and common sense showed that Judah, far from being the center of the world, would have to remain a little province in a great gentile order."[145] Daniel Elazar dates the end of the Davidic line's inner-worldly status as the royal family of the Jews even earlier, to the Babylonian exile and its aftermath. By that time, he writes, "the monarchy had disappeared as a viable institution, though hope for its restoration became part of Israel's messianic dream."[146] Because the reuniting of the lost tribes of Israel with their Judahic brethren is seen as a prerequisite to the prophetic fulfillment of that dream, the quest for these tribes has, for true believers, remained an imperative.[147]

The Lost Tribes Enter Modernity: Medieval and Early Modern Claims

The discovery of peoples said to be the descendants of the ten missing tribes took on its modern form in the time of and the centuries after Columbus's voyages. To be sure, the several claims by medieval Jewish travelers to have found the tribes—for example, in the aforementioned letters of Eldad the Danite (880 C.E.);[148] in the correspondence between R. Chisdai Abu-Yusuf and Joseph, King of the Khozars (960 C.E.), in which the latter asserts that his Jewish subjects can trace their ancestry to Cusar, one of the ten sons of Togarma, whose own father was Noah's son Japhet;[149] in the travel book of Benjamin of Tudela (1173 C.E.), wherein he reports that "there are men of Israel in the land of Persia who say that in the mountains of Nishapur . . . dwell . . . the tribe of Dan, the tribe of Zebulun, the tribe of Asher, and the tribe of Naphtali, who were included in the first captivity of Shalmaneser, king of Assyria," and who goes on to claim to have visited Jewish communities in India and China;[150] in the brief mention of the "more than sixty myriads of Jews" who dwell in "Cush" by R. Petachia of Ratisbon (1187 C.E.),[151] who might have been writing about the "Falashas," that is, Ethiopian Jews who later would claim descent either from a breakaway element in the Moses-led exodus out of Egypt, the subjects converted by the Queen of Sheba after returning from her visit with King Solomon, or the lost (or strayed) tribe of Dan;[152] and in the ramblings of Elijah of Ferrara (1434 C.E.), a veritable second Eldad, a traveler to Egypt, Damascus, and Jerusalem, who not only asserted that he had heard of a Jewish kingdom in India, but also reported that "a young Jew has told me concerning those men of his own country and religion who are their own masters, and owe dependance to any one . . . , [who] dwell among a great nation called Habesh [Abyssinia], . . . make a show of Christianity . . . [but] are constantly at war with [Christians] and only now and again with other Jews . . . ; [who] live upon an island situated near the river Sambation; the tribe of Manasseh liv[ing] opposite them . . . , [while] the tribes of Dan, Naphtali, Gad, and Asher [reside beyond the river], . . . Issachar . . . in a province occupied by themselves alone, . . . Simeon to the extreme South . . . , Zebulun and Reuben . . . on . . . [opposite] banks of the Euphrates . . . , and . . . Ephraim . . . to the south of Babylon"[153]—did keep the apocalyptic prophecy of an eventual discovery and reunification alive in European and Central Asian centers of Jewish life. Christian concerns in this period were different—seeking routes to Cathay[154] and hoping for an anti-Moslem alliance with the fabled kingdom of Prester John.[155] But Columbus's voyages and the five-hundred-year period of exploration and European penetration of Africa, Asia, the Americas, and Oceania opened up hitherto untried vistas and venues toward which the divinely inspired quest for the lost tribes might be redirected.

Although after 1492, the search for the Lost Tribes tended to shift, moving into the "New World" of the Americas and toward the farther reaches of Africa, China, and India, the premodern position held that the lost tribes were in the Near East and Central Asia. To be sure, the Bible lands and the provinces of Central Asia would continue to have a claim as places of settlement of the Lost Tribes of Israel, or of other Jews descended from the ancient Hebrews. But, as Albert Einstein and Erich Kahler insisted in the *Princeton Herald* of April 14 and 21, 1944—in a spirited reply to Philip K. Hitti's earlier testimony before the House of Representatives' Committee on Foreign Relations, in which he had opposed the Wright-Compton Resolution calling for a reconstitution of Palestine as an independent and democratic Jewish commonwealth—some Hebrews had never left their original homeland, despite the several forced exiles imposed by the Assyrians, Babylonians, Seleucids, and Romans. And the descendants of these Jews, they argued, rather than any lost tribes remnant, provided the historical as well as a contemporary basis for a

Jewish claim to the land that had been overrun by Moslems and Christians over the last fifteen centuries:

> . . . [A]fter the Babylonian captivity the second great period, a true renaissance, of Jewish Palestine began, leading on the one hand to the elaboration of the Palestinian Talmud and, on the other, to the birth of Christianity from Judaism. . . . It was as late as A.D. 429 that the Jewish Patriarchate in Palestine was abolished.

Moreover, Einstein and Kahler, neither of whom subscribed to the lost tribes thesis, went on to observe:

> Jewish communities persisted in Palestine uninterruptedly throughout the ages. In the tenth century the Arab writer, Mukadassi, complained about the predominance of the Jewish population in Jerusalem. From the fifteenth century on, the city of Safed in Upper Galilee became a flowering Jewish intellectual center where the mystical philosophy of the Kabbalah was taught and perfected. It lasted until it was wiped out by the Turkish governor in the seventeenth century. Spanish Jews, after their expulsion, sought refuge in their homeland of old; messianic movements in the eighth, seventeenth, and eighteenth centuries aimed at the liberation and reestablishment of Jewish Palestine. and constantly from all over the world Jewish individuals who felt their end approaching made pilgrimages to the Holy Land to die and be buried on its sacred soil.[156]

Many of the Hebrews who did go into exile had migrated into the interior of Central Asia. Chaim Raphael observes, "The Jews who moved into these eastern regions at different times became heavily involved in the worlds of their host countries stretching from the Caspian to the Far East, and seem to have lost many of their direct links with the Jewish world of Persia." "But," as noted earlier, he quickly adds, "they all claimed to be descended from the Lost Ten Tribes."[157] According to Paul Johnson, "[L]egends connect the arrival of the Jews in Armenia and Georgia with the Ten Lost Tribes of the despoiled northern kingdom of Israel."[158] Nor does the charge of forgetfulness of Jewish rituals effectively eliminate the possibility that some of these Central Asian Jews are either faithful or faithless persons of lost tribes' lineage. Not only did Ezekiel's prophecy state that the remnants of the lost tribes might forget their religion and yet remain redeemable, but also Louis H. Feldman's careful study of pagan views on Jewish unity and diversity indicates that most gentile writers erroneously supposed that "all Jews think and act alike, so far as their religious beliefs and practices are concerned, whether in the Land of Israel or in the Diaspora," thus, in effect, failing to distinguish those lost tribespersons who adhered to the original religion from those who had acculturated, converted to another religion, or become secular. For those who believe in their survival, Central Asia cannot be ruled out as a place of settlement of the descendants of the lost tribes.[159]

Documenting the time of arrival of Jews in Central Asia proper and its contiguous areas is difficult.[160] Some Jews of Uzbekistan claim that Bukhara, their place of settlement for untold centuries, is in fact the city of Hador to which the Assyrians had exiled the lost tribes of Israel in 721 B.C.E.; while archaeological excavations have found no structures datable earlier than 500 B.C.E.; and the Apocrypha Book of Esdras, written sometime between 150 and 50 B.C.E., claims that Persian Jews migrated to Asareth (i.e., Bukhara) sometime after Cyrus issued edicts allowing some Jews to return to Jerusalem (538 B.C.E.),[161] Jews living in or near Tbilisi, Georgia, are knowledgeable of ancient manuscripts, supported by archaeological finds, that show a Jewish settlement there as early as the first centuries of the Common Era.[162] Azeri Jews, hailing from areas around Baku and Quba in Azerbaijan, live in mountainous areas, are usually called mountain Jews, and boast of a centuries-long heritage and a special variant of the Iranian Indo-European languages, employing some Hebrew words, called Yat.[163] Among the Jews flown to Israel as a result of the recent crisis in Chechnya were Ilya Nissimov and his family, erstwhile Tat speakers, who pointed out that their compatriots had maintained *brit mila* and *bar mitzvah* traditions in spite of the Stalin era's hostility to the practice of Jewish rituals.[164]

Jews from other areas of Russian Asia appear to have had later arrival dates, speaking in some cases to migrations from the West, and, for that reason, not relatable to lost tribes' descent. Ivan the Terrible (1533–1584 C.E.) was the first czar to order an expulsion of the Jews from Muscovy, an order that was repeated for Jewish traders who would not convert by Czar Fyodor (1676–1682), extended to apply in all Russian cities by Catherine I in 1727, and carried out against 35,000 Jews by her successor, Elizabeth. Later, with the first partition of Poland in 1772, a large number of Jews, many of them probably descended from those who had been expelled from Spain in 1492 and Portugal in 1497, came under Russian control. In 1791, Catherine II restricted Jewish residency in the provinces in which Moscow and Smolensk are located, creating the conditions for development of the Pale of Jewish Settlement from which, a century later, Jews would flee to the United States, Western Europe, and, in some cases, the *Yishuv* in Palestine.[165] Jewish settlement in and around Kiev and the Ukraine dates from the breakup of the Khazarian kingdom in the tenth century.[166] A Jewish traveler from Tortosa, Spain, Ibrahim ibn Jakub, writes in 965 C.E. of visiting Krakow, which had already become a place of asylum for Jews from the West, but the major movement of European Jews into

Poland took place later, from the twelfth to the fifteenth centuries.[167] Lithuanian Jews looked to Grand Duke Gedeyminus for their settlement in that country. He had established a Lithuanian state open to Jewish settlement in the fourteenth century; within two centuries Vilnius became a thriving center of Jewish culture.[168]

The Lost Tribes in the Twentieth Century

Five centuries later, in 1940, Chiune Sugihara, Japan's consul in Kaunas, Lithuania, would issue hundreds of transit visas to thousands of Lithuanian Jews who used them to travel east across Russia into Manchuria and eventually to Japan and Shanghai, safe from the horrors of the Holocaust.[169] Two rabbis, representing the Jews of Shanghai, then under Japanese occupation, would be told by Shinto priests that their followers would be protected from the Holocaust because they are members of a sect of ancient Shintoism that had been brought to the biblical Hebrews by their leader Moses, a sometime traveler to Japan,[170] and because the Japanese population is descended from one of the lost tribes of Israel.[171] Four decades later, the so-called Falasha of Ethiopia were declared to be the lost tribe of Dan and eligible to enter Israel under that state's law of return. At the present time, the Lemba of Zimbabwe and the Menashe of India have been unsuccessful in prosecuting their separate claims to be lost Jews having the same right to enter Israel as the Ethiopian Jews. Although the Jewish-Indian theory—holding that the American Indians are descendants of the lost tribes of Israel—no longer exerts any authority over Native Americans, Jews, or gentiles,[172] the anti-Jewish Christian Identity movement continues to put forward its claim to be the true Israelite descendants, and other peoples of what was once known as the Third World appear to be waiting in the wings to announce their own lost tribes' heritage. Embedded in the esoteric history of the Judaeo-Christian civilizations of the Occident, the lost tribes continue to play their only occasionally recognized and always intermittent role in both the praxes of modernity and in its postmodern epistemology.

CHAPTER FIVE

Postmodernism and the Construction of Ethnocultural Identity

The Jewish-Indian Theory and the Lost Tribes of Israel

> The destiny of the Jewish people . . . has unfolded in such a way that it possesses a world history of its own in the literal sense of the word.
> —SIMON DUBNOW (1860–1941), *World History of the Jewish People*

> What a difference between cinder and smoke: the latter apparently gets lost, and better still, without perceptible remainder, for it rises, it takes to the air, it is spirited away, sublimated. The cinder-falls, tires, lets go, more material since it fritters away its word; it is very divisible.
> —JACQUES DERRIDA, *Cinders*

> Without mortality, no history, no culture—no humanity.
> —ZYGMUNT BAUMAN, *Mortality, Immortality and Other Life Strategies*

"What we call serious criticism," writes Sanford Budick in a discussion of the crises attending the current interest in alterity, "is occasioned when something formerly considered significant has been lost or cut off in our understanding, so that a separation (or clarification) and decision must be made."[1] Of such things said to be cut off and long missing, one may include the fates, real and imagined, of the lost tribes of Israel, that is, the tribes of Reuben, Simeon, Dan, Naphtali, Gad, Asher, Issachar, Zebulon, Ephraim, and one-half of the tribe of Manasseh. These tribal groups comprised the biblically identified Hebrew denizens of the northern kingdom of Israel who were exiled and dispersed from their homeland when it was conquered and despoiled by the Assyrians in 722 B.C.E. From that date forward, the mystery of the disappearance of the ten tribes from history has inspired very few scholarly inquiries but much questing in search of its solution.

Modernist Jewish historians, as well as most secular investigators of antiquity,[2] appear to have accepted as unchallengeable truth a conclusion that severs from the annals of the peoples descended from Judea (i.e., the kingdom that did not succumb to the Assyrians) the oblivion into which the ten tribes are alleged to have sunk. As Erich Kahler (1885–1970) put it, "The Assyrians, who . . . destroyed the North Kingdom, . . . carried . . . the vanquished into exile. The majority of them . . . dispersed and . . . merged with other populations, sharing the fate of many peoples and realms which perished in the turmoil of human history."[3] For Kahler, it is the later exile from Judea that convokes the beginning of a Judaic community as well as the onset of anti-Jewish modernity: "The characteristic and recurring hostility toward Judaism has its origin in the decisive downfall of 586 B.C. For the fall of Judea as an independent state means the rise of Judaism."[4] It was the Babylonian rather than the Assyrian exile, Kahler asserts, that gave the Jewish community its peculiar coherence—"This community . . . began to establish itself on a new symbolic plane without losing its connection with the old tribal cult, with the promised homeland, and, indeed, with the advent of a concrete day of fulfillment."[5]

However, religious prophecy holds that the ten tribes must have survived, and that one day they will be reunited with the descendants of their Judean coreligionists in a reconstituted Jewish state. Ancient Zion had been the geocultural center of a theocratically driven civilization established by the Hebrews, a patriarchically organized people. At an earlier time, that people had fled Egypt under Moses and, after wandering in the desert for forty years, the Hebrews defeated the peoples of Canaan, settling on a land vouchsafed to them by God.[6] As settlers they were not inclined to become permanent bedouins. As a leading scholar of the latter, Anatoly M. Khazanov, has observed, "There is no reason to look upon the inhabitants of the steppe, [including such peoples as] the . . . ancient Jews, . . . as real nomads."[7] Rather, they remained a spiritual, land-rooted peoplehood, who, since the beginning of their diaspora, are in quest of a return to their homeland.[8] To sacred historians, the ten tribes—[here, I transpose words describing the effects of the later Roman assault on Hebraic culture onto the alleged response of the earlier exiles from the Northern Kingdom]—are credited with having carried the "culture of the Land . . . into the great Diaspora, where it was preserved in the minds of Jews who for [more than] two thousand years truly inhabited a cerebral version of the Land."[9] That "cerebral version of the Land" and its putative representatives are the topic of this investigation.

The Texts of Israelite Survival

In one sense, the present study is a particularistic elaboration of Tamar Garb's postmodern approach to *The Jew in the Text* in that, like Garb, I seek "to focus attention on a number of specific instances in which a complex, sometimes contradictory construction of Jewishness, Jewish history, or Jewish memory either forms the central theme or motif of a work or problematizes its very mode of address."[10] However, whereas Garb and her colleagues drew their conclusions from the many and varied representations of Jews in the nineteenth- and twentieth-century Occident, I have turned my attention to the "texts" proclaiming a post-biblical and non-Occidental Jewish presence that is hidden away in the modern world. The present study examines the conjectures, histories, and theosophies of those who see the descendants of the lost ten tribes of Israel in the countenances, culture, and color of seventeenth-century Ecuadorean Indians. In the centuries since that time other peoples have been singled out as descendants of the ten tribes—for example, the entire nation of Japan, or alternatively, its imperial rulers, various peoples of Africa and Asia, and the self-proclaimed "British Israelites." But these are only a few of the numerous peoples said to descend from the people exiled from the northern kingdom. In all of these assertions two basic theses are being proclaimed: (1) a prophetic promise and eschatological prediction are about to be fulfilled in defiance of insurmountable odds; (2) a peoplehood of antiquity has persevered in a separate diaspora[11] that parallels that of the Jews in the Occident.[12] Moreover, in the contexts in which Israelite ancestry claims are put forward—for example, identifying such peoples as copper-colored South American Indians, the imperial family if not the entire nation of Japan, American priests of British Israelite Christian Identity, or others from various parts of the African and Asian world as epigoni of the long-lost Israelites—there are also to be found pursuits of a decidedly inner-worldly and secular character: In the case of the Ecuadorian aborigines, an attempt to influence Lord Cromwell and gain the repeal of England's ban on Jewish immigration. For others there are different worldy concerns: In the case of the Japanese nation, the rescue of thousands of European Jews from the Nazi holocaust; that of the British Israelites Christian Identity movement, the murder of Medgar Evers, attempts on the lives of American Jewish leaders, and the formation of the Aryan Nation; that of the several Afro-Asian designates, the right to settle in the modern state of Israel. In the present chapter, only that of the Ecuadorean Indians will be discussed. The others will be part of this author's subsequent studies.

The Charisma of Nonlinear Time and Space

Assertions of lost Israelite identity entail an instantiation of the ambivalence contained in Fredric Jameson's conceptualization of "disjunctive social time."[13] Jameson's idea has been reframed by Homi K. Bhabha: "There is, on the one hand," Bhabha observes, "a recognition of the interstitial, disjunctive spaces and signs crucial for the emergence of the new historical subjects . . .

However, . . . Jameson disavows the temporality of displacement which is, quite literally, its medium of communication. For Jameson, the possibility of becoming historical demands a containment of this disjunctive social time."[14] In the cases of the several putative inheritors of lost tribes identity, however, the disjunction involves a displacement of both social time and social space,[15] as well as a "containment" that somehow attaches the newly recognized identity onto the corpus of conventional history. All this is made difficult by the claim that the habitats at which one or another of the remnants of the lost tribes are alleged to reside consist not only of specific places of landed settlement, but also of such "non-places" as, in Mormon belief,[16] to take an outstanding example, on an unknown planet, in an undiscovered cave or volcano, or at the North Pole, thus making these tribal survivors, if nothing else, an appropriate topic for the "anthropology of supermodernity,"[17] and a strategic situs on which to construct alternative ethnocultural maps of meaning.[18]

The ten tribes of Israel have been lost from—and lost to—conventional modes of secular temporal historiography. They thus present those scholars who enquire after them with a special problem: how a prophetic cosmology of survival, remembrance, and ultimate reunification can be fitted into the widely accepted and conventionalized knowledge of events past and present.[19] In fact, however, the sense of *duree* that stands behind claims of the continued existence of Israel's lost tribes belongs not to what Maurice Natanson once referred to as "Big History"[20]—that is, the metanarratives that postmodernists claim to have evicted from their place in hegemonic Occidental scholarship—but rather to what Carl Becker noted is the "kind of history that has [the] most influence upon the life of the community . . . [:] the history that common people carry around in their heads."[21] Such modes of history have their own tracks of time,[22] their own topologies of space,[23] and these do not—and need not—necessarily correspond to the accepted linear or cyclical, time-and-space dimensions of authorized histories. At present, in the case of the lost tribes of Israel, the spatiotemporal accounts and conjectures of their allegedly living descendants partake of a dual cosmology—one, inner worldly, for example, entitling those such as the Beta Israel of Ethiopia,[24] who are recognized as legitimate heirs of the ancient Hebrew peoplehood (or, more generally, to be authentic Jews), to settle in the modern state of Israel under its "Law of Return";[25] the other, eschatological, fulfilling biblical prophecy and heralding the coming of a messianic age.[26] In either perspective, understanding the present entails interpreting the past, that is, grasping the nomothetic through the prism of the idiographic.[27] And, whether inner worldly or esoteric, each perspective maintains a belief in destiny, in a particular teleology. The latter belief at first seems to stand against the postmodern opposition to and deconstruction of preordained futures, but, ultimately—eschatologically, that is—embraces what Mikhail N. Epstein has described as the central temporal feature of the futurology of the *nouvelle vague:*

> The future was thought to be definite, attainable, and realizable; in other words, it was given the attributes of the past. Postmodernism, with its aversion to utopias, inverted the signs and reached for the past, but in so doing, gave it the attributes of the future: indeterminateness, incomprehensibility, polysemy, and the ironic play of possibilities . . . Postmodernism announced an "end to time," but any end serves to open at least a crack in time for what is to come after and, thus, indicates the self-irony of finality, which turns into yet another beginning.[28]

The quest for the lost tribes of Israel focuses on one or another present-day peoplehood, prismatically perceived as a survival of a lost past, and serving to predict and fulfill a foreordained future.

However, each time a specific claim of lost tribe identity is put forward, it produces what the sociological historiographer Frederick J. Teggart called an "intrusion."[29] An intrusion operates on conventional history by challenging its spatiotemporal horizon, forcing into liminality a hitherto buried consciousness that the latter's pre-given unquestionableness can no longer be accepted as such;[30] or with the same effect that an ethnomethodological experiment is likely to have on its unwitting subjects[31]—namely, it interrupts the flow of happenings as they are understood in the prevailing but implicit hermeneutic of everyday life and brings to the surface of perception an epistemologically piercing moment. In the case of the lost tribes, the veil of history is torn and its less-than-secure bases exposed. From that moment—often experienced as crucial, decisive, or a turning point—a reconfiguration of both history and historiography—one that incorporates or coopts the newly recognized lost tribes—is, at the very least, entertainable. As we shall see in what follows, recognizing a people as one or all of the lost tribes of Israel is one of those rare but significant moments that thematizes the idiographic horizons of the *Lebenswelt*[32]—that requires a reconceptualization of past, present, and future. Indeed, such an event opens a fissure in the spatio-temporal world, or widens one that has already been noticed but uncontained.

The Indians of the Americas as Lost Israelites

Christopher Columbus's fifteenth-century Caribbean encounter with the people we now know as Tainos[33] introduced a crisis in biblically based European cosmology. That crisis could only be resolved by insisting that these "Indians," as Columbus miscalled them, be regarded as descendants of some prehistoric migrants from Eurasia and/or Africa,[34] that is, the land-base from which humankind had originated. Although over the centuries since Columbus's voyages there have been many claimants to the title of Amerindian forefatherhood—and at least one hypothesis of reverse migration from ancient America to Asia, Africa, and Europe[35]—one that had a brief but portentous effect on future events was presented in epistolary form to a Protestant divine on November 25, 1649, by the rabbinical leader of Amsterdam's Jewish community, Menasseh ben Israel (1604–1657).[36] The letter—replying to the storm of curiosity that had arisen in England and the Netherlands over Menasseh's earlier recounting of the story brought to him by Aaron Levi de Montezinos, a crypto-Jew, to the effect that one part of the remnants of the lost tribe of Reuben now dwelt beyond the Cordillera mountains in the interior of the Spanish colony of New Granada (Ecuador) and that the tribe of Joseph lived on an island nearby[37]—promised publication of a treatise in which the learned rabbi would "handle of the first inhabitants of America which I believe were of the Ten Tribes; moreover, that they are scattered also in other Countries, that they keep their true Religion, as hoping to returne againe into the Holy Land in due time."[38]

Thus, in this letter is contained each of the elements of a historical-hermeneutic intrusion: A disputed thesis of ancient Jewish history is offered not only as factual, but also as proved to be so by the proffered fact that at least one of the tribes had survived expulsion, global dispersion, and the travails of over two thousand years of exile with its culture and belief system still intact. Further, the prophetic promise of homeland return and redemptive reunification with both the other surviving Israelite remnants as well as the descendants of the people derived from the southern kingdom, the latter in diaspora since 70 C.E., seemed about to be fulfilled. In its seventeenth-century appearance, the "Jewish-Indian theory"—that would reappear in the eighteenth and nineteenth centuries and have disparate effects on aspects of Jewish,[39] Christian,[40] and secular political thought and praxis[41]—also provided the basis and the occasion for Menasseh ben Israel's bold attempt to reshape England's immigration policy. In force since 1290 C.E., an English royal edict had banned Jews from its soil.[42] Menasseh's version of the Jewish-Indian theory thus became an (unsuccessful) instrument for bringing about the revocation of a centuries-old discriminatory statute—a feat the Amsterdam rabbi nearly accomplished by inserting both Jewish and Christian eschatologies into Cromwell's secular national policy considerations.

Menasseh's book-length version of the lost tribes' history not only incorporated Montezino's Ecuadorean Indian thesis into the religious cosmology on the matter, but also took care to allow for a diasporic dispersion to have placed the several long-lost tribes in virtually every part of the world. Thus, after asserting that "I . . . doe finde no opinion more probable, nor agreeable to reason, then that of our Montezinus, who saith, that the first inhabitants of America, were the ten Tribes of the Israelites, . . . who . . . (as God would have it) hid themselves behind the Mountaines Cordillerae," Menasseh went on to observe that, in his own disquisition on the subject, "I [shall] also shew, that as they were not driven out at once from their Country, so also they were scattered into divers Provinces, sc. into America, into Tartary, into China, into Media, to the Sabbaticall River, and into AEthiopia."[43] Their supposed dispersion over most of the earth was of crucial importance to Menasseh's twofold purpose—to divulge new proofs that biblical prophecy was being fulfilled; and to argue that only England's edict prohibiting Jewish immigration stood in the way of their biblically foretold global dispersion. Once completed, the world-wide Jewish diaspora would herald the beginning of the much hoped-for messianic era.

As to the first issue, prophetic eschatology, Menasseh pointed out that he could "prove that the ten Tribes never returned to the second Temple, that they yet keepe the Law of Moses, and our sacred Rites; and [that he could predict with confidence that they] at last shall return into their Land, with the two Tribes, Judah and Benjamin; and shall be governed by one Prince, who is Messiah the son of David."[44]

However, in order to succeed in his political, this-worldly goal, the repeal of England's anti-Jewish immigration edict, Menasseh sought to insert his religio-cosmological time-and-space hermeneutic of the ten tribes into conventional and contemporary English historico-political beliefs and practices. Moreover, he appeared to be ecumenical in his outlook, merging Judaic with Christian messianic prophecies in a manner that would win the support of Oliver Cromwell's Puritan regime. In this regard Menasseh was aided not only by the fact that in England he was already regarded as "the principal exponent of Jewish science,"[45] but also by a parallel development of the "Jewish-Indian" theory among Protestant divines and English missionaries to the New World. There was, in addition, growing support among Cromwell's Puritan admirers for the exhibition of a greater tolerance toward the once-despised Jews, "the people of God,"[46] than was then being expressed by their Spanish Catholic rivals for an American imperium.

While such English ministers of the gospel as Thomas Thorowgood and John Durie took to embellishing their own view that the Indians of the Americas were Jews—making contact with Menasseh and adding their support to his thesis, but perceiving it as an added proof of their own belief that the Jewish Indians were divinely destined to receive the blessings of conversion to

Judaism's successor religion, Christianity—Menasseh found the lynchpin for his own practical project in the homiletic he put forward as the appropriate Christian, as well as Jewish, interpretation of a prophecy found in Daniel 12:7: "When he shall have accomplished to scatter the power of the holy people, all these things shall be finished."[47] However, precisely because it was possible to translate the phrase "scatter the power" to "breaking the power,"[48] Menasseh could not rest his case on the ambiguity contained in that biblical utterance. Hence, he turned to a verse in the Book of Deuteronomy, 28:64, wherein it is written, "And the Lord shall scatter thee among all people, from one end of the earth even unto the other."[49] Seizing upon this phrase and combining it with that of the prophecies in the Book of Daniel, Menasseh contrived an argument that held that Cromwell's Puritan republic was the land referred to by the Hebrew Deuteronomic term *Kezeh ha-Arez,* often translated into French as "*angle-terre,*" or the "end of the earth," that is, "England." As Menasseh presented the matter, now that Montezino had found Jews among the Indians of the New World, only the admission of Jews into England was necessary to fulfill the Lord's promise of a completed global Jewish dispersion, the prelude to the coming of the messianic age.

Building upon this thesis, Menasseh was eventually able to convince Lord Cromwell to convoke a council to deliberate on the matter of the repeal. The council did not act in the way he had desired, however, and Cromwell, though he sought to connive at it in a different way, never issued the proposed edict of repeal.

Nevertheless, Menasseh's proposal proved to be prescient. His petition was an early appeal not only for toleration with respect to Jewish entrance to England—which, incidentally, was granted to the Jews in 1663, after the restored monarch bestowed it on them in gratitude to those other Dutch Jews who, opposed to Menasseh's approach, had aided the deposed Prince Charles during his period of continental exile[50]—but also for a communally based form of surveilled civil rights. For Menasseh had employed his Jewish-Indian thesis to request that Jews be readmitted to England not merely as alien settlers but as a communally recognized people equal to others in English law. To secure these rights, he proposed, "That all laws against them should be repealed; that the principal public officers . . . be made to take an oath to defend them; that public synagogues . . . be permitted in all parts of the English dominions, as well as cemeteries outside the cities for the burial of the dead; that they . . . be granted free full liberties of trade; and that the privilege of internal jurisdiction (subject to the right of appeal to the civil judges) . . . be conceded to the heads of the community for the time being."[51]

Further, and in a promise of fealty to the English polity, Menasseh's petition to Cromwell required that those Jews who chose to emigrate to England would "swear allegiance to the government and . . . [allow themselves to] be kept under the strictest surveillance."[52] Despite his twentieth-century biographer's belief that what Menasseh was proposing "was one of those closely controlled, semi-autonomous communities of the sort tolerated in . . . Hamburg or Leghorn,"[53] and that if his petition had been granted, "with the slightest modification in public opinion, the Ghetto might have been introduced in all of its German or Italian severity,"[54] it is worthy of note that—Menasseh's petition having failed to be accepted—the very same debate over Jewish identity, loyalty, religion, and destiny that had marked and marred Cromwell's councillors' sessions[55] was renewed in England in the nineteenth century as a part of that country's determination to remain a "Christian" nation and its leaders' worry over the effects of increasing tides of Jewish immigration from eastern Europe.[56]

English suspicion of the Jews continued through the first half of the twentieth century. England would be in the forefront of those Occidental polities that did little to save continental Jews from the Nazi holocaust.[57] Indeed, England's World War II Jewish policies spoke loudly about, but did nothing to ameliorate, the plight of Jews then desperately in search of the kind of haven that Menasseh had sought so earnestly—and had sought to build on the basis of an extraordinary claim of a Jewish connection to the pre-Columbian aborigines of America. In fact, while England and America dawdled, in fascist Italy[58] and militaristic Japan[59] efforts to rescue Jews from the terror of Hitler's Holocaust proved quite effective.

The Jewish-Indian Theory in America

Although the Jewish-Indian theory proved neither necessary nor sufficient to effect Menasseh's immigration project, once having been enunciated, it became sedimented in the arcana of lore about the Israelites. However, Menasseh was not the originator of the claim that ancient Jews had somehow gotten to America; rather, he was the first Jew to adapt it to Jewish sacred and secular interests. The theory appears to have originated among Iberian commentators on the encounters of Columbus and later Spanish conquistadores with the aborigines of America and the Caribbean.[60] Menasseh's treatise on the subject went through numerous editions and several translations; *The Hope of Israel* having appeared in English as recently as 1901 and in Spanish in 1929.[61] If nothing else, its continued popularity calls attention to the instability of racial and ethnoreligious categories of classification that are still in use and that have become grist for the postmodernists' critical mill.

But, as Simon Schama has pointed out, "Unstable identities are history's prey."[62] And such has been the case with the Jewish-Indian theory. In the centuries since Menasseh's death, it has been revived intermittently, almost always in service to Jewish or Christian eschatological as well as mundane secular interests. Thus, in 1775, in the most well known instance, James W. Adair, an eighteenth-century historian of the American Indians, put forward no less than twenty-three arguments in support of his claim that the aborigines of Florida, with whom he had lived for several years, were descendants of the lost tribes and that, because of this, their territory ought to be wrested from Catholic Spain and its anti-Jewish Inquisition by means of an Anglo-Indian alliance.[63] To evangelical Protestants, seeking converts among the Indians, as Bernard W. Sheehan has pointed out, "Coupling the Indians with the Jews yielded obvious theoretical advantages . . . [For, since] the European man had his spiritual origin in Israel, it would certainly improve the anomalistic situation of the Indian to find his historical beginnings there."[64]

However, biblical exegetes among the missionaries to New England worried over the contradictions that a close reading of their sacred literature seemed to suggest. Insistent on their belief in a Puritan variant of what is now known as flood ethnology,[65] pious evangelists of colonial New England knew that the Indians could not be autochthonous to America, but they worried over whether the aborigines they encountered were descendants of the accursed son of Ham[66]—and, therefore, perhaps beyond salvation—or whether, as offspring of the long-lost tribes of Israel, they might be unwitting instruments of a much sought-after millennium.[67] Ingenious casuistries seeking to affirm or set aside a Jewish-Indian genealogy were written and preached throughout the seventeenth century, some linking the American aborigines to Scythians, others to Judaeans, and still others seeking to give them either a Semitic origin or an absolution from the Hamitic curse.[68] One paradigm initially proved to be attractive—designating the Indians as "Canaanites," thus Hamitic in origin, Canaan being the patronym of the accursed son of Ham, who was said to be the progenitor of the seafaring Phoenician people.[69] However, while such a perspective might speak to the Puritans' self-conceived mission as biblically directed conquerors in service to the settlement of the "New-England-Israel," a new Promised Land, a Hamitic identification of the Indians opened up the question of whether the "accursed" aborigines were to be subjugated and ostracized, or made whole again by being drawn into the commonwealth of converted believers.[70]

Ultimately, however, neither the Jewish-Indian thesis nor the Canaanite-Indian genealogy could be made commensurable with the aims and interests of either the Puritan divines or their more materialist-minded settler coreligionists. Cotton Mather, a subscriber to the belief that the Indians were unsalvageable Scythians, was, as John Canup observes, "reluctant to honor them by assuming that they were the long-lost Tribes of Israel, the ancient people of God [who] would have to be gathered in before the climax of Christian history."[71] As a matter of fact, Canup concludes, "When Cotton Mather thought of Indians, he thought more often of Satan than of Christ."[72] Sacvan Bercovitch, who holds that the lost tribes identification of Native Americans was not as prevalent among the Puritans as some others have supposed, claims that "by the time King Philip's War broke out the Indians were unequivocally identified with the doomed 'dark brothers' of Scripture—Cain, Ishmael, Esau, and above all the heathen natives of the promised land, who were to be dispossessed by divine decree of what really belonged to God's chosen"[73]—that is, the Puritan settlers.

However, in the nineteenth century, it was precisely their continuing anomalous situation in America that gave rise to disparate programs directed at their redemption through a renewed lost tribes identification. The North American tribe selected most prominently for either salvation-through-conversion-to-Christianity or reclamation-via-Judaism was that of the Cherokees. Exemplary of the former approach were the efforts of Elias Boudinot (1740–1821), a sometime member of Thomas Jefferson's cabinet and the founder of the American Bible Society. In 1816, Boudinot published his premillenial magnum opus, *A Star in the West,* proving by means of comparing evidence of language, customs, traditions, and religious practices that there existed a more than coincidental cultural similarity between the contemporary Cherokees and the ancient Israelites.[74] As Israelite descendants, the "Indians are perfect republicans," he observed, "they will admit of no inequality among them but what arises from age, or great qualifications for either council or war."[75] They were also ripe for evangelization. To this end, Boudinot adopted and converted a young Cherokee man, Buck Watie, who in turn married a white woman, took the name of his adoptive father, and rose to become the controversial go-between and remarkably accommodating negotiator during the struggle over Cherokee removal.[76] Regarded as a traitor to his people, the younger Boudinot was assassinated by members of his tribe on June 22, 1839.[77] Although the descendants of the Watie-Boudinot family would continue to play important roles in Cherokee politics, in later years the Cherokee-Israelite theory seems to have lost its significance in both Indian and Protestant circles.[78]

In the same era, a Jew, Mordecai Noah (1785–1851), an erstwhile U.S. consul in the Barbary States during James Madison's presidency—who had been recalled from his post in April 1815, because, in Secretary of State James Monroe's cryptic account, "it was not known that the Religion which you profess would form an obstacle to the exercise of your consular function"[79]—made the decision to end his coreligionists' diaspora by establishing a Jewish homeland on American soil. Although the modern emancipation of the Jews had been announced by Napoleon a decade and one-half earlier—when the future emperor had paused twenty-five miles away from Jerusalem to urge that, "Israelites arise! Now is the moment . . . to claim your political existence as a nation among nations!"[80]—the major result in America had been a Protestant call for a new Christian crusade to the Holy Land: "Rise, American ambassadors," cried Albany's Chapel Street Presbyterian pastor, John McDonald, "and prepare to carry the tidings of joy and salvation to your Saviour's kinsmen [i.e., the Jews] in disgrace."[81]

Having begun to encourage an increase in Jewish immigration to America upon his return to the United States, and aware of other Jewish attempts to develop enclaves in Florida and west of the Mississippi River, Noah proposed that the New York legislature permit him to establish "a colony for the Jews of the world," a homeland that, given his surname, he not coincidentally called "Ararat," on Grand Island, a 17,000-acre tract in the Niagara River. His petition attracted the interest of the German *Verein für Kultur und Wissenschaft der Juden*[82] and, in its early years of development, that society and other European and American Jews began to invest capital in the scheme.[83] But Noah's conception of Jewish identity encompassed more than the Jews of Europe. To the dedication ceremony of his ultimately abortive plan to carry forth, in a hitherto unimagined way, the project envisioned by the biblical prophets of zionism[84]—held on September 15, 1825, in the city of Buffalo's Episcopal Church of St. Paul—Noah invited Red Jacket as well as several other Indian tribal chiefs, explaining that he fully subscribed to the belief that they and their fellow tribesmen and -women were descendants of the ten lost tribes of Israel and, as such, were, like the Jews from Europe, being called to become full-fledged members of the immediately proclaimed "Jewish nation [that he had established] under the auspices and protection of the constitution and laws of the U. S. of A."[85]

The Jewish-Indian Theory in Postmodern Thought

At the present time, the claim that the Indians of the Americas are descendants of the lost tribes of Israel has for the most part been relegated to folklore and to the "little histories"[86] that exist at the edges and in the interstices of a complex culture. Yet, the thesis that the lost tribes are still living somewhere in the modern world has not entirely disappeared, nor has it been altogether disavowed. Recently, for example, Pierre Vidal-Naquet, while recounting his life as a Jew under France's pro-Nazi Vichy regime, recalled "making the acquaintance of an austere and mystical lady from Dieulefit who belonged to a famous family of pastors, the Atgers. She explained to me at length that the ten tribes of Israel had spread across the world, including Denmark, as its name, which came from the tribe of Dan, proved."[87] Even more recently, Bernard Lewis, a noted authority on the history and sociology of Jewish-Muslim relations, in the course of a wide-ranging commentary on how the designation and classification of the continents and their peoples are sociocultural constructions that have become legitimated through widespread usage and acceptance, admitted, "I do not know at what stage or by what processes the descendants of the Aztecs and the Incas came to understand and accept their identity as Americans."[88] But, whatever the stage or process, the credence given to their identification as Jews, and more particularly, as descendants of the lost tribes of Israel, is, at present, quite insecure. Indeed, it has been removed from most serious discussions of either people and has become a source of bitter humor, most pointedly in Mel Brooks's 1974 film, *Blazing Saddles*.

However, it is not altogether a departure from its locus in culture to find the Jewish-Indian theory today to be a feature of dark comedy. For, in all of its usages, the thesis that there still exists a cultural peoplehood that conventional and secular historians insist could not have survived exile and dispersion acts to ironize and displace the accepted limits of the latter claim. In America, where the canon of its authenticated history has only begun to be called into question by the protagonists of a multiethnic multiculturalism[89]—but where the older "Jewish Question" no longer occupies as central a place as it once did in either modernist or proto-postmodernist works of scholarship—an older situs of the expression of Jewish mordant humor,[90] Hollywood,[91] becomes one venue for raising the issue of the theory's relevance and meaning, its place in the time-space continuum. Some of today's movies, perhaps less so than television, speak to "that rupture-point in human history [that has emerged] between the decline of the now-passé age of sociology and the upsurge of the new world of communications."[92]

About this situation, Homi K. Bhabha has observed, "the national culture comes to be articulated as a dialectic of various temporalities—modern, colonial, postcolonial, 'native'—that cannot be a knowledge that is stabilized in its enunciation."[93] But, as Mel Brooks's film illustrates, it is a kind of knowledge that can be articulated in the form of comedy, in the supposedly "unspeakable images"[94] that unresolved ethnicity has evoked.

Employing a satire on the Jewish-Indian theory, *Blazing Saddles* provides its viewers with a postmodern glimpse of a culture that is simultaneously modern and traditional, colonial and postcolonial, national and fragmented, with peoples who are mainstream and marginalized—a pastiche, a collage. The "entire film," observes Lester D. Friedman, "reverberates with the Jewish sense of alienation that leads Brooks to focus on the problems faced by outsiders in the Old West, those segregated by race, color, or religion."[95] In a memorable scene, Brooks essays a complex variant on what Herbert Marcuse once called the desublimation of repression,[96] presenting a band of Indians, whose chief is portrayed by Brooks himself in "redface," speaking Yiddish to one another. Compounding this send-up of the Jewish-Indian theory, Brooks's Indian parodies what is, in fact, the common epithet used when American Jews talk amongst themselves about American blacks. "Schwartzers?" his Indian inquires incredulously as he and his men come upon a wagonload of African Americans being transported across the plains. One critic has interpreted that scene to be benevolently universalizing: "black and white interchange—and, at bottom, all men—even Indians are secretly Jews."[97] But, American Indians had been said to be Jews for hundreds of years. So also had the so-called Falasha (now called Beta Israel) of Ethiopia, the inhabitants of Kaifeng, China, the people of Japan, the Pathans of Afghanistan, the Shin-Lung people on the Burma-India border, the Knanites in southern India, the Pachucans of Mexico, and many others.[98]

Perhaps the sociological lesson of *Blazing Saddles,* a message of some aspects of postmodernism, is that all our systems of classification are simultaneously necessary and arbitrary—in fact are ethnomethodological experiments that always suffer from the fact that there is no escape from Garfinkelian rules, only one of which is "let it pass."[99]

Conclusion

The lost tribes of Israel have passed through and beyond most of the peoples of the world. They epitomize a combination that Simmel had not foreseen—a permanent synthesis of traveler and stranger,[100] a wandering body of Jews that reminds us of how malleable our conceptions of time, space, and character—and peoplehood—are. "Thus," observes Rudolf Glanz, "the wandering Jew . . . filled the full function of the Jew in American folklore, namely, being a known phenomenon to provide a standard to be applied to the unknown that so often seemed to pose a threat."[101] With *Blazing Saddles* the unknown comes into its own. "Somehow," writes Lester D. Friedman, "it seems comically appropriate that the West's most conspicuous outsider, the Indian, should speak in the tongue of history's traditional outsider, the Jew."[102]

In effect, once having been ensconced in *Blazing Saddles'* postmodern comic frame, the debate over whether the Jewish-Indian theory has any validity has entered the realm of what Jean-Francois Lyotard calls the *differend:* "a differend would be a case of conflict between (at least) two parties that cannot be equitably resolved for lack of a rule of judgment applicable to both arguments."[103] The query, "Are (some or all) American Indians descended from the lost tribes of Israel?" cannot be given an unequivocal answer, one, that is, that would satisfy both a rational modernist historian and a New Age postmodern investigator. For, as David J. Hess has pointed out "New Agers incorporate and rework the research of anthropologists, physicists, philosophers, and other scientists and scholars to legitimate a discourse that also sanctions crystal healing, channelers, astral bodies, goddess religion, and other beliefs and practices generally associated with popular culture."[104] Jewish eschatological esoterica, or at least that part of it that quests for the lost tribes, like so much else of what modernist secularists consider paranormal, has become a part of that popular culture, a part, that is, of the "nostalgic aesthetic of postmodern movies known as *a la mode retro.*"[105] Like Karl Marx's quest to discover the real Napoleon III,[106] Mel Brooks's postmodern placement of the lost tribes of Israel in Hollywood's American West has turned mythic history into mundane farce.

PART IV

Cinematic Routes to Malaise

CHAPTER SIX

Social Reality as Theater

Dramas, Narratives, and the Postmodern Challenge

> . . . all this life of mortal men,
> what is it else but a certain kind
> of stage play? Whereas men come
> forth disguised one in one array,
> another in another, each playing
> his part . . .
>
> —ERASMUS, *The Praise of Folly*

Alfred Schutz's suggestions about the intersubjective aspects of one type of literature, drama,[1] have inspired this sociologist to rethink the matter in terms of a dialogical inversion. Whereas Schutz proposed to elucidate the sociological aspects of literature, including drama, I propose to reconsider aspects of the theater in relation to the drama of social reality. My remarks are especially oriented to recent postmodern challenges to the epistemological status of both the humanities and the social sciences. In brief, I shall argue that precisely because of the postmodernist perspective, the methods and outlook associated with dramatism, including but not confined to those contained in the remarks of Schutz, provide an appropriate perspective with which to investigate social action. Moreover, the dramatistic approach to social action that I shall present here, derived from earlier studies I carried out with Marvin B. Scott,[2] also speaks to some of the major dilemmas posed by poststructuralist and postmodernist critiques and offers a resolution of them. That resolution could be employed to rescue sociology and the other social sciences from the demise (i.e., "decentering," "deconstruction") that the *nouvelle vague* seems to promise to, or portend for, them.[3] But first, some observations on postmodernism.

Language, Meaning, and Drama: Positions

Among the illusions that Jacques Derrida (1930–) claims plague Occidental thought is that of spatiotemporal boundedness. "Derrida," observes Madan

Sarup, "argues that phonocentrism-logocentrism relates to centrism itself—the human desire to posit a 'central' presence at beginning and end."[4] Centrism is, it should be noted, a feature of *positionism,*[5] an orientation overlooking conceptualizations of space, time, and I would add—out of consideration for the sociologist William Graham Sumner's (1840–1910) contribution of the term *ethnocentrism*[6] to the lexicon of centrism—of manner, or generalized attitude. (Positionism, I should point out here, is the orientation that stands at the base of the anchor points of "territoriality" and "time tracks" in Scott's and my *Sociology of the Absurd.*)[7] And the problematics of positionism affect everything, including, especially, truth. "By itself," Derrida observes, "the expression 'limits of truth' can certainly be understood . . . as the fact that the truth is precisely limited, *finite,* and confined within its borders."[8]

What are those borders of truth? For such postmodernists as Jacques Derrida, Fredric Jameson, and Michel Foucault, these borders arise out of their variously posited theses that the modernist conception of meaning, that is, the connection between words and things, the signifier and the signified, has been irrevocably broken. A wall of epistemology keeps them apart from one another. "Thus," as Derrida once put it, "I have regularly marked the turn by means of which the word 'signifier' leads us back to or retains us in the logocentric circle."[9] In addition, and to destabilize the conventional sense of meaning even further, Derrida introduces the "undecidables," that is, "unities of simulacrum, 'false' verbal properties . . . that can no longer be included within philosophical (binary) opposition, but which, however, inhabit philosophical opposition, resisting and disorganizing it, *without ever* constituting a third term, without ever leaving room for a solution in the form of speculative dialectics."[10] (Appropriately, Derrida selected the Greek word "Pharmakon" as an ideal-typical "undecidable," for it can mean both "remedy" and "poison" and thus in its duality can both cure and kill.)[11] Finally, there is Derrida's collapse of past and future into an ever-present presence, indicated in his commentary on his own neologism, "*differance*": "It is because of *differance,*" he observes, "that the movement of signification is possible only if each so-called 'present' element, each element appearing on the scene of presence, is related to something other than itself, thereby keeping within itself the mark of the past element, and already letting itself be vitiated by the mark of its relation to the future element, this trace being related no less to what is called the future than to what is called the past, and constituting what is called the present by means of this relation to what it is not: what it absolutely is not, not even a past or a future as a modified present."[12]

For Derrida, differance (with an "a") refers to the spatiotemporal simultaneity of "differing" and "deferring," and this dynamically equilibrating simultaneity, in turn, invites a veritable instauration of both philosophy and philosophy's contribution to a critique of binary oppositioned conceptualization in social science: "Thus," he writes, "one could reconsider all the pairs of opposites on which philosophy is constructed and on which our discourse lives, not in order to see opposition erase itself but to see what indicates that each of the terms must appear as the *differance* of the other, as the other different and deferred in the economy of the same . . . , [e.g.,] culture as nature different and deferred, differing, deferring; all the others of *physis—techne, nomos, thesis,* society, freedom, history, mind, etc.—as *physis* different and deferred, or as *physis* differing and deferring."[13] On this point Derrida concludes—and I will return to this issue in my discussion of Schutz's contribution to dramatism *infra*— ". . . in this way we may see the site of a reinterpretation of *mimesis* in its alleged opposition to *physis.*"[14]

Whereas Derrida holds out the possibility of a development of a renewed philosophy and a new kind of social science, Fredric Jameson's adaptation and elaboration of Jacques Lacan's conceptualization of schizophrenia is far less sanguine about any instauration of either science or society. There is still room for both space and time to operate in Derrida's world of undecidables and *differance,* but for Jameson postmodern space and time have outpaced "the capacities of the individual human body to locate itself, to organize its immediate surroundings perceptually, and cognitively to map its position in a mappable external world."[15] Hence, for Jameson, there is a special kind of spectatorship for the postmodern viewer of a work of art or *kitsch*—Jameson's example is Nam June Paik's stacked or scattered television screens exhibiting dyssynchronous sequences of images—a role for the beholder (to use Schutz's term)[16] that transcends and, perhaps, confounds the latter's (that is, Schutz's) formulation of the microsociological situation that is likely to prevail when the "prescientific" beholder gazes at or hears and sees the work of an *auteur:* "The postmodern viewer," Jameson observes, ". . . is called upon to do the impossible, namely, to see all the scenes [in Paik's video display] at once, in their radical and random difference . . . and to rise somehow to a level at which the vivid perception of radical difference is in and of itself a new mode of grasping what used to be called relationship: something for which the word *collage* is still only a very feeble name."[17]

Derrida's formulations of the objectives of "deconstruction" and "differance" have inspired such African American postmodern investigator/critics and authors as Henry Louis Gates Jr. and Toni Morrison, respectively, to search out (in the case of Gates) the traces of "blackness" that are hidden beneath the racially mixed Jean Toomer's claim that he and his fiction represent the transcendence and overcoming of a single racial identity,[18] and to uncover (in the case of Morrison) the hitherto unnoticed traces of "blackness" in nineteenth-century novels that set off the manifest presentations of "whiteness."[19] Jameson's synthesis of schizophrenia, space, and time under the terms of the postmodern condition, on the other hand, appears in its designation of *collage* to demand recognition of a liberation of difference from contradiction—namely, difference perceived for its own sake.

With the advent of Michel Foucault's observations about the relationship of authorship to authenticity, and both of these to hegemonic authority, there is a certain parallel with, as well as a significant departure in epistemological attitude from, Schutz's thesis about "anonymity."[20] In effect, Foucault—and, before him, Roland Barthes[21]—had elaborated upon—and sought to dismiss—the kind of statement about an author's role in giving meaning to a drama that Schutz had made in reference to both the music and the scenario of Mozart's operas: "Mozart," Schutz had observed, "does not merely communicate to us the beholders, the objective meaning that the situation has within the context of the plot . . . He shows us, in addition, the different meanings that the same situation has to each of the characters involved in it . . . [I]n Mozart's hands such a typified situation becomes unique and concrete, individual and atypical by the particular meaning it has for each of the participant persons."[22] And, in effect in anticipation of Derrida's comment about the relationship of *mimesis* to *physis,* Schutz concludes, "It could rightly be said that *Mozart's dramatic art is rather a representation of the basic structure of the social world than an imitation of nature.*"[23]

In bringing together the "omniscient" subjectivity of the author with the objectivity of his or her product—that is, the narrative, scenario, screenplay, musical drama, etc.—Schutz had sought to resolve certain problems of intersubjectivity that, unresolved, could have so thickened the proscenium separating author/actor from reader/beholder that understanding would have been inherently and irresolvably problematic. In this regard, Schutz pointed out that for the drama to be understood by those who beheld it, certain preconditions would have to be present: "(a) the interpretability of speech or gesture of the individual actor who, again, is symbol for the hero whom he presents to the audience as well as to an interpreter; (b) the understandability of all relations among all persons who constitute the substance of the drama; (c) the possibility of vicariously experiencing the spatial-temporal development of the acting on the stage; (d) the possibility that all the factors mentioned can be thought of as a means of expression or as symbols of that idea which determines the specific character of a given drama."[24]

However, it is precisely these four preconditions of understanding that have been recently re-rendered problematic, not only by the onset of the postmodern condition, but, even earlier, when Aron Gurwitsch critically appraised aspects of Schutz's seemingly sanguinary ideas about intersubjectivity.[25] In 1944, Gurwitsch had fixed a critical eye on certain aspects of Schutz's formal sociology as these were presented in the latter's seminal essay, "The Stranger: An Essay on Social Psychology."[26] Seizing upon their common experience as refugees and exiles from Nazi persecution, Gurwitsch disputed what appeared to him to be Schutz's uncritical privileging of the stranger's bland and conformist social adjustment to modernity[27]—(e.g., Schutz's statement that "the adaptation of the newcomer to the in-group . . . is a continuous process of inquiry into the cultural pattern of the approached group. If this process of inquiry succeeds, then this pattern and its elements will become to the newcomer a matter of course, an unquestionable way of life, a shelter, and a protection. But then the stranger is no stranger any more, and his [or her] problems have been solved.")[28] Gurwitsch disagreed:

> According to you, the stranger is every person who changes his surrounding world for certain reasons . . . But the situation of the immigrant of the last ten years is different. He had no choice . . . The specific characteristics of this curious being . . . don't allow themselves to be simply formalized, and the crises that this type lives through are incommensurable with those fundamentally harmless problems of adapting which you describe. . . . [W]e find ourselves in new surroundings, and we soon discover that we are on another planet . . . If . . . categories such as "pattern of behavior" are to be universally applicable, the result is a positively dreadful picture of man. In this case man is an *animal psychologicum et sociale,* trainable, a being with certain reactions which one can modify by using certain techniques . . . I will never accept that for man the important thing is a well-oiled operation, that it is all a matter of making a smooth functioning possible via *adjustment.*[29]

Gurwitsch's objections to Schutz's formulation of the "adjustment" problems of the stranger arose, I believe, because he thought he had detected in his friend's analysis a departure from his usual stance—viz, that an element of the naturalistic philosophy that had so recently elevated nihilism and relativism to paramountcy in the psychological and sociological sciences had somehow crept into Schutz's discussion. That turn in social thought, Gurwitsch believed, had shifted the basic conception of every member of humankind from that of being an *animal rationale* to that of existence as a mere vital being.[30] Once perceived as the latter, it followed, so Gurwitsch argued, that "every human action will forever be what it was in its most primitive form: simple reaction, behavior, produced by the functioning of the organism and conditioned by exterior stimulations."[31] Moreover, there followed from such a perspective an even worse consequence—a vulgar pragmatism wherein "the whole value of an idea consists in answering the need for satisfaction; and therein lies the sole reason, necessary as well as sufficient, for preferring one idea to another."[32] Under such an epistemological regime, Gurwitsch went on to point out, "we are in a world where only opinions (*doxai*) exist; . . . [and, on] such a basis there is possible a 'tolerance' which, to be exact, would better be called complete indifference."[33] Opposing this trend, which he regarded as ethically pernicious as well as philosophically unsound—(Gurwitsch argued "that the principles on which totalitarianism rests are the same as those which may be discovered at the base of the psychological naturalism and relativistic philosophy")[34]—Gurwitsch called for the restoration of the "classical conception according to which . . . the combination of the terms *animal* and *rationale* indicates the profound duality of human nature and the highly problematic character of man's existence."[35] Schutz would not disagree with this exhortation.

My point here is neither to reopen nor resolve the particularistic Schutz-Gurwitsch debate over the character of the stranger's social adjustment. It is clear, as Lester Embree has shown,[36] that Schutz's understanding of the actual problematics entailed in getting at either an ordinary person's or a scientist's comprehension of actions, relationships, and situations could not be obtained by positing a conformity, that there "is always [the] great danger of mistaking 'meaning' of one sort for another."[37] Indeed, just as Gurwitsch had rejected the naturalistic image *animal psychologicum et sociale,* so Schutz rejected the sociologist Talcott Parsons's replacement of "subjective events in the mind of the actor . . . [with] a scheme of interpretation for such events, accessible only to the observer," noting that "the only question Professor Parsons never asks is, what really does happen in the mind of the actor from his [or her] subjective point of view."[38] What I intend, rather, by introducing a reference to Schutz's and Gurwitsch's famous debate, is to elaborate on my own argument, namely, that the postmodernists lean toward an uncritical acceptance of what they call the postmodern condition, a condition that both Gurwitsch and Schutz fought so valiantly to oppose. In the event, the very preconditions that Schutz had held are necessary for the beholder to understand a drama are being undermined. Indeed, in the worst-case post-Saussurean scenarios of the postmodern philosophy, they are trapped inside Nietzsche's prison-house of language.[39]

In an earlier study, I proposed a different interpretation of the Schutz-Gurwitsch debate. I pointed out "that both sociology and social reality have shifted [away] from recognizing a general condition of possible and, indeed, probable inter-subjective understanding to one . . . [recognizing] the extreme difficulty, if not the unlikelihood, of the latter."[40] I went on to assert that "concomitant with that shift is the coming into interaction of the condition of perceptual vision unmediated by mutuality,"[41] and that in terms of phenomenological spatialization, the *Umwelt* of Schutz has given way to that which Gurwitsch perceived with such apprehension.[42] As matters have turned out, the postmodernists seem to have come to a similar conclusion, but they express their convictions on the matter in terms related to their critique of the entire legacy of the Age of Reason, of their reduction of its message to a discussion of the incommensurability of "texts" and "intertextuality." At the same time, for such avant-garde dramatists as Richard Schechner, there is in both dramatic texts and everyday life the realization of a theater of the absurd,[43] out from which proscenium, the actors, still in character, have burst, confronting an audience who are also actors in their own irremediably absurd dramas of social reality. Ordinary life and Peter Weiss's play, "Marat\Sade," interpenetrate,[44] and the *animal rationale* trembles.

Coming to Terms with Postmodernism, Schutz, and Gurwitsch

Inverting the Problem: From Resource to Topic

How shall we respond to this latest crisis in the human sciences? To begin with, social scientists ought to adapt a paraphrase of Marx's eleventh thesis on Feuerbach to their work if the sociological disciplines are to persevere. Marx had lamented over the fact that "the philosophers have only *interpreted* the world in various ways; the point, however, is to *change* it."[45] For contemporary social scientists, the matter is different. It calls for a less elegant version of the eleventh Feuerbachian thesis: The philosophers have formulated the logics of the world; the point, however, is to look into the world(s) and see how humans live and interpret their own lives and those of their consociates, contemporaries, predecessors, and successors.[46] For this procedure to come about, the social scientist must stand much of the conceptual and perceptual apparatus of the social sciences on its head—must, that is, convert the resources hitherto employed *for* investigation into the topics *of* investigation.

What this means in the instant case is that the claims about the situation in which we are, perhaps unwillingly, participating, put forward by its postmodern "philosophers" (e.g., Derrida, Jameson, Foucault, Baudrillard, Lyotard, and Lacan), must be regarded not as accurate depictions of what is in fact the case, but, rather, as only probabilistic and hence testable hypotheses about the condition and character of human beliefs, conduct, outlooks, and *Weltanschauungen* of people(s) in the world. These basic aspects of life are performed in and on the several and varied *Umwelten* that constitute the arenas of their actions and interactions. It is to these that the social scientist must repair, having bracketed the postmodern descriptions of them. This is no small point; for altogether too much of twentieth-century modernist social science has proceeded in the exact opposite manner than is being presented here.[47] When, for example, sociologists presume that society exists *sui generis*—namely, that its law of motion is analogous to that of an organism, that its denizens are creatures of the kind of socialization that Parsons described and both Schutz and Gurwitsch deplored, that unusual behaviors and out-of-the-ordinary conduct are signs of "deviance," and that social changes are absorbed by society as outcomes of its inherent "dynamic equilibrium,"[48] that is, slow, orderly, continuous, and teleological processes that regularly reestablish "stability in the midst of change"[49]—they beg the fundamental question for which the discipline was founded: "how is society possible?"[50] Moreover, it is necessary for conventional, especially positivist, sociologists to take seriously the counsel offered to them a quarter century ago by Peter McHugh when he observed:

> Sociology . . . is responsible not just for its substantive discoveries but for having created the very possibility of them, because it has created itself. Sociological truth, as with any other kind, exists only because sociology has generated its own ways of conceding truth. It is not an aggregation of private people sensing individual objects, but a public, rule-guided, and institutionalized canon of social procedure.[51]

The problem, however, exacerbated by the postmodern critique, is that a dispute reigns over *what* rules of procedure ought to prevail in sociology and *whether* any rules are operant in society. It is my contention that dramatism and the dramaturgic method (associated with such names as Kenneth Burke and Erving Goffman, but drawing upon the dramatistic phenomenology of Alfred Schutz) are appropriate here because, unlike the procedures appropriate to positivism, functionalism, and their several variants, these meet a basic requirement of science: They are faithful to the nature of their subject matter.[52] That is, faithful, if and only if the subject matter of sociology is taken to be the person and group capable of "performing."

Dramatism and the Investigation of the Topic

It has become a commonplace of sociological postmodernism to announce the "death of the subject."[53] (For these mourners at the funeral not only of the "subject" but also of social science itself, this death is the sequel to Barthes's announcement of "the death of the author.")[54] Postmodernism's thanatology of the subject, however, is, as I see it, based on an error of interpretation—namely a denial of the modern subject's capacity to be an effective agent in the postmodern world. In fact, as Pauline Rosenau is at pains to show, the postmodern image of the subject corresponds to that of the individual dwelling in the midst of a lonely crowd, and committed to acting in service to the aims and agonies of what used to be called the Protestant ethic. "They understand him/her to be 'puritanical' and overly preoccupied with 'self-authentication.' S/he pursues a 'righteous' life of 'self-denial.'"[55] Although, as Rosenau concedes, some postmodernists seek to raise up a new subject from the ashes of the old one's cremation—namely, "S/he will be a decentered subject, an 'emergent' subject, unrecognizable by the modernists, empiricists, and positivists. S/he will [have] . . . a new nonidentity, focused not on the 'Great Men' of history, but rather, on daily life at the margins. This subject will reject total explanations and the logocentric point of view that implies a unified frame of reference, but s/he need not oppose all dimensions of humanism"[56]—they agree on the dis-appearance of the one that preceded it.

The dramatistic perspective reverses all of this. It begins with asserting the literal truth of Shakespeare's passage in *As You Like It* that "all the world's a stage." It goes on to point out that each culture provides a "treatment" for the "script" of life, the "scenes" and "acts" of which are "written" and/or "performed" by individual or collective social "actors," who also "direct" or are "directed" in their performances, "criticized" by themselves and by their "audiences," and choose or are commanded either to replay their "part" again and again, to perform their "role" only occasionally, or to "close" the drama and begin a new one.[57] The analytical components of dramatism have been developed by Kenneth Burke:

> For there to be an act, there must be an agent. Similarly, there must be a scene in which the agent acts. To act in a scene, the agent must employ some means, or agency. And it can be called an act in the full sense of the term only if it involves a purpose . . . These five terms (act, scene, agent, agency, purpose) have been labelled the dramatistic pentad. [58]

In postmodern thought the agent (i.e., the modern "subject") is deemed incompetent and unworthy to perform; the scene (i.e., the situation) is said to be without a single unambiguous meaning; agency (i.e., the means to carry an action to completion) is declared to be inefficacious; and purposes are alleged to be disconnected from any possibility of accomplishment.[59] Thus, as Baudrillard proclaims, the social has come to an end, and social science (i.e., a science of the social) is said to be impossible.[60] Or, as Keith Tester has concluded on the basis of his investigation into what he calls *The Life and Times of Post-Modernity:* "In . . . more concrete hermeneutic terms, this means that post-modernity can be taken as the intimation of a transcendence of all the modern establishments of universality."[61]

What a sociological dramatism offers to these pessimistic theses is an epistemological turnabout. In effect, I argue that in their descriptions of the postmodern condition, these advocates have mistaken the topic to be investigated for the theorem used to investigate it. A special instance of this error is to be found in their assumption that the "subject" is dead. The error is a double one. First, postmodernists have assumed that a "subject" who lacks perfect control over his/her actions, or who has less than perfect knowledge of his/her condition, or who is a victim of prejudice, discrimination, oppression, or some other form of victimization, is diminished in, or "decentered" from, full "subjecthood." But modernist social scientists had never attributed such "perfections" of socialization to those who constituted the "subjects" of their investigations. To give three examples that could be multiplied by many more: Robert E. Park, building on Georg Simmel's concept of the "stranger"[62] (as had Schutz in his essay of the same title),[63] developed a conceptualization of the "marginal man"[64] that in turn was elaborated upon by Everett Stonequist[65] and, since, has sparked a considerable number of researches on the social psychology, sociology, and political aspects of the lives of those who are products of two cultures but members of neither.[66] And, Aron Gurwitsch has introduced the term *marginal consciousness* to designate the third domain of the field of consciousness, the one that "includes data which, though co-present with, have no relevancy to the theme"; the theme is "that which engrosses the mind of the experiencing subject, or . . . which stands in the 'focus of his [or her] attention.'"[67] Herbert Blumer, building on the pragmatic philosophy of George Herbert Mead, established the perspective known as symbolic interactionism that holds, among other things, that "human group life is necessarily a formative process and not a mere arena for the expression of pre-existing factors."[68] Symbolic interactionism rests its claims on the fact that the "human individual . . . has to cope with the situations in which he [or she] is called on to act, . . . construct and guide his [or her] action . . . , [but, Blumer is careful to point out that he or she] may do a miserable job in constructing . . . [that line of] action."[69] Finally, Kenneth E. Bock, whose most recent work catalogs the many debilitating effects that the concept "human nature" has had on both historical and social scientific studies, seeks nothing less than a restoration of human agency to the center of humanistic investigations.[70] "The attempt of modern students of society to apply methods of natural science in their work has done much to sustain and elaborate the Western belief in human impotence —in this case a belief that people are incapable of deliberately and rationally shaping their social and cultural life."[71] While rejecting the antihumanistic claim that people "are pawns caught in a game where the moves are controlled by impersonal forces,"[72] Bock calls for an "open image of humanity"[73] that recognizes simultaneously, the theses put forward by Pico della Mirandola[74] and Samuel Butler. Bock paraphrases the medieval philosopher, proposing that "humans . . . should regard themselves as capable of anything,"[75] and he goes on to assert that "even in small matters of daily conduct we can be so puzzled and embarrassed about what we should do that we see the point of Samuel Butler's quip about life being 'like playing a violin solo in public and learning the instrument as one goes on.'"[76] In sum, then, the first error made by the postmodernists with respect to the "subject" is that they have transmuted a normative judgment about the character and condition of the subject into an epistemological claim and then made that claim the resource *for* their investigations rather than the topic *of* them.

A second error of the postmodernists follows from the first. It consists in begging the very question of research. Having denied the possibility of a subject, that is, an agent capable of engaging in purposeful action in the accomplishment of a task—in, effect, "deconstructing" and, hence, discarding not only positivism and functionalism,[77] the leading paradigms of sociology during the past half century, but also the Burkean pentad, they make social science virtually impossible. However, although Richard Rorty's holding of the mirror of science up to nature[78] revealed that there was no reflection (and, thus, he was able to refute positivism's claim to provide either a "copy" or an "image"[79] of society), and Lyotard's and Foucault's investigations of the circle of signifiers in language rendered representation impossible[80] (in effect, reducing functionalism's metaphor of society-as-organism at the very least, to a problematic status) there still remains, as Rorty noticed, the possibility, indeed, the necessity of narratives, as he put it, of having a philosophy without mirrors, of continuing the conversation.[81]

Rorty did not tell us the form that these narratives should take. But, drawing on Schutz's commentaries, and on the works of such scholars as Burke,[82] Goffman,[83] Berger,[84] Harré,[85] Schechner,[86] Turner,[87] Evreinov,[88] and Lyman and Scott,[89] the case can be made that dramatism holds out much promise and resolves many questions. Specifically, and in contrast to the postmodernists' *a priori* presumption about the "subject," a dramatistic perspective requires that the investigator look into the social world(s) as it/they actually exist, regarding what happens as dramas of social reality and seeking to discover, *inter alia,* whether the postmodern condition is in fact a feature of people's lives.[90] The "subjects" of these investigations are the ordinary as well as the extraordinary actors in the scenes of everyday life. It is to be discovered, not assumed in advance, whether and to what extent they possess and present whole and integrated, or segmented and discordant selves (i.e., "roles" and "parts") in their interactions; whether individual and collective behavior is or is not guided by a uniform set of rules, (i.e., a "scenario"); how individuals "write," "re-write," and "perform" in the "scripts" (i.e., the "text")[91] of life that conform or deviate from the "pre-text";[92] how and to what extent and with what effect individuals and collectivities are able to "direct" and serve as "critics" and "audiences" for their own life-dramas and to partake of those "scripted," "cast," and "directed" by others.[93] Schutz tells us that "the technical task characteristic of the drama . . . [is] to present to the spectator, immediately and without interpretation, relations between humans through their acting and speaking within a specific spatial-temporal frame."[94] Dramatism evokes in the social scientist the recognition that s/he is a spectator/actor in whatever drama of life has been chosen for study, and that the actors in the scene(s)—including him/herself, if the study is to meet the reflexive requirements of *theoria*[95]—are presenting immediately and with whatever common-sense interpretations they bring to bear on their own as well as any other's conduct, the relations that prevail amongst them, and that the scientist's task is to apprehend these and re-present them in terms of what Schutz once referred to in reference to the sociological task of symbological hermeneutics as "dual interpretability."[96]

In light of the claims of postmodernism, one should take care to notice Schutz's admonition that "it can no longer be taken for granted that 'positing the symbol' occurs in the same life form in which 'symbol interpretation' occurs."[97] Moreover, what a sociological dramatism, chastened but not deterred from its task by the postmodern critique of epistemology, can do is translate Schutz's thesis—namely, the positing of humans as inhabitants of a spatiotemporal, that is, dramatistically analyzable, *Lebenswelt*—(one that includes not only those physically co-present, but also the contemporaries, predecessors, and successors relevant to the scene(s))—in which the "objects . . . are homogeneous, independent of me, endowed with specific qualities and self-sufficient"[98]—into a testable hypothesis.

Especially valuable for such an investigation will be "The Social Stratification of Language," Schutz's Lecture XVI, delivered on January 12, 1953, in his as yet unpublished series entitled *Problems of a Sociology of Language*.[99] There, Schutz tells us that "language is not only a linguistic phenomenon," and that the "speaker-and-listener situation is a paradigmatic sociological phenomenon."[100] And, I would add, this is especially the case for a dramatistic sociology that conceives of the world in the absurdist tradition developed by Lyman and Scott, that is, the perspective that holds that the world makes no ontological sense, but whose *Lebenswelten* and *Umwelten* are always (or, almost always) meaningful to their denizens.[101] And, Schutz reminds us, the social scientific investigator will have to pay attention to such phonocentric/logocentric/gestural matters of "text" (to borrow from Ricoeur's and Schechner's dramatistic lexicon) as "slang," "taboo words," "loan words," and the vocabularies of subjugated peoples and ethnoracial minorities.[102]

In relation to those who have been victimized and stigmatized one type of dramatistic sociology is demanded by those postmodernists who seek to elevate to "subjecthood" such subjugated peoples as African Americans, Asian Americans, Hispanic Americans, Native Americans, women, homoerotic sexual preference groups and individuals, and the physically challenged.[103] Postmodernists seek to privilege the texts of these victims over those of their victimizers. However, Schutz pointed out, in effect, giving particularistic guidelines to those who choose to investigate the dramas of life enacted by the marginalized, "there is some indication that nation, race, and culture have different meanings for in-group members and for out-group observers . . . . . . The inner speech form includes orientation in space and experience of time . . . The linguistic group is a sociological phenomenon."[104] Schutz's approach has many advantages, not the least of which is the fact that widespread dissemination of the findings of a dramatistic sociology of subjugated and oppressed peoples would do much to move the latter out of their aforementioned perceptual place at the margins of what Gurwitsch called the majority groups' field of consciousness, providing in the event, the accomplishment of a postmodern imperative.

Toward a New Dramatistic Sociology

Schutz's commentaries on the sociological aspects of literature give added weight to a burgeoning dramatistic epistemology. Although dramatism is traceable to Aristotle, and, later, to its reinforcement in the kinds of social analyses carried out from the sixteenth through the eighteenth centuries, it was set aside in the name of various schools of materialist science in the nineteenth and early twentieth centuries and did not reemerge until Kenneth Burke revived it and systematized its orientation and method.[105] With the antifoundational critique of the postmodernists posing yet another and more serious crisis for the much-embattled social sciences,[106] it is a matter of great significance to investigate how and whether it, or any form of social science, can survive. Schutz's dramatistic sociology, even when it posits certain features of the *Lebenswelten* and *Umwelten* that Gurwitsch regards as questionable, offers guidance in such an investigation—one that would topicalize the claims of postmodernists and establish the epistemological space wherein such an investigation could take place. Moreover, one such project of this kind could focus directly on those who dwell at the edges of any hegemonic group's field of consciousness and whose scenarios of life are not only spatiotemporally limited provinces of finite meaning,[107] but also socially, culturally, economically, and/or politically marginalized.[108] In other words, a dramatistic sociology that drew on Schutz's and Gurwitsch's approaches, as well as those of the classical and contemporary dramaturgical thinkers, could look directly into the truth claims[109] put forward *a priori* by the subject/subjugated-oriented postmodernists. Moreover, such a perspective could bring the "Other" more clearly within purview of the perceptual field of academic and, perhaps, social consciousness.[110] As Michael D. Barber tells us, "Schutz's work, by placing at the foundation of the sociology of knowledge the never-to-be-intellectually mastered otherness of the Other, challenges the sociologist's self-centered interpretations and invites him to acknowledge his [or her] discipline's own horizons and begin anew the infinite task of understanding the Other."[111]

Schutz has given us the challenge; now let us begin the response.

CHAPTER SEVEN

Cinematic Ideologies and Societal Dystopias

Filmmaking in the United States, Japan, Germany and the Soviet Union, 1900–1996

> The drama and novel live by words. How much of this noblest vehicle of thought can the photoplay conserve in its domain?
>
> —HUGO MÜNSTERBERG, *The Photoplay*

> In Italy, for thirty years under the Borgias they had warfare, terror, murder and bloodshed, but they produced Michelangelo, Leonardo da Vinci and the Renaissance. In Switzerland, they had brotherly love, they had five hundred years of democracy and peace—and what did they produce? The cuckoo clock.
>
> —HARRY LIME (Orson Welles), *The Third Man*

> History goes round and round, and eventually gets somewhere. Like a corkscrew.
>
> —PAUL BERMAN, *A Tale of Two Utopias*

Introduction

A social scientific as well as sociopolitical approach to cinema and other media studies has been in the making for several decades. Hugo Münsterberg's *The Photoplay,* published in 1916, not only provided an early form of a *geisteswissenschaftliche Psychologie,* but also called for a nationalization of this art form in behalf of ensuring the cultural edification and moral uplift of the masses.[1] More than two decades later, worry over the allegedly evil influences that movies might be having on America's young people led to the largely censorious Payne Fund Studies.[2] Of these, the more libertarian analyses—

unrecognized at the time and still neglected landmarks in the development of the disciplines of sociology and social psychology—were those of Herbert Blumer[3] and Philip M. Hauser,[4] the former of whom would later assert that popular films provide "a reaffirmation of basic human values but an undermining of the mores."[5] In 1946, the Weber scholar, J. P. Mayer, authored a sociology of film that asserted that "the emotional, non-rational impact of films, particularly of feature films, shaped in the widest sense 'political' opinions."[6] An anthropologist, Ian Charles Jarvie, has gone further, producing studies that focus on the multifaceted relationship of films to society,[7] the variety of roles that movies play in social criticism,[8] and the presentation of a distinctive philosophy of film.[9] Although intellectuals have for at least two centuries bemoaned the supposedly harmful effects of popular culture on the masses,[10] at present, the entire curriculum of moving picture and related cultural studies is being challenged for its alleged Eurocentric and patriarchal biases by the new (anti-) paradigm, critical postmodernism.[11] However, it is worth noting that, sparked by the pragmatic perspective, the nature, role, and effects of ideologies, including those of the Occident, had become a part of media studies and criticism soon after the Second World War had ended and the Cold War had begun.[12]

Studies of national cinema are only now emerging in relation to the struggles over art, craftsmanship, ideology, and ethnic, gender, and class perspectives. In the United States, where this trend flourishes, there have appeared, to name but a few of many: Kevin Brownlow's comprehensive reconsideration of the silent era's social conscience films and their attitude toward sex, violence, prejudice, and crime;[13] Tom Conley's insightful examination of the subtle manner in which screenplay writing melds history and modifies ideology;[14] Lee Lourdeaux's discerning filmographies of four Irish and Italian cinematographers in America;[15] J. Hoberman's path-breaking *Bridge of Light: Yiddish Film between Two Worlds;*[16] several revisionist analyses of the role of Jewish filmmakers and studio heads,[17] as well as the shifting imagery of the Jew in American plays and films;[18] reexamination of the role that racism has played in the cinematic depictions of African American[19] and Afro-British[20] men and women; revision and republication of Parker Tyler's[21] and Vito Russo's[22] studies of how homosexuality has been treated by Hollywood; the many film studies examining women's roles and introducing a cathectic-centered feminist perspective on moviedom;[23] remarkably innovative readings of the meanings entailed in such novel-to-screenplay Hollywood (and, later, British) genres as monster and vampire films;[24] and J. P. Telotte's reexamination of the experimental narrative pattern in *noir* films of the 1940s and 1950s,[25] as well as his studies of Val Lewton's fantasy films[26] and the techno-value tensions in seven decades of science fiction movies.[27]

Nor have film studies avoided analyzing the political and economic culture in which Hollywood's cinematography developed. Lary May has explored how Hollywood films resonated with the shift in the United States from Victorian ascetic constraints to urban consumer orientations.[28] In 1971 Eric Bentley documented thirty years of a congressional committee's quest to uncover "un-American" activities in the mass media, a quest that resulted not only in "permanent exclusion from one's chosen field of employment, social ostracism, divorce, and voluntary exile . . . , [but also] premature deaths from 'natural' causes and from suicide."[29] In February 1978, longtime film critic Andrew Sarris concluded the title essay of his film commentaries on the relationship of politics to American cinema with a denunciation of McCarthyism, the House Un-American Activities Committee, witch hunts, sectarian self-righteousness, and the movie moguls who caved in before the censorious superpatriots. However, he then took a different tack, observing, "When I look at *Watch on the Rhine* and *The North Star,* in which good leftists solemnly teach themselves the historical necessity of killing fascists and even obstacle-creating opportunists in cold blood, I conclude that the left has little to teach us about liberty or justice."[30] In contrast to Sarris's view, Terry Christensen has argued, on the basis of his survey of more than two hundred American films—including the anti-fascist *Watch on the Rhine* (1942), which he praised for its "quality and subtlety,"[31] and the Russophilic *The North Star* (1943), that *Time* magazine had hailed as a "cinemilestone . . . , but [that] the Hearst press [had] dismissed . . . as communist propaganda"[32]—that the basic political message of Hollywood's cinema is "that politics is corrupt."[33] In effect, Christensen's outlook discounts any ethical reason for movie heroes to participate in America's politics unless, as Norman K. Denzin sees it, the hero is a lone outsider determined to overcome or bypass the particular instance of corruption that is revealed in the screenplay.

Denzin,[34] a postmodern sociologist-cum-cineast, has given a new reading to the sociopolitical issue, presenting no less than six factors that support his basic thesis—namely, that the narrative structure of Hollywood's political films focuses on the rebellious reformer as outsider and tends to emphasize private woes rather than public issues as the basis for political action. (While the German social scientist Max Weber distinguished between the ethical responsibilities of science and the less-than-honorable power struggles that are inherent in politics,[35] it was the American sociologist C. Wright Mills who advised future social scientists "that many personal troubles cannot be solved merely as troubles, but must be understood in terms of public issues,"[36] that is, that Hollywood's version of the hero was that of a true political activist.) Denzin's thesis proceeds stochastically: (1) In America there is no longer a grand metanarrative that could move a collectivity to action; in its place there is the mythologized individual (misfit, outcast, stranger, or other type of marginalized person) who stands and fights alone.[37] Nevertheless, (2) "the revolutionary political rebel is a dying species in the postmodern, bureaucratic and multinational corporate world"[38] because (3) the populace has "been lulled into complacency by [an] official history that the power elite has written."[39] However, (4) Hollywood's screenplays, "by placing the protagonist outside the social, outside the passive collectivity, . . . sustain the fiction of a division between the public and private, perpetuating the myth that they are incommensurable and mutually antagonistic."[40] Moreover, by presenting (5) issues of public policy, national security, and law enforcement—in a "dizzying display of electronic, panoptic wizardry"—Hollywood films depict democracy as little more than a "carnival . . . without a director."[41] Ultimately, because of his irremediably faulty "gaze,"[42] (6) the socially as well as self-isolated hero, along with the spectator in the theater audience, is forced to admit that there is "a fatal flaw in [the] epistemological framework that says certain truths can always be discovered if one is objective and has the right tools of observation."[43] (This last point is illustrated in *D.O.A.* [1949] in which the hero—an accountant—plunges into a limbo land of criminalized absurdity in order to find out who has fatally poisoned him and why.[44] But it is belied in the more recent *Lone Star* [1996] in which the hero—a sheriff—conducts a veritable sociological investigation to uncover the facts behind a twenty-year-old murder and in the process discovers that, unknowingly, he has been long involved in an incestuous affair.)

Denzin's pessimistic outlook is all the more pertinent when compared, on the one hand, with Ralph Willett's earlier and more conventional critique of cinematic politics—especially the politics of race—(". . . in the insecure social climate of the postwar period, audiences were prepared to accept liberal films . . . only if they provided the reassuring confidence which was difficult to find either in business or in domesticity")[45] and, on the other, with recent postmodernist Inez Hedges's sanguinary conclusion on the political-cinematic possibilities for gendered minorities—(". . . women, . . . race, class, and culture . . . will be the major issues of the 90s . . . [D]isruptive language, dual narration that lets the spectator in on the thoughts of the characters, the marking of the arranger as nonwhite and non-male, performative space . . . are partial solutions to the need for films to operate outside of conventional norms . . . And, since our [film] language reflects our reality its transformation can help to transform our world as well.").[46] In the sociopolitics of cinema, it would seem, Akira Kurosawa's 1950 masterpiece, *Rashomon*—with its multiplicity of mutually contradictory retrospectives on the same event[47]—has proved to be prescient.

Cinema Across Time and Space

The recent critical appraisal of European, Asian, African, and Middle Eastern movies has enlarged the opportunities for comparative film analysis, but most studies are still confined to a single nation's movies.[48] Cross-national comparisons have not yet found a neutral standard on the basis of which to make valid comparisons, leaving the several state-centered, ethnonational studies to be suggestive of possible developments. Genre approaches, for example—well developed among cinema scholars in the United States[49]—bid fair to overleap national boundaries and become multinational and multiethnic in scope. Within the United States, genre analysis has proliferated a classification of film types—not only distinguishing among comedies,[50] musicals,[51] westerns,[52] crime,[53] and *noir*[54] movies, but also generating studies of African American,[55] Asian American,[56] Hispanic,[57] Native American,[58] women's,[59] and gender-[60] or age-specific[61] films. Still other classificatory schemas in use in the United States organize their critiques around eras of filmmaking,[62] or such genres as the once-fearful, later-comic gothic and horror movies,[63] the proto-pastoral, vintage-American small-town story,[64] cinematic celebrations of American wars,[65] especially World War II;[66] and, once a film star had become president of the United States, various analyses of whether and how his former career had affected the manner and politics of his leadership and his public policies,[67] and, reversing the theme, looking into how his presidency had affected the making of movies.[68]

Historians of Hollywood's films have tended less to compare American movies with those made in other countries than to treat the domestic film industry as one whose products depict the somewhat disorderly but nevertheless progressive evolution of a nation of immigrants, steeped in innocence and ethnocultural division,[69] through eras each reflecting a particular paramount sociocultural value—"the working-class antipretentiousness of the Nickelodeon Era, the middle-class materialism of the Silent Feature Era, the positivism and populism of the post-Depression Studio Era, the apparent retreat from political problems of the postwar Transitional Era, the rebellious, anti-Establishment pessimism of the Hollywood Renaissance"[70]—until the 1990s, when the arrival of the postmodernist movement seemed to threaten the very idea of such a trajectory at both base and superstructure.[71]

The sudden end of the Cold War, bringing to an end Hollywood's versions of the paranoid style in American politics,[72] for example, movies depicting juvenile delinquents, mad scientists, horrible beasts, or aliens from outer space as surrogate or crypto-communists,[73] not to mention its "realistic" stories about the "red menace" to America,[74] has unstrung the ideologically dependent movie makers[75]—no doubt only temporarily. One postmodern thinker, unacknowledgedly reminiscent of Hollywood's function as a "dream factory,"[76] envisions all of the United States in terms of moviedom's "field of dreams"—the title of a motion picture (1989) in which the spirits of dead baseball players materialize and convince a down-on-his-luck Iowa farmer to turn his depleted agricultural land into a baseball diamond, promising that "they (i.e., the public, the fans) will come" and, presumably, that those who do come will pay to see this innovative take on the privatization of farm subsidy—a situation, this critic believes, that forces each American into anguishing over what is, in fact, a Hobson's choice: ". . . one who sees will be torn between the two sides of vision—between a herd call toward tyrannical normalcy and a minority-based, sagacious truth from beyond."[77] An even bleaker future for America and its newly enhanced techno-filmic representations is presented by two scholars aiming with their acerbic critique to undermine what they regard as the pretensions of modernity.[78] With a neo-Veblenian irony, expressed through a cybertech vocabulary coupled with a religious fervor, Arthur Kroker and Michael A. Weinstein envision

> A virtual millennium of pure tech, Year 2000 is driven by the cold seduction of digital dreams. Really a return in hyper-garb of the age of Christianity . . . , St. John the Baptist is on the Net, and this time he is wearing a Nintendo power glove and cyberware scanning eyes for announcing the coming of the newest California hyper-Messiah of the day. Pure Tech churns personal histories into cyber-dust, twisting and turning the always failed search for a stable personal identity on which to hang one's hopes . . . A recycled culture for the Remake century glitters before us like a neon mirage on the shimmering desert landscape. A virtual sign without virtue for a millennium that opens on the screens of cyber-culture as the triumph of artificial intelligence, but without the intelligence of artifice.[79]

Where once Hollywood produced a plethora of social problem movies calling attention to unresolved issues in such domestic matters as crime, delinquency, poverty, marriage, the family, moral failure, penology, mental illness, political corruption, and the dangers from home-grown or foreign fascism,[80] the perspective of at least one postmodern sociologist, Angela McRobbie, deprecates all such films as products of a politically contrived "moral panic" designed, usually, to serve conservative interests and punitive ends.[81] According to Norman K. Denzin, "Traditional, realist, narrative cinema, like traditional ethnographic sociology, tells only one version of the story, a version which has a zero degree of textual politics."[82] In refusing to "perpetuate the illusions that stories have happy endings, that heroes always prevail, that the private is sacred, and that in the end man and woman will be joined in peaceful bliss,"[83] movies, such postmodernist cineasts as Denzin argue, are attempting to raise the political temperature.

Passion, Politics, Racism, Zionism: Films in South Africa and Israel

However, the fires of political, social, and moral controversy arising over popular, racially tolerant films made in South Africa under *apartheid,* or movies sympathetic to "Oriental Jews" and to Palestinians in Israel, needed no added intensification from the postmodern torch. Beset by state censorship, limited state subsidies, government crackdowns, not to mention difficulties in international marketing and overseas distribution, South Africa's apartheid-era movie makers tended to produce Afrikaans films, designed to please white audiences and emphasizing "the cultural traumas resulting from urbanization," endorsing "back to the homelands" pictures, made for blacks, and reinforcing the ideology of "grand apartheid," that is, the total and irrevocable separation of the races.[84] During the era that ended with the inauguration of Nelson Mandela as president, in both feature and documentary films, the South African "government and its para-statal bodies [were] constantly looking for ways to promote intergroup relations in terms of apartheid social relations."[85]

"Israeli cinema," observes Ella Shohat, "has been relentlessly 'Eurotropic' in the main, spurning any authentic dialogue with the East."[86] In such interracial Romeo-and-Juliet screenplays as *A Very Narrow Bridge* (1985), to take a prominent example, Laila, the "Juliet" of the plot, does not die; instead, she "is forced to cross the Allenby Bridge to Jordan, but promises to return, leaving the future dialogue, here allegorical of the larger Israeli/Palestinian dialogue, under a question mark."[87] Shohat calls for a cinematic response to that larger question in what she calls "polyphony." "True cinematic polyphony will emerge, most probably," she concludes, "only with the advent of political equality and cultural reciprocity among the three major groups within Israel—European Jews, Oriental Jews, and Palestinian Arabs."[88] At this writing, the possibility of such a polyphony has receded in the face of the yet-unresolved Palestinian issue and the continuing Arab-Israeli conflict.

Films under Fascism: Japanese and German Cinema

Perhaps no arena of film studies has documented the effects of state control and ideological conformity more than that concerned with cinematic productions made during the time of Japan's military dictatorship and before, during, and after Germany's Nazi era.

JAPAN

In the late 1930s, with the military regime's expansion of control over nearly all aspects of Japanese society, that nation's already well-established film industry could not escape from complying with what began as "requests" and soon became censorious controls and propagandistically directed edicts.[89] In April 1939, patterned after the Nazi *Spitzenorganisation der Filmwirtschaft,*[90] the Japanese government set up film controls and began issuing edicts, of which that of 1940 established a leitmotif that, with ever-more strictness, would be enforced throughout the war years:

> National movies of healthy entertainment value . . . showing persons ready to serve are hoped for. Comedians and vaudeville satirists will be restricted if they overdo this comedy. Slice-of-life films, films describing individual happiness, films treating the lives of the rich, scenes of women smoking, drinking in cafes, etc., the use of foreign words, and films dealing with sexual frivolity are all prohibited. Films showing industrial and food production, particularly the life in farming villages, should be presented.[91]

Despite the rigid surveillance of the newly created Censorship Office of the Home Ministry,[92] and the directives by the Cabinet's Office of Public Information, however, a few Japanese filmmakers did find ways to circumvent the government's censors. "As pressure upon directors became stronger," Donald Richie observes, "some made a strategic retreat into history, where they would be allowed a bit more freedom . . . Other directors pursued their own interests . . . , insofar as they were allowed to."[93] Still others utilized the government's edicts to criticize war-induced frauds and profiteering. Thus, in the midst of the Second World War, *Hana Saku Minato* (*The Blossoming Port,* 1943), the first film made by Keisuke Kinoshita—whose distinguished postwar career would become the subject of a fruitful debate over whether his later films are excessively sentimental[94]—relates a tale of two confidence men who deceive a small coastal town's citizens into backing a fraudulent shipbuilding firm;[95] while Kimisaburo Yoshimura's ambiguous *Nishizumi Senshacho-den* (*The Story of Tank Commander Nishizumi,* 1940) inserts into its war and conquest theme the eponymous officer who not only overcomes hierarchical codes of conduct and fraternizes with conscripts and enlisted noncoms, but also befriends noncombatant members of the enemy, aiding a Chinese woman in distress.[96] Nevertheless, in the film's tragic *denouement,* the humanitarian officer is shot in the back by a dying Chinese soldier.[97] Such humanistic or sociologically critical films were in the minority, of course,[98] but they illustrate how ethically motivated movie makers could find ways to evade the censors and avoid harsh persecution.

Government censorship of films did not end with Japan's defeat in 1945. In one of its most flagrant instances after the American Occupation had begun, General Charles Willoughby, head of Supreme Commander Douglas MacArthur's Intelligence Section, banned socialist movie maker Kamei Fumio's *The Japanese Tragedy* (1946) after Prime Minister Yoshida Shigeru had complained to him about the movie's critical attitude toward Emperor Hirohito's wartime role.[99] Having agreed to keep the emperor on the throne, the occupation authorities felt obliged to cover up any blame he might otherwise have incurred for starting and encouraging Japan's undertaking of an imperialist and cruel war. "As long as the emperor lived," observes Ian Buruma, "Japanese would have trouble being honest about the past."[100]

In 1949, General MacArthur saw to it that *Eirin* (the Motion Pictures Code of Ethics Committee, composed of six representatives from Japan's six major film studios) was empowered to regulate movies.[101] During the years immediately following the surrender, Japanese film directors either grudgingly acquiesced to the new regulations or acknowledged that a new set of values was emerging. Thus, they sometimes made films that described a dismal present but looked hopefully toward a happier future (e.g., Akira Kurosawa's *Subarashiki Nichiyobi* [*One Wonderful Sunday*], 1947),[102] or treated Japan's defeat as a liberation from unprogressive feudal values (e.g., Yasujiro Ozu's uncharacteristically harsh *Kaze no nake no mendori* [*A Hen in the Wind*], 1948).[103] A few years later, Japanese filmmakers began to produce movies that were critical of society (e.g., Keisuke Kinoshita's *Karumen Junjosu* [*Carmen's Pure Love*], 1952), or to honor democratic and antiracist attitudes (e.g., Tadashi Imai's *Kiku to Isamu* [*Kiku and Isamu*], 1959), the latter type of cinematographers seeking, so one unforgiving critic claims, to absolve themselves, allegorically, for the propagandistic motion pictures they had made during the war.[104]

Japan's film industry revived, however, and for nearly three decades thrived, often with historical or allegorical *chambara,* that is, sword-fighting samurai screenplays[105] made by the tripartite oligopoly of studios—Shochiku, Toho, and Toei—until the late 1980s, when they virtually ceased to make anywhere near the number of films they had produced in the recent past.[106] A new generation of independent filmmakers started employing allegorical stories of sex as a cinematic way to criticize Japanese society. *Eirin*'s censorship had been occasional and sporadic, but, after the Occupation had ended and the new wave developed, it began to operate in cooperation with the police and public prosecutors. Seeking to suppress independently made *roman poruno* (i.e., literature-based pornographic) films, *Eirin* eventually censored Nagisa Oshima's *Ai no Corrida* (*In the Realm of the Senses,* 1976), bringing about his trial and subsequent critical book-length response.[107] At this writing, it is clear that the feminist variant of the postmodern critique, with its emphasis on the subjugation of women, has reached Japanese film commentary. Thus, while Oshima valiantly fights for his and fellow cineasts' right to film their unique artistic visions free of censorship,[108] Sandra A. Wawrytko argues,

> Modern Japanese cinema may be said to hold up a mirror that reflects an intermingling of elements from Japanese society, past and present, . . . these celluloid images should not be hastily mistaken for a true reflection of reality —either traditional or modern . . . As the artistic products of male directors, the films display varying degrees of sensitivity to the plight of Japanese women as victims of vastly inequitable gender roles . . . However, . . . their works represent attempts by men to portray and interpret what, for them, is an essentially alien experience—living as a woman in Japanese society.[109]

Ironically, given her interest in having Japan's films present a true reflection of Japanese societal reality, Wawrytko proposes that the mirror through which such a reflection will be presented should be "that provided by the primal Shinto role models of women and sexuality that preceded Confucian and Buddhist trepidations."[110] For such a role model she nominates the mythical Ame no Uzume, who successfully tempted the Sun Goddess Amaterasu—who will become the matriarchal ancestress of Japan's unbroken imperial line—from her isolation in a cave by performing "an erotically suggestive dance"[111] and, later overcame Saruto-hiko's blocking of the descent onto the earth of Amaterasu's grandson, Ama-tsu-hiko-ho Ninigi no Mikoto, destined to become Japan's first emperor, by exposing "her sexual organs to him." "These actions," Wawrytko believes, "demonstrate the perception that female sexuality was a form of power that was neither suppressed nor rebuked, but valued."[112]

In Oshima's hardcore, sensually violent Franco-Japanese film, *Ai no Corrida* (*In the Realm of the Senses*)—on the other hand, culminating a filmmaking career that had been characterized by a series of movies emphasizing true but perhaps unattainable freedom as a cruelly expressed liberation from every form of societal constraint (e.g., *Ai to Kibo no Machi* [*A Town of Love and Hope*, 1959]; *Seishun Zankoku Monogatari* [*Cruel Story of Youth*, 1960]; *Nihon no Yoru to Kiri* [*Night and Fog in Japan*, 1960]; *Shiiku* [*The Catch*, 1961]; *Hakuchu no Torima* [*Violence at Noon*, 1966])[113]—a sensually besotted man (Tatsuya Fuji) is willing to gratify a woman's (Eiko Matsuda) sexual desire by allowing her to strangle him to death at the height of their ecstatic love-making. After killing him, the woman cuts off his penis.[114] In light of Wawrytko's gender-specific postmodern critique, then, a new question arises in relation to Oshima's and other Japanese male cinematographers' venture into pornographic variations on the *nimaime* genre (e.g., Oshima's *Ai No Borei* [*Empire of Passion*, 1978] in which a woman and her lover are haunted by the ghost of her murdered husband until an appropriate retribution for the crime is obtained):[115] Is the modern version of Ame no Uzume to be seen as appropriately represented by Sadao Abe, the sexually aggressive murderess in *Ai No Corrida?* If so, will it be possible to build the kind of community, one based on sexual freedom, that Oshima's films sought as a replacement for Japan's feudal, militaristic, and sexually repressive society?[116]

Germany

Since 1945, analyses of German films have been Janus-headed, that is, seeking foreshadowings of Nazism in Weimar's cinema, or unreconstructed visions (or revivals) of Hitler's "contributions" in the postwar films. During the early years of the Weimar era the German film industry aroused admiration for its surrealistic artistry and superb craftsmanship, but, later, these films received criticism and denunciation either for the fascistic and antisemitic uses to which that art and skill were put, or for their adumbrations of Nazism. Indeed, although the matter has been disputed by critics in cinema studies,[117] Siegfried Kracauer's claims about the symbological content of one of that era's most famous feature films, Robert Wiener's *Das Cabinett des Dr. Caligari* (*The Cabinet of Dr. Caligari,* 1919)—

> The dreamlike reasoning [of the film] penetrates Dr. Caligari to the core by conceiving of him as a counterpart of [tyrannical Roman emperor] Valentinian and a premonition of Hitler. Caligari is a very specific premonition in the sense that he uses hypnotic power to force his will upon his tool—a technique foreshadowing, in content and purpose, that manipulation of the soul which Hitler was the first to practice on a gigantic scale.[118]—

are not without historical as well as sociological value.[119]

Kracauer's dichotomous division of Weimar's film genres is fruitful, perceiving Germany's films of that era as, from 1918 through 1924, expressionistic and phantasmagorical, and, then, from 1924 through 1929, following the settling of the inflation and monetary questions,[120] as "realistic."[121] The onset of the latter genre was also almost coincidental with the takeover of Germany's major film studio, UFA, by Alfred Hugenberg, a political reactionary[122] and media magnate who in 1928 called for a "consolidation of the right" in order to bring to an end what he called the "trash" of parliamentary democracy[123] and who, on February 2, 1933, would appear in the reserved balcony of the Ufa-Palast am Zoo with Hitler and Franz von Papen at the premiere of UFA's gift to the new *Führer* and Third Reich Chancellor, *Dawn,* a film steeped in Nazi ideology and dedicated to the memory of the six thousand sailors drowned and one hundred German U-boats sunk during World War I.[124]

Kracauer believes that "*Caligari* exposes the soul wavering between tyranny and chaos, and facing a desperate situation: any escape from tyranny seems to throw it into a state of utter confusion."[125] It is a thesis perhaps unintentionally reaffirmed cinematically in F. W. Murnau's (1888–1931) thanatological fantasy of vampiric love and female sacrifice, *Nosferatu* (1921–22) with Max Schreck's (1879–1936) unforgettably menacing portrayal of "Count Orlock," the blood-and-sex-seeking villain, suggesting an antisemitic subtext;[126] and with Fritz Lang's (1890–1976) *Dr. Mabuse der Spieler* (*Dr. Mabuse the Gambler,* 1922), and the Nazi-banned sequel, *Das Testament des Dr. Mabuse* (*The Last Will of Dr. Mabuse,* 1932–33), the first depicting "the world in which we all live . . . , hovering between crisis and convalescence, leading somnambulistically just over the brink, in the search for a bridge that will lead [us] over the abyss";[127] the second, putting into the mouth of the insane megalomaniacal criminal, Dr. Mabuse, the very words that characterized Nazi ideology.[128] Rudolf Klein-Rogge (1888–1955), who portrayed Dr. Mabuse in both films, captured the sociocultural malaise under which the arch-criminal thrived: He, Dr. Mabuse, is "the exponent of the decaying Europe, armed with the dangerous knowledge of the civilization of his continent. He rises consciously in order to strike a breach into the moral uniformity of his time but less for the sake of material advantage. He wants to be a guiding force, a creator, if only in destruction. In a word, his objective is power, which in our time has been transferred from the individual to the collective."[129] Or, more directly, as Dr. Mabuse says in *Dr. Mabuse, der Spieler,* "We must plunge the world into an abyss of terror."[130] And, in the first of the two films, Mabuse not only merges the individual into the mass by successfully disguising himself as nine different characters and by hypnotizing his victims such that they will even commit suicide at his behest, but also is so cunning and so powerful that the forces of the police and the army must be combined in order to destroy his infernal criminal syndicate.[131] As a foreshadowing of Hitler, Lang's first Mabuse film was all too prescient.

When, in 1924, museum director Gustav Hartlaub took note of *die neue Sachlichkeit* emerging in Weimar's popular arts, he was referring "to the general feeling in Germany of resignation and cynicism after a period of exuberant hopes."[132] One cinematic practitioner of the new wave, Georg Wilhelm Pabst (1885–1967), presented a film that caught its immiserating theme: *Die Buchse der Pandora* (*Pandora's Box,* 1929).[133] Transposing the myth explaining how evil spread over the earth into a tale of female lust and serial murder, Pabst directed the American actress Louise Brooks (1906–1985) in the title role of a prostitute. The film's finale, as recalled by Brooks, is a worthy tribute to the equation of sex with death that characterized *die Neue Sachlichkeit:* "It is

Christmas Eve, and she is about to receive the gift that has been her dream since childhood: death by a sexual maniac."[134]

Concomitant with its emphasis on *Lustmord*—the apotheosis of which, perhaps, occurs in Fritz Lang's *M,* depicting the child-killer Beckert (Peter Lorre), who, according to Maria Tatar's interpretation of his confession in the film's *denouement,* "is driven by the need to commit acts that will end by unleashing maternal rage to punish him for his craven sexual desires"[135]—films of both of Weimar's genre periods evidenced "a distinct racist strain."[136] In such popular features as *Die Herrin der Welt* (*Mistress of the World,* 1919) and *Der Mann Ohne Namen* (*The Man without a Name,* 1921), "Caucasian heroes do in Orientals, Arabs, and Black Africans at a frenetic pace";[137] while the "Asiatic barbarism of the Huns is given undue emphasis in *Die Nibelungen*"[138] (*The Dwarf Children of the Mist,* 1924). Orientals and Africans are differentiated in the films' stereotypy: in Lang's *Spione* (*The Spy,* 1928), "Asians are involved in underworld enterprises, but then so is nearly every other character in the film."[139] "Negroes appear frequently . . . , usually as bowing, scraping servants or as entertainers,"[140] but in an episode in *Der Wüde Tod* (*Destiny,* 1921) a black is a "hired killer."[141] However, the racist theme is muted in this cinematic fantasy in which a personified Death pursues the heroine throughout time and space—a Moslem city, Renaissance Venice, China—until she sacrifices her own life to save an infant.[142]

But, it is the Jew who is the demonized enemy in Germany's cinema and, indeed, the Jew is depicted as the enemy of civilization itself in several Weimar-era films. Paul Wegener's remake of his 1913 film about the Kabbalistically evoked liberator of the Jews,[143] *Die Golem Wie er in die Welt kam* (*The Golem Who Came to Life,* 1920),[144] shifts the theme from the earlier screenplay—that of the clay monster's unrequited love for his maker's daughter—to one that seems to say that Reason alone cannot be effective in putting down Kabbalist Rabbi Loew's berserk homunculus once it has been awakened.[145] When, in August 1919, the Düsseldorf audience rioted at the showing of *Die Gelübde der Keuschheit* (*The Vows of Chastity*), "the anti-Semitism evoked . . . was evidently a result of the common notion that all the 'enlightenment' films were [being] produced by money-hungry Berlin Jews." Soon after, the movie was prohibited from being presented in theaters in Frankfurt am Main, while cinema owners in Kassell went even further, agreeing "to show no more 'Aufklarungsfilme' in their movie houses."[146]

But perhaps the single most representative legacy of Weimar's ambiguous cinematic thematic, and of its relation to Germany's treatment of the Jewish question, is to be seen in the career trajectories of two of the leading actors in *The Cabinet of Dr. Caligari,* Werner Krauss (1884–1959) and Conrad Veidt

(1893–1943). Krauss had had the title role in *Caligari* and went on to enact the part of "Springfield Jack," that is, Jack the Ripper, in *Das Wachsfigurenkabinett* (*Waxworks,* 1924). Willing to make propaganda films for the Nazis, Krauss, who after the war claimed he had attempted to avoid the job, played five Jewish characters in a film toward which Joseph Goebbels took a special interest, *Jud Süss.*[147] As "Rabbi Loew Süss," as well as his cunning henchman, Süss Oppenheimer's secretary, "Levy," Krauss participated in what was arguably the most fiendish of the Nazi's cinematic accompaniment to the regime's war on the Jews. Released in 1940, *Jud Süss* was shown wherever Jews were about to be deported to the East. It was, as David Welch observes, a movie that "contributed to the radical anti-Semitism already prevalent in Germany and [it] facilitated the way for the evacuation of the Jews."[148] During the Four-Power Occupation of Germany, Veit Harlan (1899–1964), who directed *Jud Süss,* was twice tried but not convicted for "crimes against humanity," of which *Jud Süss* was one. Between 1950 and 1958, he directed nine films. Krauss, along with Emil Jannings (1882–1950)—"Professor Umrath" in Joseph von Sternberg's *der blaue Engel* (*The Blue Angel,* 1930)—were blacklisted in the postwar years. Ferdinand Marian, who had played the title role in *Jud Süss,* committed suicide over feelings of guilt for his part in that picture. When, a few years later, Krauss attempted to make a comeback on the dramatic stage in Switzerland, street riots erupted.[149]

Conrad Veidt, on the other hand, whose portrayal of the somnambulist "Cesare," would long remain with the audiences of *Caligari* and would haunt him for the rest of his life,[150] went on to appear, as "Ivan the Terrible," with Krauss, in *Das Wachsfigurenkabinett*[151] and once more with him, as Baldwin, "the best fencer in Prague," who sells his soul to the devil and ends up fighting his mirror-image doppelganger in the E. T. A. Hoffman-reminiscent *Student vom Prague* (*Student from Prague,* 1926).[152] Veidt would make several more films in Germany, but with the rise of Nazism, and despite a promise of security for himself and his half-Jewish wife from Joseph Goebbels, Hitler's minister of propaganda,[153] he fled the Nazi state for England. There he appeared in several movies, among them *The Wandering Jew* (1933), a milder version of *Jew Süss* (1932),[154] *Dark Journey* (1937), *The Spy in Black* (1939), *Contraband* (1940), and as "Jaffar" in *The Thief of Baghdad* (1940). Moving to America, Veidt reprised his well-established doppelganger role, this time in *Nazi Agent* (1942), in which he essayed the parts of both the nefarious spy and the latter's anti-fascist twin brother.[155] But it was as the thoroughly evil Gestapo Major, Heinrich Strasser, in the 1943 film *Casablanca* (a picture directed by the Hungarian emigre cineast Michael Curtiz [Mihaly Kertesz, 1888–1962], and whose cast included such refugees from Nazism as Peter Lorre, Paul Henreid, Marcel

Dalio, and Madeline LeBeau)[156] that he gave his most unforgettable portrayal of the dogmatic Nazi—a matter confirmed by the fact that in later years, when *Casablanca* was shown in postwar but not thoroughly denazified Germany, all "references to Nazis were cut, including every scene involving Conrad Veidt's Major Strasser."[157] As Siegbert Salomon Prawer observes, "Conrad Veidt went to Hollywood where the parts he was given included the sinister Nazis whom he played so well . . . In real life, . . . it was Werner Krauss who sold himself to the Nazis and Conrad Veidt who shared the lot of German Jews that managed to escape the holocaust."[158]

In Hitler's Germany, the film industry became an agency of Nazi propaganda, under the firm but not always total[159] control of Joseph Goebbels, who held the position of *Reichminister für Volksaufklärung und Propaganda* and headed the *Kulturfilmstelle* of the *Reichsfilmkammer.*[160] State authority over the production and presentation of films was strengthened with the passage of the censorship bill (February 16, 1934), about which a government press release announced: "Hitherto film censorship has been negative. Hereafter, the new State will assume entire responsibility for the creation of films. Only by intensive advice and supervision can films running contrary to the spirit of the times be kept off the screen."[161] The chapter titles of David Henry Hull's *Film in the Third Reich* provide a pithy summary of the conversion of what was once a private artistic enterprise into a medium of ideological propaganda: "1934: Goebbels Shows His Teeth"; "1935: Interlude"; "1936: Goebbels Abolishes the Critics"; "1937: Goebbels Absorbs the Industry."[162]

Nazi conquests extended the cultural as well as the political domain of the Third Reich. In France, to take the most important instance, there exists to this day a fierce debate over whether, under Vichy compromises, the ultimate survival of the French cinema industry was purchased at too great a price.[163] The wholesale eviction of Jewish actors, directors, and theater owners;[164] the emergence of a so-called new French school of cinema during the Nazi occupation;[165] the sacrifice of artistry and conscience for money (or, in some cases, as a cover for anti-Nazi resistance activities carried on in other venues);[166] and the many acquiescences to the Vichy government's or to Goebbel's directives[167] has led at least one critic to assert, "That the French cinema survived at all is an accomplishment—unless one considers that the cinema survived because two of the most odious regimes in history wanted it and aided it to survive."[168]

In Goebbel's plans for the supervision of Nazi Germany's media of information, the film industry was considered to be of the highest importance. Convinced that, on the one hand, "To be perceived, propaganda must evoke the interest of an audience and must be transmitted through an attention-getting communications medium," but, on the other, that "propaganda to the home front must create an optimum anxiety level" and "facilitate the displacement of aggression by specifying the targets for hatred,"[169] the Reich's propaganda minister "was attracted to films because they were easier to make and mould and because they reached much wider audiences than live theatre."[170] In strikingly dramatic documentaries, for example, *Triumph des Willens* (*Triumph of the Will,* 1935), Leni Riefenstahl's paean to Hitler,[171] *Olympia* (1938), her kinesthetic ode to ancient Greece's transition to Nazi Germany,[172] and Fritz Hippler's scathingly antisemitic *Der ewige Jude* (*The Eternal/Wandering Jew,* 1940)[173] as well as in such feature films as Goebbel's *Antikommintern*-sponsored, NSDAP-distributed *Friesennot* (*Frisians in Peril,* 1935)[174]—providing a harrowing tale of rape and murder in the context of the plight of the Volga Germans under Bolshevik tyranny—and in the previously mentioned film, Veit Harlan's anti-Jewish *Jud Süss* (*Jew Süss*), 1940—in which Werner Krause's portrayal of "the grasping Rabbi Loew was so convincing that he asked Goebbels to announce publicly that he was not Jewish but a loyal Aryan merely playing a part as an actor in the service of the State"[175]—Goebbels did achieve what he had set out to do. However, in spite of his attempts at a film-industry *Gleichschaltung,*[176] or, perhaps, because one of his principles of propaganda—namely, "Propaganda cannot immediately affect strong counter-tendencies; instead it must offer some form of . . . diversion."[177]—allowed clever filmmakers a way to circumvent his directives, some cinematographers and actors avoided participating in "national interest" pictures, confining their cinematic activities to making seemingly innocuous comedies or apolitical musicals.[178] But, open cinematic resistance to Hitler or Goebbels did not arise. Jewish players, writers, and directors were evicted from their positions in the industry; those who failed to find asylum abroad or special protection in Germany perished in the death camps.[179] Fritz Lang's *Das Testament des Dr. Mabuse,* despite Goebbels's ban on its showing and Lang's later claims to its anti-Nazi theme,[180] "betrays," Krakauer observes, "the power of Nazi spirit over minds insufficiently equipped to counter its peculiar fascination."[181]

The fascination with Nazism did not fade from Germany's movie screens in the postwar years. The victorious Allies' efforts at denazification did not last long and were by no means thorough.[182] But, the interest in revisiting the Nazi era cinematically seems to go beyond undying commitment, unbearable shame, unresolved guilt, or unabashed nostalgia, although each figures in the half century of German movies since the first postwar film, Wolfgang Staudte's *Die Mörder Sind Unter Uns (The Murderers Are among Us),* was screened in 1946.[183] Indeed, it was an obsession of mixed motives and ambivalent feelings. *Die Mörder*'s screenplay, the first of a series of so-called "Trümmerfilme" ("rubble films"),[184] reduced virtually all of the issues that would constitute Germany's *Vergangenheitsbewältigung* ("coming to terms with the past") to a personal problem, relieved by love. As summarized by the Reimers, the plot

> revolves around the postwar lives of Susanna, an idealistic young woman who has been released from a concentration camp; Mertens, a cynical doctor who is tormented by memories of the war; and Bruckner, an ex-Nazi officer and now an increasingly successful industrialist. Bruckner murdered women and children in a Polish village, a crime that Mertens witnessed, and the doctor is now intent on killing Bruckner, thereby making him pay for his past. Susanna's love for Mertens cures him of his cynicism. She also helps him to realize that his plan to punish the industrialist without the benefit of a legal trial would not serve the future. With Bruckner behind bars, the story ends on the statement that only a trial conducted in the full light of a free society will bring justice to the people who were wronged.[185]

This movie's happy ending, Reimer and Reimer observe, was "a mainstay of classic cinema [and] takes viewers beyond the scars and helps them recognize that brighter days lie ahead."[186]

However, Anton Kaes holds a different view. He believes that *Die Morder*'s "appeal to the legal system makes little impression primarily because it does not inevitably follow from the film's dramatic structure; it seems tacked on."[187] During the first years of the Four-Power Occupation of Germany, as Kaes points out, a "'political quarantine' [of Germany's filmmakers] . . . inhibited an open political analysis of the conditions, mechanisms, and consequences of National Socialism."[188] In its place, the *Trümmerfilme* makers evaded "[q]uestions about right and wrong, guilt and atonement . . . [by adopting] a predominantly existentialist-humanist approach, obscured by the psychology of love stories, or diverted into appeals to Christian forgiveness."[189] Moreover, to some members of the audience, there might have been a subtler message, serving a different function, in the "rubble films," as well as in those produced later, revisiting (and revising) Hitler's biography,[190] the Holocaust,[191] and the role of the German people during the Nazi era.[192] According to Mark Koenigil, "If a film offers . . . a new idea, a novel type of realism, it will not be understood by those accustomed to maintaining a sordid attitude. To the sadist, who cannot give vent to his feelings, only—after all, we can't all be Hitlers and Himmlers—the darkened theatre represents their field of action. For two hours their suppressed instincts come to the fore and there they can remain, associating themselves with the film."[193]

Postwar Germany's cinematic *Vergangenheitsbewältigung* proceeded through six subgenres before the Cold War had come to an end and the two Germanies had become one.[194] In many ways the East and West German film industries' multifaceted quest for an understanding of the Hitler era, their debates over whether the German people or only the Nazi leaders were responsible for the concentration camps, the genocides, and the war, and their inquiries into how long if, at all, and in what ways, the recent past is to be remembered, has its parallel in the *Historikerstreit* carried on by the nation's historians during the same period.[195] While German historians sought a diachronic space somewhere between aporia and apology,[196] reappraisal and repression,[197] at the same time seeking to take or to ward off moral responsibility for the Holocaust,[198] or to document a negative symbiosis between Germans and Jews,[199] the nation's cinematographers went in quest of the culprits (e.g., Peter Lorre's brilliantly pessimistic portrayal of those who could not be forgiven: *Der Verlorene* [*The Lost One,* 1951][200]); in exoneration of the obedient but nondoctrinaire German soldier, (e.g., Paul May's three-part *08/15,* [1954–1955], following the wartime career of an infantryman as he moves from private to lieutenant, from training in Germany to fighting on the Russian front, all the time questioning his Nazi superiors' authority but performing excellently as a soldier—a picture that, as the Reimers notice, gives such a soldier "all the classic virtues of war—bravery, honor and patriotism . . . [but] depicts neither darkness nor despair nor a dictatorship that tried to destroy the democratic world,"[201] and that Kaes believes "distinguished between the honest soldier and the unreasonable, despicable regime, and thus succeeded in intensifying already prevalent apologist tendencies");[202] in examination of whether the Allies' insistence on unconditional surrender prolonged the war, deterred "good Germans" from opposing Hitler and the Nazis, and cost both German and Allied lives (e.g., Eberhard Fechner's *Winterspelt,* 1977, in which an American officer rejects a German commander's offer to surrender on the eve of the Battle of the Bulge because such an abject act "offends the military sensibility");[203] in caricaturish reconstruction of the Nazis (e.g., Kurt Hoffmann's *Wir Wunderkinder* [*Aren't We Wonderful,* 1958], a comedy whose pastiche structure foreshadows postmodernism but whose scenario gives the impression that the Nazis drew their membership and support largely if not solely from the lumpenproletariat of prostitutes, fools, and buffoons);[204] in search of a reason to repress the memory of, or obtain absolution from, the crime of genocide (e.g., a number of films explored and often romanticized the issues, beginning with *David* [1978] and continuing with *Das Boot ist Voll* [*The Boat Is Full,* 1980], *Der gelbe Stern* [*The Yellow Star,* 1980], *Charlotte* [1981], *Regentropfen* [*Raindrops,* 1981], *Es ging Tag und Nacht, liebes Kind: Zigeuner (Sinti) in Auschwitz* [*It Went On Day and Night, Dear Child: Gypsies in Auschwitz,* 1981–1982], *An uns glaubt Gott nicht mehr* [*God Does Not Believe in Us Anymore,* 1982], Heinz Scheik's fictionalized docudrama *Die Wannseekonferenz* [*The Wannsee Conference,* 1984], *Bittere Ernte*

[*Angry Harvest,* 1984], *'38—Auch das war Wien* [*'38—Vienna before the Fall,* 1986], and the improbable but apparently true story of Jewish Salomon Perel's adventures as *Hitlerjunge Salomon* [*Europa, Europa* 1991]);[205] and to inquire over whether remembering the Nazi era was important, and if so, for what purposes (e.g., Christian Herrendorfer's *Hitler: Eine Karriere* [*Hitler, A Career,* 1977] a docudramatic film version of codirector Joachim Fest's 1973 bestseller, *Hitler, eine Biographie,* which Jean-Paul Bier insists has made Hitler into a political savior who "had given national dignity back to the Germans, . . . solved the unemployment problem, and . . . reestablished in the hearts of millions of Germans a feeling of law and order.").[206]

Perhaps the ultimate cinematic legacy of the Hitler era is to be found in the movies made by Rainer Werner Fassbinder (1946–1982), whose brilliant career as an iconoclastic filmmaker was cut short by suicide. As Reimer and Reimer point out, "Fassbinder's films . . . are like morality plays in which the mistakes of the past are paraded in front of the viewers to help them recognize what he views as the repressive (or fascist) tendencies in German society, a theme that runs through all his movies."[207] For some of Fassbinder's movies, such illicit forms of sex and romance as both age and racial miscegenation (e.g., *Angst essen Seele auf* [*Fear Eats the Soul,* 1973] in which Ali, a thirty-year-old Moroccan *Gästarbeiter* marries a German janitress at least twenty years his senior, and, for their honeymoon dinner, at her request, takes her to a restaurant that was a favorite of Hitler's);[208] male homosexual prostitution (e.g., *Faustrecht der Freiheit* [released as *Fox and His Friends,* 1974]); and lesbian love affairs (e.g., *Die Bitteren Tranen der Petra von Kant* [*The Bitter Tears of Petra von Kant,* 1972]), thematized the sense of alienation and loss felt by Germans born after the war.[209] Fassbinder claimed that he had sought to depict "how the 1950s shaped the people of the 1960s" in order to compensate for the fact that people like himself, born in 1945 or after, "didn't learn much about German history in Germany."[210] Fassbinder's proposal for a television film to be based on Gustav Freytag's nineteenth-century novel *Soll und Leben* was rejected by the director of the West German network on the grounds that using Freytag's work to "come to terms with the historical phenomena of anti-Semitism and anti-Slavism is subject to too many risks and misunderstandings."[211] Shifting his filmic focus to the problems faced by those widowed in the war, those who provided morale to German soldiers, and those who live under the opiate of Nazism, Fassbinder made three films (*Die Ehe der Maria Braun* [*The Marriage of Maria Braun,* 1978]);[212] *Lili Marleen,* 1980[213]; and *Die Sehnsucht der Veronika Voss* [*The Longing of Veronika Voss,* 1981])[214] that, as Sklar points out, "centered on women's lives as markers of social and psychological struggles in the postwar period."[215] As I have observed elsewhere, "Fassbinder's Germany, as a rearmed ally of the West, is a not yet morally reconstructed society, possessed by a culture whose peculiar century-long bourgeois heritage has not yet exorcised its worst demons. [At the time of his death, June 10, 1982, his hope] that his films would upset the widespread complacency . . . as well as cure the amnesia that permitted too many Germans to forget the past, had not been fulfilled."[216]

Cinema of a Failed Revolution: The Soviet Union, 1919–1991

In 1993 there appeared what is undoubtedly the first English language edition of a history of filmmaking during the seventy-three-year existence of the Soviet Union.[217] Dmitry and Vladimir Shlapentokh treat the whole of Soviet cinema in terms of the relationship between the constraints imposed by Marxist-Leninist ideology and the realities of political, economic, cultural, and social life under communism. The Shlapentokhs have the benefit of working with a closed but hitherto unanalyzed case history: the disintegration of the Soviet Union having written *finis* not only to *the* revolution, but also to the latter's popular-culture cinema of revolution. In this respect, their investigation not only provides a comprehensive account of an era and its cinematic representations, but also permits a reconsideration of earlier accounts and critiques, especially those steeped in excessive appreciation and uncritical support of the then-prevailing ideology.

Historically speaking, a film industry had in fact already begun to flourish in the cities of Czarist Russia at the turn of the century. By 1917, there were four thousand theaters in the nation, and, under such French-influenced directors as Evgeni Bauer (1865–1917), these had developed what Robert Sklar describes as "a distinctive style featuring a carefully lighted and decorated mise-en-scene, slow movement, and tragic endings."[218] Apparently Lenin had a great appreciation for the uses that could be made of what he regarded as "the most important of the arts";[219] for he signed the decree nationalizing the movie industry in 1919.[220] Its principal task, according to Anatoli Vasilevich Lunacharskii, founder, with his brother-in-law Alexander Bogdanov (Malinovskii), of Russia's "Proletarian Culture" movement and Lenin's appointed commissar of Enlightenment, was propaganda,[221] the supervision of which was put under his control in *NARKOMPROS,* the *Narodnyi Kommissariat po Prosveshcheniiu* (*The Commissariat of Enlightenment*),[222] and *Goskino* (*The State Committee of Cinematography*).[223] Although the Shlapentokhs claim that "for all intents and purposes, . . . the Soviet movie industry was built by Stalin,"[224] Richard Pipes has taken note of the fact that "during the Civil War, private as well as state-owned [film] studios concentrated on the production of propagandistic shorts (*agitki*), usually less than 30 minutes long . . . [and] shown in regular movie theaters and in agit-trains that crisscrossed the country."[225] Pipes offers the intriguing thesis that, since "a major purpose of Communist propaganda was arousing violent political emotions against the regime's enemies,"[226] the pioneers of the new Soviet cinema took their cinematographic cues from the works of the American director D. W. Griffith, whose film *Intolerance* (1916) had been smuggled into Moscow in 1919, and who, it was rumored, had been invited to become the commissar of the burgeoning Soviet film industry.[227] However, although the Soviet director V. I. Pudovkin (1893–1953) would praise Griffith's *Way Down East* (1920) for its depiction of "landscape as character,"[228] Sergei Mikhailovitch Eisenstein (1898–1948) would deny that Griffith had utilized *montage tropes*—the central innovation of Soviet cinema in the 1920s—in his films.[229] For that technique, Sklar credits the Soviet director Lev Kuleshov (1899–1970).[230]

A sense of how more than one ideological critique is entailed in any discussion of the relation of Soviet films (or, for that matter, any nation's films) to the problematics of truth is illustrated by comparing with one another three of the critical commentaries on Sergei Mikhailovitch Eisenstein's classic *Bronenoset Potemkin* (*The Battleship Potemkin,* 1925).[231] Such a comparison will in the present essay serve as a synechdochical critique of the Shlapentokhs' illuminating study. The Shlapentokhs recognize that there are at least five types, or classes, of reality: Ontological Kantian, individual psychic, institutionally created, artistic, and scientific—and that these types "interact with each other at the phenomenological as well as ontological levels."[232] Their concern, however, is for the most part limited to indicating how Soviet ideology impacted on cinematic versions of Russian reality. Although it is a thesis of the Shlapentokhs' study "that the official dominant ideology, or the ideology supported by state apparatus, . . . distorts reality much more than other ideologies,"[233] and that "movies created by directors ideologically critical of the current regime are, as a rule, considered by us to be more factually accurate than are movies created by the apologists of the current regime,"[234] analysts of *Battleship Potemkin*—a film made by a director sympathetic to the revolutionary ideology that had become regnant in Russia—have shown, in effect, that more than distortion in the name of a particular ideology is at stake in questions about this movie's historical accuracy or its cinematic truth.

Eisenstein's cinematography of the 1905 mutiny aboard the battleship Potemkin exemplifies his use of *montage,* or "montage tropes," as he liked to call them, a quick succession of short scenes, usually of the same event, depicting it from different vantage points in momentary time and visual space.

Montage is alleged to give a scene a heightened sense of realism to which the movie's audience can respond both appreciatively and in an emotionally appropriate manner.[235] The Shlapentokhs are content to treat Eisenstein's cinematic recreation of the abortive 1905 revolt on the battleship Potemkin as one in which "the director followed the tradition of revolution era movies"[236] and to say no more. However, although Sklar argues that "few have come close to matching the intricacy and delicacy of Eisenstein's montage,"[237] a narrative historian of cinema and a postmodern feminist film critic have focused, respectively, on serious errors of fact and a less-than-sensitive gender perspective in *Battleship Potemkin,* distortions, that is, that must give one pause when considering the reliability of Eisenstein's own statement on the artistic principles to which he was committed:

> To dig, to dig, to dig.
> To enter, penetrate, bury myself in every
> crack in the problem, seeming to go
> always deeper and deeper and to come
> nearer to the core of it.
> There is no assistance to be sought from
> anywhere else.
> Except not to hide what has been found: to
> bring it into the daylight—in lessons,
> in printing, in articles, in books.[238]

But, perhaps, not in films. For, according to D. J. Wenden, who has compared the historical accounts of the ultimately unsuccessful mutiny on the Potemkin with Eisenstein's filmic retelling of it, there are numerous factual mistakes in the latter.[239] Wenden does not excoriate Eisenstein for these mistakes, however; rather, he insists, "Eisenstein's variation from the truth, or failure to tell the whole truth (as he knew it) are not necessarily sinister or reprehensible . . . To . . . make a film that would appeal to unsophisticated Russian audiences, Eisenstein had to change and simplify the confused story of the mutiny."[240] Judith Mayne is less forgiving.[241] To this postmodern feminist critic the sophistication of the movie audience is not a matter of central concern. Rather, she regards Eisenstein's usage of *montage* as the employment of one more artistic procedure rooted in the "polarity of activity versus passivity, with the attendant implications of mastery and creative remolding, [implications] that lend themselves easily to the critique of binary opposition that has been central to feminist examinations of culture and theory."[242] Specifically, Mayne is able to locate the setting for a gender-based binary opposition in the film's famous "Odessa steps" scene. "It is" she writes, "as if the Odessa-steps sequence, with its frenzied movements and its predominance of female bodies, functions as

Potemkin's dark continent, from which the film emerges into the bright light of abstraction, homogeneity and revolutionary brotherhood—into, that is, a world populated once again exclusively by men."[243] Nor will Mayne exonerate other Soviet film directors from her charge that they foisted a basic gender discrimination on the screen: "It is perhaps tempting to argue that this troublesome representation of female agency has more to do with Eisenstein's particular disposition toward women than with the sexual politics of film narrative in the Soviet Union. I would argue, rather, that Eisenstein's visions of the sexual contours of revolution offer a representation 'in amazingly bold relief' (to borrow from Lenin's description of Tolstoy) of a dynamic that emerges in many Soviet films of the period."[244] For Mayne, the technical agency of that dynamic is *montage* itself, especially as developed by such male Russian cinematographers as the aforementioned Kuleshov,[245] Eisenstein, and the extraordinarily prolific maker of such films as *Three Songs of Lenin* (1934), Dziga Vertov (1896–1954).[246] "[W]hether male or female, these cinematic creatures evoked by Kuleshov and Vertov attest to montage as a means of mastery, as power over the raw material of individual fragments of film."[247] And, as Mayne concludes in an afterword to her investigation of silent Soviet movies, "Whether it be the disruptive female presence which hinders the growth of class solidarity in *Strike,* the inaccessibility of the woman to the realm of metaphoric representation in *Mother,* the containment of the woman within the boundaries of both the image and the past in *Fragment of an Empire,* or the affirmation of maternity as an alternative to male hegemony in *Bed and Sofa,* the woman question echoes throughout Soviet film practice as a nagging reminder that the female body does not always fit neatly into patterns of narrative cinematic or ideological opposition."[248]

Mayne's argument serves to remind us that critiquing films in terms of a single, hegemonic, dominant ideology thesis runs the risks associated with employing a focus that is too narrow—one that is likely to miss aspects of both ideology and resistance, as well as sociocultural inadvertencies that somehow creep into the picture and are also on screen. Perusing the investigation of Soviet movies conducted by the Shlapentokhs, for example, a reader is given a rapid-fire survey of seven decades of films made in the Soviet Union. It is a tour that surveys the entire era of filmmaking, but one that rarely halts to examine a single movie in depth, or as particularly representative. Ultimately one feels one has been treated to a chapter-by-chapter montage of trailers (what to American audiences are called previews), each of which links a decade or so of films to the vicissitudes of ideology under Lenin, Stalin, Krushchev, Brezhnev, and Gorbachev. To their credit, the Shlapentokhs give us details about the tensions that divided ideological opinion and cinematic representation over such issues as nationalism and Russophilism,[249] ethnic minorities,[250] youth,[251] and the Jewish question.[252] But it is a basic thesis of their book that "only with the death of Stalin and the disappearance of mass terror were film makers (as well as other intellectuals) able to create their own ideological vision of the world."[253] Thus, the center of their book is the era of Stalin's rule, dominated by their argument that his tyrannical hegemony made any cinematic opposition or critique virtually impossible.[254]

With the advent of *Glasnost* (1986–1988), the central administration of Soviet movies began to lose force, but conservative local and regional commissars took up the task in their areas of control, forbidding the showing in Omsk, Krasnodar, Tomsk, Kiev, and Stavropoɪ[255] of S. Snezhkin's *Chrezvychainoie sobytie raionnogo mashtaba* (*The Extraordinary Event of District Importance,* 1988), a film exposing the moral defalcations of Komsomol leaders. Moreover, in these freer final years of the Soviet regime, filmmakers still could not undertake a comparison of Stalinist totalitarianism with Nazism.[256] With greater freedoms emerging in the age of *perestroika,* Russian movie makers dared to produce pictures that criticized bureaucrats (e.g., *Pervyi paren* [*The Top Guy,* 1986]),[257] sympathized with victims of anti-Semitism (e.g., *Moi Dorogoi Edison* [*My Dear Edison,* 1986]), portrayed alienated youth (e.g., *Igry dlia detei shkol'nogo vozrasta* [*Games for Teenagers,* 1986]), revealed the operation of class differences (e.g., *Soblazn* [*Seduction,* 1987]), explored juvenile crime (e.g., *Legko li byt'molodym* [*It's Not Easy to Be Young,* 1987]), and revised once again the image of the masses, this time with contempt (e.g., *Nash bronepoezd* [*Our Armored Train,* 1989]).[258]

However, during the next three years, a deep pessimism appeared in Russian films, accompanied by a rejection of moral values (e.g., *Nebesa obetovannyie* [*Chosen Heaven,* 1991]), a positive consideration of nihilism (e.g., *Astenicheskii sindrom* [*Asthenic Syndrome,* 1990]), and a quest for refuge from the troubles of this earth in outer space (e.g., *Dom pod zviezdnoi kryshei* [*The House under the Starry Sky,* 1991]).[259] The final years also witnessed a rise in the number and content of crime films—attributing criminality to one's class position (e.g., *Moie imia Arlekino* [*My Name Is Arlekino,* 1988]); establishing the noble mobster as an antihero type (e.g., Vory v zakone [*Thieves in Law,* 1988]); suggesting that organized crime in Russia is more powerful than the state (e.g., *Shtemp,* 1991); but also asserting that organized crime and the government are intertwined (e.g., *Korruptsia* [*Corruption,* 1990]).[260] Social problem films, not unlike those that were made in the United States in the 1930s, began to depict marginalized people for the first time—prostitutes (e.g., *Interdevochka* [*Intergirl,* 1988]); drunkards, drug addicts, beggars, loafers (e.g., *Smirennoie Kladbishche* [*Humble Cemetery,* 1989]); sexual exploiters (e.g., Malen'kaia Vera [*Little Vera,* 1988]); the suicide-prone (e.g., *Sobachii pir* [*Dog's Feast*] 1990]);

emigrants (e.g., *Passport* [*Passport,* 1990]); and Jews (e.g., *Popugai govoriashchii na idishe* [*The Parrot That Speaks Yiddish,* 1990]).[261] Ultimately, the last of the Soviet film makers began to revise and reverse the secular pantheon of heroes and villains such that the killing of the Romanovs, the hostility toward rich landlords and the bourgeoisie—indeed, in which the very bases of the Revolution—were now called into question (e.g., *Tsareubitsa* [*The Tsar's Murder,* 1991]; *Umirat ne strashno* [*To Die Is Not Frightening,* 1991]; and *Dukhov den'* [*The Day of the Ghost,* 1991]); religious martyrs are restored to honor (e.g., *Pustynia* [*Desert,* 1991]); Stalin is treated as a monster, a criminal, and a liar (e.g., *Puteshestvie tovarishcha Stalina v Africu* [*Stalin's Trip to Africa,* 1990]; *Pokhorony Stalina* [*Stalin's Funeral,* 1990]; *Piry Valtasara ili noch' so Stalinym* [*Valtasar's Feast or the Night with Stalin,* 1989]; *I chert s nami* [*And to Hell with Us,* 1991]); the realities of the Gulag are depicted (e.g., *Kholoidnoie leto 1953* [*The Cold Summer of 1953,* 1987]); and in which intellectuals are regarded with a decided ambivalence (e.g., *Taxi-bliuz* [*Taxi-Blues,* 1990]).[262]

From prerevolutionary days, Russian films had specialized in presenting tragic endings.[263] In a sense, the disintegration of the Soviet Union in 1991 had been prefigured in the USSR's basic cinematic theme—the film that ends abruptly and sadly, without resolving the problem that had first set the scenario in motion. "The last Soviet movies," the Shlapentokhs observe, "presented Soviet life, and even life in general, in extremely pessimistic ways."[264]

In the final years of the short-lived Gorbachev era, a revival of the horror film, best represented by Evgeni Iufit's *Papa, ded Moroz umer* (*Papa, Santa Claus Is Dead* 1991), transvalued the deep sense of despair into occult necrorealistic phantasmagoria: That movie, note the Shlapentokhs, "is filled with degenerates, vampires, and corpses who make love to each other."[265] The picture's title, indicating the death of Santa Claus, when contextualized within its vampire-filled scenario, seems to illustrate a thesis developed in Perkowski's study of Slavic folk beliefs, namely, that the mythical bringer of toys to children on Christmas Eve and the demonic nosferatu who, whenever he can, will drain their blood "embody a polar opposition to one another."[266] For, as Perkowski goes on to explain, "Santa Claus, with origins in the infant Christ and St. Nicholas, represents good, while Dracula the Vampire, with origins in the Slavic folkloric vampire and Vlad Tepes, represents evil."[267]

With the death of Santa Claus, the vampire is given a new lease on life. By the same token, within the world of defunct Soviet communism, the death of Marxism is followed by the reemergence of the cinematic vampire and the vampire state.[268] This, in turn, suggests that folkloric myths have not been thoroughly exorcised from the Slavic mind by the rational philosophies of modernity and that they serve functions in addition to metaphorical critiques of Stalin and his apparatchiks. Rather, in the aftermath of communism's demise, they herald the inner-worldly resurrection of the undead Gothic spirit—a spirit that continues to haunt the surviving (and, perhaps, reviving) worlds not only of aroused militant Slavophilism, but also of liberalism,[269] capitalism,[270] and the Western Enlightenment.[271] That spirit speaks to a characteristic that is at the heart of modernity's paradox. "The vampire's *nature* is fundamentally conservative," insists Ken Gelder, "but *culturally,* this creature may be highly adaptable."[272] Just as an individual, educated under the tutelage of George Herbert Mead's philosophy of a worldly minded self, incorporating within his or her own outlook a sense of the constructibility as well as the malleability of ideologies, can see into both the culture of his or her own *Umwelt* as well as that of the "Other," and act on that perception,[273] so the vampire, in Gelder's opinion, "can be made to appeal to or generate fundamental urges located somehow 'beyond' culture (desire, anxiety, fear), while simultaneously, it can stand for a range of meanings and positions *in* culture."[274] But whereas Mead expected such a cosmopolitan self to look empathically on the life and customs of the "Other," the vampire employs the same ability to commit the greatest of evils, namely, "The vampire is . . . evil, devoid of any moral code; he stands outside—and therefore threatens—all normal society; he drinks blood; he kills without mercy; and still worse he is capable of the final and most inhuman of acts—transforming his victims into equally horrific creatures—a unilateral decision that no mere human under his power is strong enough to prevent."[275] The Shlapentokhs pass lightly over and make no deep interpretation of Iufit's mordant film, preferring to close their study with the argument that "the Soviet experience shows that movies in general are doomed to distort reality in one way or another, even if many film makers try to be as objective as possible,"[276] and an invitation to "future historians to compare films and film makers from the Soviet and the post-Soviet epochs."[277]

Perhaps one such film historian will see in *Papa, ded Moroz umer's* screenplay a foreboding adumbration of the revolt in Chechnya and the atrocities in former Yugoslavia, and note that while Marxism might be so rotted that only a skeleton of its old form remains—the dry bones evidence constituting, in occult folk culture, that "the dead body is finally safe [from vampiric corruption] and that the living are out of harm's way"[278]—the nosferatu of revived nationalism has returned as its bloody-minded successor.

Concluding Remarks: Dystopia as the End of Cinematic Ideology?

The disintegration of the Soviet Union has been followed by a revival of the claim that ideology no longer functions to drive regimes, direct policies, and deliver socioeconomic critiques. The original version of the thesis in fact limited the definition of ideology to Marxism and situated the domain of its decline in the West.[279] The revised thesis, coming in 1989, after the Cold War had to all intents and purposes come to an end, extended the definition of ideology to embrace fascism as well as communism and enlarged its domain to include eastern Europe and the successor states of the USSR.[280] "The triumph of the West, of the Western *idea,*" Francis Fukuyama announced in 1989, "is evident first of all in the total exhaustion of viable systematic alternatives to Western liberalism."[281] Five years later, only slightly chastened by the barrage of criticism, left, right, and academic, that had greeted his original *pronunciamento* and its book-length sequel, he insisted that "we are at a unique juncture in history when, most people would admit, liberalism does not have any serious competitors. There is only 'one language,' that of liberal democracy."[282]

Yet, there are two "inconvenient facts," as Weber would have called them,[283] that mar Fukuyama's sanguinary thesis. The first is one that he will not acknowledge as significant—the rise of virulent and in some cases fascistic ethnonationalisms not only in the successor states to what was once the USSR, but also in much of the erstwhile "Third World" countries and in the Western democracies.[284] Fukuyama holds that his thesis is "normative" and, hence, not entirely dependent on empirical proofs: for example, "[F]ascism may be winning politically in Serbia, but no one (even I would guess, in Belgrade) sees Serbia as an attractive generalizable model for the future."[285] In his most recent work, Fukuyama seems to have tossed empiricism and the world of documented facts away altogether; for he writes, "The collapse of communism and the end of the cold war have not, as some commentators have asserted, led to a global upsurge of tribalism, a revival of nineteenth-century nationalist rivalries, or a breakdown of civilization into anomic violence."[286] Few, however, can give credence to this statement.

As Fukuyama now sees the matter, the triumph of democratic, liberal, market-oriented political economies is dependent on a resurgent "social capital," a commodity which he defines as "a capability that arises from the prevalence of trust in a society or in certain parts of it," one that is "usually created and transmitted through cultural mechanisms like religion, tradition, or historical habit."[287] Trust, in turn, is defined in what cineasts would call a Capraesque manner. It "is the expectation that arises within a community of regular, honest, and cooperative behavior, based on commonly shared norms, on the part of other members of that community."[288] While some may read in this a claim that there has occurred a return to Tönnies's conception of precapitalist *Gemeinschaft,*[289] in Fukuyama's political philosophy, trust, as social capital, is a basic feature of Fukuyama's version of capitalist culture. "The concept of social capital," he writes, "makes clear why capitalism and democracy are so closely related. A healthy capitalist economy is one in which there will be sufficient social capital in the underlying society to permit businesses, corporations, networks, and the like to be self-organizing."[290] In his "Reflections," however, Fukuyama concedes that "what empirical fact can do . . . is to give us [a] greater or lesser degree of *hope* that the normative statement is true."[291] If one uses the cinemas as an indicator of end-of-ideology Germany, Japan, Russia, and the United States, however, there seems little representation for anyone's claim that the storehouses of social capital are near full or that hope is in the ascendancy. Francis Fukuyama, meet John Doe!

The second "inconvenient fact," so well illustrated by the cinema studies just recounted, is the sense of sociocultural despair that at the same time seems to be so prevalent in cultural expressions, electoral and nonelectoral politics, and in the several violent insurgencies going on in various parts of what might be called the new world disorder. Fukuyama blames this pessimism on his postmodern critics who as he sees it, believe "that no ground exists, either for an original cognition or for liberal democracy itself," and whose position is "politically, morally, and humanly intolerable."[292] Nor is Fukuyama's latter worry without merit. But this works against his own sanguinary thesis. The late Leo Lowenthal (1901–1993), a lifelong student of mass and popular culture and a member of the original Frankfurt School, told Emilio Galli Zugaro in May 1985:

> This so-called postmodernity is a pseudo-philosophical orientation that would base itself—I think without justification—on Nietzsche . . . Of course some of their representatives, in their irrational, pseudo-romantic stance, have become harbingers of fascist or National Socialist ideologies . . . Of course, one shouldn't moralize. These aren't evil people. But in my opinion they're victims of a desperate situation in which the impatience, the expectation that something has to happen—even if it means that nothing at all should happen—overwhelms the rationally advisable attitude of waiting, of critical thought.[293]

The despair at the end of the Cold War may suggest a corollary to Lowenthal's point: all of these years there has been an unrequited waiting: "Waiting for Lefty," "Waiting for Godot," awaiting Jesus, looking for the Messiah, and so forth. That the millennium is not yet come around—especially when, as in the United States, there is expectation that Americans are dwelling in the true "redeemer nation,"[294] or, as in Germany and Japan, where their participation in World War II had the expectation of a fulfillment of their dreams of world hegemony;[295] or, as in the Soviet Union and other Marxist regimes, where history was perceived not only as unidirectional but also as favorably disposed toward realization of their versions of a communist political economy and culture—can evoke intense frustration and lead to anger and ennui. And each of these in turn can be a spur to action—or to lethargy. Reflecting as early as 1946 on the failure of Marxism to become the ideology that would lead "the people" to establish the "realm of the Free and Equal," Weber scholar and cinema critic J. P. Mayer asserted, "A new universal belief, integrating all classes and their aspirations, guiding 'the people,' must be formulated."[296] In the four decades since he wrote those words, no such belief has been proclaimed.

Mayer had hoped that "such a belief, if it can establish itself, may perhaps be accompanied by the re-emergence of a new popular theatre and cinema."[297] He had, in 1946, looked to England to provide a religio-liberal solution to the central problem of modernity, the problem that neither Marxism nor fascism had resolved: "We can therefore hope that England will succeed in establishing the new social integration of all classes, which the present world crisis demands and which, according to the mediaeval Christian Catholic analogy, assigns to each social group its positive function in society. In this way only can freedom of the individual be reconciled with the administrative and organisational needs of the modern mass state."[298] However, if we take a popular American film of 1996, *Independence Day,* as representative of the American, and, possibly a global sociopolitical outlook, we will see a querulous confirmation of Immanuel Wallerstein's recent observation that the "destruction of the Berlin Wall and the subsequent dissolution of the U.S.S.R. . . . , celebrated as the final triumph of liberalism as an ideology . . . , marked *even more* the collapse of liberalism and our definite entry into the world 'after liberalism'"[299]—truly an end of ideology.

Independence Day, although made in Hollywood, presents a post-liberal world situation in which the entirety of the planet earth is threatened with imminent destruction by attackers in city-size space ships capable of wiping out virtually the whole of the human race and all its accomplishments. It is a movie illustrative of what Walter Laquer has called "Postmodern Terrorism," except that Laquer is speaking of real-life-and-death, not reel-life-and-death, happenings.[300] The space invaders are not allegorical representatives of the Soviet menace, or of Middle-Eastern terrorists, or American militia militants; rather, they speak to a nameless post–Cold War nemesis, terror itself. As Joseba Zulaika and William A. Douglass observe, "The evil other of the Cold War being moribund, we will no longer be taken [by the makers of thrillers] to Checkpoint Charlie or be presented with a cast of KGB villains . . . [W]e confront the new exemplar of inscrutable wickedness, the latest perpetrator of ultraviolent gore."[301]

Independence Day makes clear that millions of people from every densely inhabited place on earth are killed by the spaceships' employment of a ray of destruction that inflicts massive damage on both the substance and symbols of the post–Cold War global scene—on the White House, the Empire State Building, and, for the most part offscreen, on similar structures and icons in Moscow, Berlin, Tokyo, and other of the globe's principal cities. Somehow, for reasons unstated in the film but perhaps because it evokes the lingering memory of America's victorious survival in the recently completed Cold War, it falls to the United States to provide both the personnel and the technics needed to save the world. However, the film invokes a peculiarly narrow vision of heroic individualism in its depiction of the eventually successful counterattack (which, it must be said, manages to save only a fraction of the earth's population, and of these, only those who live in remote and unsettled areas). The "victory"—such as it is—is managed by a motley crew of hastily assembled misfits of every stripe: A feckless president of the United States who climbs into the cockpit of a plane to lead the last battle (Bill Pullman); a socially awkward, unhappily divorced Jewish scientist-technician who figures out how to stop the attackers (Jeff Goldblum); his father, an unacculturated orthodox Jew who leads terrified children of different races and religions in Hebrew prayers as the final enemy attack is about to begin (Judd Hirsch); a half-crazed drunk who executes a suicidal flight into the enemy's spaceship when all else has failed (Randy Quaid); and a happy-go-lucky African American airborne fighter pilot (Will Smith) well integrated into his military unit (all of whom but him are killed in the first encounter with the space marauders) and living off-base with his girlfriend, a divorced mother (Vivace Fox), who risks his life in the final air battle to deliver the *coup de grace* to the enemy. "According to Nostradamus," Laquer reminds us, "a great King of terror will come from heaven in July, 1999."[302] According to *Independence Day,* if he comes, we will be saved, if at all, not by any institutional arrangements springing from such ideologies as nationalism, Marxism, fascism, or liberalism—but by the united and coordinated efforts of those who have been depicted as society's outsiders. The plot of *Independence Day* is, in effect, a dialectical inversion of, and an ironic commentary on, Max Weber's concluding remarks in one of his final addresses to German students:

> Certainly all historical experience confirms the truth—that man would not have attained the possible unless time and again he had reached out for the impossible. But to do that a man must be a leader, and not only a leader but a hero as well . . . And even those who are neither leaders nor heroes must arm themselves with the steadfastness of heart which can brave even the crumbling of all hopes.[303]

In *Independence Day,* an uncharismatic president,[304] an ungainly, secular Jewish laboratory technician,[305] an Orthodox Jew who appears as an anachronistic refugee from Louis Wirth's *The Ghetto,*[306] a hopelessly mad alcoholic who has traversed far beyond the stations of the lost,[307] and—*pace* Julia Kristeva[308]—a merry black jet pilot who only wants "to kick ET's ass,"[309] not only muster the requisite steadfastness of heart, but lead the few survivors, that is, the rest of us, on to victory—saving what little is left of the perhaps irrevocably shattered world. After it is over, and the space invaders destroyed, there is no "utopia glimpsed beyond the nightmare of an as yet unfinished modernity."[310] *Sic transit gloria mundi.*

PART V

Beyond *Gemeinschaft* and *Gesellschaft*

CHAPTER EIGHT

Community

A Theoretical Perspective on Its Dilemmas, Contradictions, and Possible Future

> Citizenship is not a cure for spiritual malaise but spiritual malaise is a roadblock to citizenship because it impairs the capacity to create the community institutions on which a civil society and a democratic culture must rest.
>
> —BENJAMIN R. BARBER, *Jihad vs. McWorld*

> Beyond the smoking rubble rises the American Jerusalem, the New Jerusalem, the New Atlantis, the New Republic, the New Deal, the New Frontiers, the New Birth of Freedom, Morning in America, novus ordo seclorum . . . [N]ever . . . complete, the American Garden will always glow beyond the river's bank, as untouched as the world on creation's first day.
>
> —MICHAEL LIND, *The Next American Nation*

Introduction

On September 3, 1995, the *New York Times* gave over a portion of its front page to an essay describing the kind of civility that prevails in Bear Creek, Washington, a walled-in private town.[1] In its depiction, the report gave new meaning to the moral philosopher Edward Tivnan's observation that "a community, by definition is a mutual protection society."[2] For, although Tivnan had qualified his statement by asserting that "communities have a moral obligation to protect their weakest, poorest and unluckiest members,"[3] the citizens of Bear Creek have acted as if their entire membership is under permanent siege. In Bear Creek:

> Four private guards man the entrance gates 24 hours a day, keeping the residents . . . in a nearly crime-free bubble. And should a dog try to stray outside its yard, the pet would be instantly zapped by an electric monitor.[4]

Although most homes in Bear Creek cost from $300,000 to $600,000, the Bear Creek phenomenon is widespread in the United States and is by no means confined to the wealthiest classes.[5] "What is different now," writes *New York Times* reporter Timothy Egan, "is that a big portion of middle-class families, in non-retirement, largely white areas of the country, have chosen to wall themselves off, opting for private government, schools and police."[6] Mary Gail Snyder, a researcher of the burgeoning gated community movement, has perceived in these developments a protean character affecting the provenances of territoriality:[7] "What we're doing," she claims, "is privatizing our public space."[8] For, in its constitutive sense, the human community is a configuration of socially constructed space, and of the relation of such spatial formations to the following: the separation of that which is public from that which is private; the moveability of boundaries of social and interpersonal interaction; and the persistence of primordial, pigmental, epidermal signifiers as designators of a category that can be employed to segregate one human group from another.[9]

Bear Creek represents but the latest redirection taken in the centuries-long search for a viable mode of localized social cooperation. It manifests itself in this instance as a tripartite turn: toward personal security and away from individual freedom; toward ethnically homogeneous interaction and away from contact and accommodation with the ethnoracial multiverse; toward a strictly prescribed limitation on communicative contact and against any sense of responsibility for those persons and groups regarded as "others,"[10] that is, those who do not belong to one's own community of ethnoracial and class consociates.[11] Harvard Law School professor Gerald Frug has contrasted the mores and social composition of the village of an earlier era with those of the contemporary gated community and found the latter wanting:

> The village was open to the public . . . The village did not have these kinds of restrictions. The village had poor people, retarded people. Somebody could hand you a leaflet. These private communities are totally devoid of random encounters. So you develop this instinct that everyone is just like me, and then you become less likely to support schools, parks or roads for everyone else.[12]

Despite their growth—the number of community associations has increased from 4,000 in 1970 to 66,000 in 1990—it is quite possible that the efforts undertaken in behalf of obtaining an exclusive and personal zone of safety will prove to have been in vain. "We have not found evidence that gated communities are any safer than a similar community that is not closed off," Mary Gail Snyder and Edward Blakely concluded on the basis of their empirical researches into the matter. "The major problem, still, is teen-age property crime."[13] Minors and their antics seem to be unavoidable. As William L.

Prosser pointed out more than three decades ago, "Children, as is well known to anyone who has ever been a child, are by nature unreliable and irresponsible people, who are quite likely to do almost anything. In particular, they have a deplorable tendency to stray upon land which does not belong to them, and to meddle with what they find there."[14] However, even if a haven from the heedless acts of youthful hellions is not ever to be found, people will have other reasons for pursuing their search for community.

The Idea and the Ideal of Community

With the efflorescence of the modern age—expressed not only by the activation of the philosophy of the Enlightenment, but also in such collateral developments as the Protestant Reformation, the rise of science, the foundation of capitalist economies, European expansion over the non-Occidental globe, and the sometimes voluntary, other times involuntary coming together of peoples of different color, ethnicity, religion, and culture—there occurred a recognition that the very shape and character of human association was undergoing fundamental change. Perhaps no social thinker captured the essence of this change more profoundly than Ferdinand Toennies (1855–1936).[15] By formulating the ideal typification *Gemeinschaft* and *Gesellschaft,*[16] he set in conceptual form a binary that was not only a processual history, but also a dichotomy that would generate one basis for the critique of modernity. Each term of that binary represents a different quality of human will (or affirmation) with respect to "social relationships, social values, and social associations"[17] as expressed in and as a relation to a specific social entity. What Toennies called the *essential will* referred to "affirmation of a social entity for its own sake"; *arbitrary will,* by contrast, to "an affirmation of such an entity because of an end, or purpose, which is extraneous to it."[18] Essential will, a source as well as a consequence of the *Gemeinschaft,* is manifested in such social entities (institutions) as personality, marriage, the family, intimate friendships, the folk community, the rural settlement, the small town; while arbitrary will, associated with *Gesellschaft,* has its locus in the modern city, in bureaucratic structures, formal organizations, and an emphasis on the primacy of the impersonal in interaction and on conduct carried out in accordance with social roles.

"All intimate, private, and exclusive living together," Toennies observed, ". . . is understood as life in *Gemeinschaft* (community)"; *Gesellschaft,* on the other hand, is society—that is, "public life—it is the world itself."[19] That the *Gesellschaft* was recent, a creature of modern civic formations, was perceived by Johann Caspar Bluntschli (1808–1881): "The entire concept of *Gesellschaft* (society) in a social and political sense . . . finds its natural foundation in the folkways, mores, and ideas of the third estate . . . Wherever urban culture blossoms and bears fruits, *Gesellschaft* appears as its indispensable organ." Moreover, he added, "The rural people know little of it."[20] "In *Gemeinschaft*," Toennies pointed out, "with one's family, one lives from birth on, bound to it in weal and woe."[21] *Gesellschaft* was quite something else: "One goes into *Gesellschaft* as one goes into a strange country," he observed.[22]

As Toennies saw the matter, *Gesellschaft* was in the ascendancy; *Gemeinschaft* in decline. Such was the trend of Occidental history once the instaurative shift in philosophical thought and social praxis, begun in the sixteenth century, had achieved epistemological, economic, and political legitimation and had decisively overcome its predecessor. One material change of great significance for this process was the dissolution of the communal tillage system, as a result of which "the pure, complete, and absolute, that is, unconditional, private landed property has eventually evolved."[23] The privatization of property, as Toennies explained, was the catalyst of capitalism and the lever that tipped the balance of sociohistorical forces toward *Gesellschaft* and against *Gemeinschaft*. "For the ownership of capital as far as . . . it is ownership of money, as a natural and general private property, stands in contrast to the natural and general communal *(Gemeinschaft*-like) property in land." On the other hand, he went on to argue, "through the combination of shares as a means to a common end arises from private property the associational *(Gesellschaft*-like) property."[24]

Hand in hand with the rise of private property went the development of "capital cities," a consequence "of the concentration of the resources of whole nations in the hands of both merchants and statesmen";[25] an increase in travel and migration; and a shift toward utilizing formalized theory and the tools and findings of science in the conduct of practical matters. The latter change was of great importance; for while the older "pursuit of the practical arts remains tied to tradition; its ways of thinking, subject to authority, . . . dogmatic, and . . . in conformity with the thoughtways of the uneducated and simple-minded masses, submitting to what has so long been a valid norm in sacrosanct doctrine," by contrast, "theory and scientific endeavor are motivated by a search for what is novel."[26] One consequence of this change was an all-out assault on customary habits. Toennies concluded, "This tendency [of people to think scientifically and put practice into line with theory] brings them into opposition to what has persevered in the traditional ways which are moving, so to speak, in a circle, while the novel forces forge boldly ahead in a straight line."[27] As the geocentric standpoint in astronomy was undermined, the animistic outlook in biology gave way to the science of iatromechanics, and the anthropomorphic perspective was replaced by mathematical models and methods.[28] All of these revolutions were accompanied by a vast expansion of urban development. One result was that more and more people began to believe that they had lost something. They had become attenuated from their erstwhile custom-bound neighbors and lifeways. They had, in greater and greater numbers, become homeless in both body and spirit. In response, they would begin to seek a return—embark, that is, on a quest for *Gemeinschaft.*

Toennies was quick to point out that there were many different manifestations of *Gemeinschaft,* and that each was becoming eroded by the forces favoring *Gesellschaft.* "There exists a *Gemeinschaft* of language, of folkways or mores, or of beliefs."[29] But such *Gemeinschaften* were not to be found in the formal associations of the modern era. "Lawyers," he noted, "may speak of domestic (*häsliche*) *Gesellschaft,* thinking only of the legalistic concept of social association; but the domestic *Gemeinschaft,* or homelife with its immeasurable influence upon the human soul, has been felt by everyone who ever shared it . . . *Gesellschaft* exists in the realm of business, travel or sciences . . . To make the word combination 'joint-stock *Gemeinschaft*' would be abominable . . . On the other hand, . . . [t]he *Gemeinschaft* of property between man and wife cannot be called *Gesellschaft* of property."[30]

Among the forces encouraging the enlargement of *Gesellschaft* over more and more aspects of life, the most significant—according to Toennies—was the ascendancy of modernist modes of patriarchy and the expansion of male authority. "[T]he realm of life and work in *Gemeinschaft* is particularly befitting to women; indeed, it is even necessary for them," he observed. For women, "the home and not the market, their own or friend's dwelling and not the street, is the natural seat of their activity . . . Also, many tasks in agriculture befit the woman and in the soundest cultures have been put on her shoulders, often however, to the point of excess. . . . Farming can be conceived as a service to nature, close to the household and immediately bearing fruit."[31]

Because commerce, rather than the family farm, had become the economic form paradigmatically associated with modernity, men, rather than women, had become the active agents of the business world. According to Toennies, profit-driven men and domestic farm women differed with respect to their qualities of will. "The will to enrich himself makes the merchant unscrupulous and the type of egoistic, self-willed individual to whom all humans except his nearest friends are only means and tools to his ends or purposes; *he* is the embodiment of *Gesellschaft.*"[32] Moreover, precisely because in the realm of business (and, in light of Max Weber's comments on the kinds of behavior associated with politics as a vocation,[33] Toennies might have added popular governance) deception is a basic element of rational action, the man, who, Toennies believed, was more willing to set aside his ethical scruples than a woman, is more apt to succeed: "The words which he chooses are calculated in terms of their effect; therefore, truthful words, when not profitable, change easily into lies . . . Thus, in a more general sense, the lie becomes a characteristic element of *Gesellschaft*."[34]

However, according to Toennies, one of the more unfortunate consequences of modernity is its assault on the hearts and minds of women, dragging them unwillingly away from hearth and home and forcing them into the lower echelons of the industrial labor force. "The masters of capitalistic production," he wrote in 1887, "find female labor especially fit for running machinery since it corresponds most closely to the concept of simple and average human labor."[35] Indeed, these capitalists believed that female labor "stands between the versatility and adaptiveness of child labor and the strength and trustworthiness of masculine labor."[36] As a by-product of her induction into factory labor, "the freedom and independence of the female . . . worker as contracting party and possessor of money will develop her rational will, enabling her to think in a calculating way . . . The woman becomes enlightened, coldhearted, conscious."[37]

For Toennies, the coming triumph of *Gesellschaft* over *Gemeinschaft* was not only a profound tragedy, but also the herald of a forthcoming crisis. Throughout his life he wondered and worried over whether it would be possible to modify, halt, or reverse the trend. As his son-in-law, the sociologist Rudolf Heberle, pointed out, Toennies opposed both Russian Bolshevism—"which destroyed all genuine *Gemeinschaft* or its survivals"—and "the National socialists'—the Nazis'—attempt to create a 'Volksgemeinschaft' by compulsion."[38] Toennies's own commitment was to a humane sociocultural reconstruction. It found expression in his "belief in a regeneration of Western society and culture through a new kind of *Gemeinschaft* based upon an organically developed combination of state and cooperative socialism."[39] Such could be achieved, he had observed in 1887, if the "future persons of capitalistic *Gesellschaft* [would] be educated to methodical, correct thinking . . . combined with the stimulation of a spirit of *Gemeinschaft*, the creation of a social sentiment, the ennoblement of the mind, and the education of the conscience."[40] Moreover, development "would naturally go in this direction if the social forces did not work against it."[41] But, alas, he pointed out, the "social forces are more interested in maintaining the conflict between moral forces and philosophies which belong to a culture of *Gemeinschaft* which is continually decaying."[42]

However, Toennies could not rely on a restoration of conscience among either entrepreneurial or laboring men. For, he believed, "In every regard the capable man of *Gesellschaft*, whether he considers himself free master of his wealth or master only of his labor power and other capabilities, is always ambitious and calculating, accepting opinions critically and using them to his advantage."[43] But, precisely because he believed that, despite its modification by her having to participate in the struggle to earn a living, the rational will suited to *Gesellschaft* was "foreign and terrible to [woman's] inborn nature,"[44] he held out hope for what the effects would be of an emerging feminine consciousness. "The analogy of the fate of women with the fate of the proletariat has been recognized and outlined long ago," he observed.[45] "Their growing group consciousness, like that of the isolated thinker," he hoped, would ". . . develop and rise to a moral-humane consciousness."[46]

The Idea of Community in American Social Thought

Although Toennies's conceptualization of the problem of *Gemeinschaft/Gesellschaft* would exert a strong influence on American social thought, its character would be modified by its passage through the Chicago School of sociology. The latter's emphasis on the dichotomous qualities of city and country life; on the positive features of primitive, pastoral, and country settlements; on the enclaves established by successive waves of ethnoracial minorities; and on the inevitable absorption of all peoples by the inexorable processes of acculturation, assimilation, and amalgamation would engender a nostalgia for those aspects of its erstwhile *Gemeinschaft* that America had lost. It would lead to various attempts to discover or recreate them in the city and to an uncertainty about whether individualism and personal freedom were worth the price in personal and social security that they exacted. For the most part—but with such notable exceptions as the public philosophy of John Dewey (1859–1952) and the sociological outlook of Robert E. Park (1864–1944) and W. I. Thomas (1863–1947)—the quest for community in America turned away from the humanistic socialism advocated by Toennies and began to move down a decidedly conservative path.[47]

Dewey, Pragmatism, and the Lost American

Although Toennies did not lose his respect for the positive effects religious belief might have on persons and groups, he perceived the trend toward *Gesellschaft* to have taken place in church bodies at the same time that it manifested itself in the secular realms of urbanization and commerce.[48] John Dewey, on the other hand, like virtually all of America's modern social thinkers,[49] could not extricate himself altogether from the Protestant outlook that pervaded the society's *Weltanschauung*. Whereas, in his final work, published in 1935, one year before his death, Toennies had numbered the active forces of social development in the modern age as urban population growth, advances in technology, the global expansion of both commerce and war, the extension of the industrial praxis to agricultural enterprise, the centralization of state power, and the more profound role that the city plays in modifying spiritual sentiments and moral development, and, on the basis of his analysis, had concluded that "pious devoutness [is] an essential trait of rural, critical thinking, of urban life,"[50] Dewey hoped to retain some aspect of Protestantism's pious morality as part of his pioneering pragmatic outlook. In this regard, Dewey's most recent biographer, Alan Ryan, points out that "Dewey's mature philosophy . . . spoke to a deeply felt need to believe that science would not undermine faith, that radicalism did not mean chaos, that a faith in individuals did not lead to wild individualism, and that a faith in community did not lead to an oppressive collectivism."[51]

Dewey's quest—toward which he directed his philosophy of democracy—was a "search for the great community."[52] Unlike those who, like Robert Redfield,[53] read Toennies's thesis as one favoring a return to or a reinstauration of the rural hamlet or the primitive village, Dewey accepted the existence of modernity, correlating his communitarianist commitment to an expanded democracy that had its locus in the industrial city.[54] Such a community, he believed, might be constructed through the rational improvement of communication and the dissemination of the enhanced communicative skills to ever-widening sectors of the populace.[55] What today we can recognize as an adumbration of Jürgen Habermas's proposals for an instauration of reasoned communicative conduct,[56] Dewey regarded as his argument in behalf of a scientifically driven new form: "associated living." Lecturing in China in 1919–1920, Dewey observed that "it was only comparatively recently that it dawned on us that the problems of associated living were susceptible to investigation and ordering [by] the same methods which had proved so useful in dealing with the objective world."[57] Moreover, he insisted, "Regarded as an idea, democracy is not an alternative to other principles of associated life. It is the idea of community life itself."[58]

For Dewey, associated living was a learnable mode of community formation, one that is suited to a civil society wherein public problems generate public interest and, in turn, interest groups. To foster the development of such a community, Dewey devoted much of his life to proposing changes in the pedagogical methods and curricular content of America's[59] and China's systems of education. While in China he had pointed out "associated living is characterized by cooperation, and . . . it is to the mutual advantage of everyone concerned in it. It is like friendship. Friends help each other, exchange knowledge and insights, with the result that their lives are richer and more meaningful."[60] However, he told his Chinese listeners that, whatever their understandings of and attitudes toward the principles of Lockean liberalism to which he subscribed,[61] there is a definite discipline required for associated living,[62] and among its absolute preconditions is the existence of a single common language for everyone to know and use.[63] However, the discipline was made to seem less harsh than others then extant by Dewey's proposal that the classroom be converted into a place for "creative dramatics";[64] while his proclamation of the current necessity for a single national language of instruction was mitigated by his belief "that at last we can look forward to a time when there will be associated living on a world-wide scale, with mankind living in a society which transcends all national and linguistic barriers."[65]

In America, Dewey's justification for implementing associated living focused on the weakness of public opinion and on how education and science might be harnessed to further the cause of a rationally administered democracy. Dewey's program in China had failed. Indeed, in Dewey's own words, it had resulted in a "tragedy of the first magnitude;" for neither he nor his Chinese disciples had reckoned with a matter about which he had hardly spoken a word—political power and military force. With militarists in charge of China's cultural and social institutions, and a civil war soon to begin, as Barry Keenan has pointed out, "Deweyan experimentalism . . . offered no strategy his followers could use to affect political power."[66] The forces holding back associated living in America, on the other hand, were of a different order altogether. They were commercialism and a widespread resistance to a pedagogically informed public philosophy. With respect to these enemies of promise, Dewey believed he had a chance to succeed.

What is striking about Dewey's approach to the reconstitution of an American community is its *Gesellschaft*-like character. Three decades before he tried for a second time to resolve America's public problems—moved by Walter Lippmann's critique of what the latter called the *Phantom Public*[67]—Dewey had attempted to socialize and upgrade public opinion with his ultimately abortive plan for a new kind of newspaper, "*Thought News.*" That newspaper would employ "philosophic ideas in interpreting typical phases of current life."[68] Years later—no issue of "*Thought News*" having ever been published—Dewey took up the problem again, lamenting over the fact that while America's "reception of new elements of population in large numbers from heterogeneous peoples, . . . and the welding [of] them into even an outward show of unity is an extraordinary feat . . . , [the] creation of political unity has also promoted social and intellectual uniformity, a standardization favorable to mediocrity."[69] Dewey had come to believe that "opinion has been segmented as well as outward behavior."[70] He worried over his observation that the "cake of custom . . . is too often flat and soggy," and that, "In spite of attained integration, or rather perhaps because of its nature, the Public seems to be lost."[71]

What had happened, he asserted, was that "the machine age has so enormously expanded, multiplied, intensified and complicated the scope of [its own] indirect consequences, [has] formed such immense and consolidated unions in action, on an impersonal rather than a community basis, that the resultant public cannot identify and distinguish itself."[72]

Dewey's proposed solution to the problem was couched in terms of the increased importance of science and a demand for an expansion of rationality. He allowed that though there once had been "a time when a man might entertain a few general political principles and apply them with some confidence,"[73] that time had passed and democratic republics could not return to it. Indeed, he went on, "The old principles do not fit contemporary life as it is lived, however well they may have expressed the vital interests of the times in which they arose . . . Men feel that they are caught in the sweep of forces too vast to understand or master . . . [and that even] the specialist . . . operates only after the event, looking backward, while meantime social activities have moved on to effect a new state of affairs."[74] The heart of the problem, as Dewey conceived of it, was one of mental and moral lag; for, as he pointed out, "Mental and moral beliefs and ideals change more slowly than outward conditions."[75] At present, he asserted, there is an unequal struggle between outmoded traditions and the scientific outlook. The former "retain their glamor and sentimental prestige in literature and religion, [while] the new ones are perforce harsh and narrow."[76] What was needed was a more expansive interpretation and, even more important, a much wider communication of the rational and scientific ideas and practices to the ordinary citizenry. "Without such communication the public will remain shadowy and formless, seeking spasmodically for itself, but seizing and holding its shadow rather than its substance."[77] America as a "Great Society" was to be "converted into a Great Community,"[78] by means of a newly reconstituted public that had been immersed in the knowledge of those "deep issues . . . which . . . can find a common denominator among all the shifting and unstable relationships."[79]

Dewey's proposals gave short shrift to the senses of emotional instability, impersonality, and *anomie* associated by so many who, with the loss of *Gemeinschaft,* found themselves mired in the realities of *Gesellschaft*. "I do not deprecate emotion," he told his students in China; "emotion is essential, but it must be under the control of intelligence if it is to contribute to the solution of fundamental problems."[80] To Dewey, the much-vaunted American sociability was a deviant sensibility, "largely an effort to find substitutes for that normal consciousness of connection and union that proceeds from being a sustained and sustaining member of a social whole."[81] Indeed, Dewey went even further, asserting that the "unrest, impatience, irritation and hurry that are so marked in American life . . . are evidence, psychologically, of abnormality, and as it is as idle to seek for their explanation within the deliberate intent of individuals . . . [so] it is futile to think that they can be got rid of by hortatory moral appeal."[82] As for the anxiety about loneliness, Dewey was adamant: "We should not be so averse to solitude if we had, when we were alone, the companionship of communal thought built into our mental habits."[83] Ultimately, Dewey called for a repudiation rather than a restoration of the old ideals of *Gemeinschaft:* "If we could inhibit the principles and standards that are merely traditional, if we could slough off the opinions that have no living relationship to the situations in which we live, the unavowed forces that now work upon us unconsciously but unremittingly would have a chance to build minds after their own pattern, and individuals might, in consequence, find themselves in possession of objects to which imagination and emotion would stably attach themselves."[84]

Dewey's endeavors in behalf of a rationally grounded democratic community did not take hold in America. Despite the fact that, or perhaps because, conservative thinkers denounced his praxiological proposals as "flattering to the presumptuousness of the modern mind," his books and essays were said to be a "mirror of twentieth-century discontent."[85] However, such discontented conservatives as Russell Kirk have complained that "veneration was dead in Dewey's universe; indiscriminate emancipation was cock of the walk," and bitterly lamented what he took to be a fact, that "the gray haze of the Utilitarian future toward which Dewey led the rising generation was not immediately repellent to a people who had submitted themselves to the lordship of sensation."[86] In actuality, Dewey's rationalistic and praxiological empiricism neither resolved the dilemmas and contradictions attending the realities of America's public philosophy nor registered for very long on the hearts and minds of those in search of a new or a restored *Gemeinschaft.* By 1982, when the philosopher Michael A. Weinstein undertook an evaluation of American classical philosophy as a moral quest, he could hear only its faint echo: "The basis for a renewal of individualism in the present day is a deepening of inner tolerance to the point at which it becomes normal and not eccentric to live with world-sickness and still to be free for commitment to limited tasks within the public domain."[87]

Montesquieu vs. Rousseau: The Chicago School of Sociology, 1913–1952

"The real problem [in the unfinished quest for community]," Robert A. Nisbet observed one year after Dewey's death, "is not . . . the loss of old contexts but rather the failure of our present democratic and industrial scene to create new contexts of association and moral cohesion within which the smaller allegiances of men will assume both functional and psychological significance."[88] At the University of Chicago's sociology department, from the time of Robert E. Park's arrival in 1913 to that of the death of Louis Wirth (b. 1897) in 1952, there flourished a scientifically driven concern to discover the bases, forms, and possible futures of community in America. The projects undertaken during the four decades were guided by opposed views on the question of how and whether community contributed to freedom and order. Broadly speaking, two opposed points of view emerged—a "Rousseauean" outlook, emphasizing the positive features of preindustrial, pastoral, and primitive *Gemeinschaften;* and a "Montesquieuean" perspective, hailing the emancipatory, individualistic, idiosyncratic, and free forms of life made possible in the urban *Gesellschaft.*

A "Rousseauean" way of thinking about America's problem of community development found its quintessential representative in the Chicago anthropologist Robert Redfield's celebration of the little community and in his favorable depictions of the folk cultures of nonindustrial peoples. Rousseau (1712–1778) had, in fact, provided a comprehensive template of savage life in his *Discourse on the Origin and the Foundation of Inequality among Mankind*[89] from which such later romantic scholars as Redfield might pick their favorite characteristics and themes. Rousseau's vision of the savage was that of a purely natural being:

> I see [he wrote] an animal less strong than some, and less agile than others, but, upon the whole, the most advantageously organized of any: I see him satisfying his hunger under an oak, and his thirst at the first brook; I see him laying himself down to sleep at the foot of the same tree that afforded him his meal; and there are all his wants supplied.[90]

As Rousseau saw the matter, savage ways of responding to "natural infirmities, infancy, old age, and sickness of every kind"[91] were at least equal to those of other animals and often as good or better than those of civilized peoples. "It is . . . observable in regard to infancy that the mother being able to carry her child about with her, wherever she goes, can perform the duty of a nurse with a great deal less trouble than the females of many other animals . . . With old men, who stir and perspire but little, the demand for food diminishes with their abilities to provide it; and as a savage life would exempt them from the gout and the rheumatism, and old age is of all ills that which human assistance is least capable of alleviating, they would at last go off, without its being perceived by others that they ceased to exist, and almost without perceiving it themselves."[92]

It was Rousseau's belief that the family had arisen as a later and salutary development of primitive culture. It, in turn, had provided the affective basis for establishing the savage community. "The first developments of the heart were the effects of a new situation, which united husbands and wives, parents and children, under one roof; the habit of living together gave birth to the sweetest sentiments the human species is acquainted with, conjugal and paternal love. Every family became a little society . . . Those who heretofore wandered through the woods . . . gradually flock together, coalesce into several separate bodies, and at length form . . . a distinct nation, united . . . not by laws or regulations, but by the same way of life, and alimentation, and the common influence of the climate . . . By seeing each other often they contract a habit, which makes it painful not to see each other always. Tender and agreeable sentiments steal into the soul, and are by the smallest opposition wound up into the most impetuous fury: jealousy kindles with love; discord triumphs; and the gentlest of passions requires sacrifices of human blood to appease it."[93]

By contrast Rousseau attributed the ills of modern society to the establishment of private property. "The first man," he insisted, "who after enclosing a piece of ground, took it into his head to say, *this is mine,* and found people simple enough to believe him, was the real founder of civil society."[94] To the pre-civil man—and to Rousseau—"the fruits of the earth belong equally to us all, and the earth itself to nobody!"[95] And to the onset of civil society and the unequal distribution of wealth, Rousseau attributed the ills—physical as well as psychical—of modern humankind:

> The extreme inequalities in the manner of living of the several classes of mankind, the excess of idleness in some, and of labor in others, the facility of irritating and satisfying our sensuality and our appetites, the too exquisite and out of the way foods of the rich, which fill them with fiery juices, and bring on indigestions, the unwholesome food of the poor, of which even, bad as it is, they often fall short, and the want of which tempts them, every opportunity that offers, to eat greedily and overload their stomachs; late nights, excesses of every kind, immoderate transports of all the passions, fatigues, mental exhaustion, in a word, the numberless pains and anxieties annexed to every condition, and which the mind of man is constantly a prey to; these are the fatal proofs that most of our ills are of our own making, and that we might have avoided them all by adhering to the simple, uniform and solitary way of life prescribed to us by nature.[96]

In order to alleviate the "numberless pains and anxieties" of modern man, Rousseauean anthropologists and sociologists sought to discover those peoples who still led a "simple, uniform, and solitary way of life"—the living representatives of nature's and the savages' true *Gemeinschaft*—and to hold them up as models for the inhabitants of civil society to emulate.[97]

Redfield drew on Toennies's binary *Gemeinschaft/Gesellschaft,* as well as on von Wiese's and Becker's sacred/secular dichotomy, to assert the virtues of

Mexican and other nonindustrial peoples' "folk cultures" and to lament the steady disappearance of the "little communities" rooted in kinship and tradition.[98] A true Rousseauean (in the way the term is here being used), Redfield opposed the lifeways, attitudes, and practices associated with Occidental urban civilization, extolling by contrast the simple and for the most part joyous communities of those nonwhite, non-Anglo peoples of the forest and the wood.[99] His wife, Margaret Park Redfield, called attention not only to the false and vulgar commercial practices of American businessmen, who had debased the already declining recognition of the debt owed to mothers by turning its observation into a commercial holiday, but also pointed out that the very need to have such a remembrance day illustrated the drop in significance of familial attachments: "Mother's Day, originally promoted by the florists, and still a source of profit to them, has its whole point in an organization of society in which parents and children lose touch with one another."[100]

Redfield went even further. His final essay, published in 1958, the year he died, abjured the techno-military advances that had assured mutual destruction to the participants in any third world war, but despaired of any attempt to halt the march of death-dealing technology. Combining his affection for pastoral life with his admiration for primitive folk culture, Redfield lamented the near disappearance of authentic communal forms in America.[101] To Redfield and those who followed in his footsteps, the values and practices associated with *Gemeinschaft*—some of which they perceived in the styles of life found in the many racial ghettoes, ethnic enclaves, and immigrant settlements that made up an important feature of the inner city in the area in which the Chicago School flourished, but which they believed to be caught up in the inexorable processes of *Gesellschaft*-oriented assimilation, acculturation, and amalgamation—represented primordial humanity.[102]

The "Montesquieuean" outlook that characterized the *Weltanschauung* of Robert E. Park was for the most part rejected by his students and disciples. Most of the latter adopted one or another urban variant of Rousseaueanism—that is, a critique of the burgeoning civil society in America that would find its authentic voice in Louis Wirth's 1938 essay, "Urbanism as a Way of Life."[103] Montesquieu's sociopolitical philosophy is still unsusceptible to a simple or single formulation.[104] Yet, whatever else one says about it, few would disagree that its positive vision is built around the characteristics of a state-and-city-centered *Gesellschaft.* Montesquieu (1689–1755) believed that the challenge of institutionalizing order in the new societies emerging in the Occident could be met by establishing rational legalism through adoption of constitutional forms of government. Unlike those authors who worried over the emerging trend away from fixed communal status and toward mass and contracted relations among men and women, Montesquieu regarded the emerging individual, as Hulliung reminds us, as "a sturdy and independent fellow, quite resourceful and capable."[105] Moreover, such a person would thrive in a civil society where a bourgeois "I" is also bound by shifting ties of interest to a non-ascriptive "we," the group or party that for the short or long haul represents his or her desires and wants. Liberty, in Montesquieu's understanding of it, is characterized by an absence of restraints, while it expresses its positive duties as "the power of doing what we ought."[106] Whereas the kinship unit, the primitive village, the ethnoracial group, and the religious body are exclusive and exclusionary, for the assimilation-oriented Montesquieu, the "gates of the polis were thrown open to merchants, laboring classes, women, slaves, and Jews."[107] There, they could multiply their associations and become even more liberated from the shackles of tradition.

For Robert E. Park, who had helped found the American branch of the Congo Reform Association, an organization that exposed the atrocities committed by the minions of Belgium's King Leopold II in Africa, and served for nearly a decade as Booker T. Washington's amanuensis, ghost writer, and observer of black life in the rural South, the city to which he moved after Washington's death, Chicago, represented the place where folk cultures would make contact with urban civilization. Out of the former's conflicts with and accommodations to the latter, there would emerge, first, "the marginal man"[108]—a product of two cultures, a member of neither—and, ultimately (but this would be a long time in coming), the individuated personage. The latter—sometimes hero, sometimes victim, sometimes survivor, sometimes indifferent to the struggle, a one among many similarly situated—would enjoy membership in a socioeconomic class and in specific interest groups that would be his or her sole sources of reference and, perhaps, solace.

In the *Gesellschaft* of civilization, Park's sociology seemed to presage that the promise of the Enlightenment—a cutting loose of the individual from the traditional ties of kinship, "blood," race, ethnicity, tradition, and religious creed that bind one too closely to the involuntary groups into which he or she had been born—would at long last be fulfilled. Park did not believe that individuals would necessarily be happier in their newfound freedom. Indeed, their lot in life might still be characterized by poverty, sickness, and deprivation, by personal misfortunes, unhappy sex lives, friendlessness, by a loss of *elan,* or by the erosion of what were once deep and satisfying relationships. Park's "real passion," recalled his student Everett C. Hughes, "was man, the struggler—and, unlike many of those who have drawn—as he did—a sharp contrast between the city and those communities where life appears to run in safer, smoother channels, Park's choice lay with the city, where—as he put it—every man is on his own."[109]

Park set down the contrasts between what he called a "family" society, built around intimate, familial, and ethnic groups, and a "territorial" or civil society, built around individuals, strangers, and impersonal economic formations:

> The familial group has primarily age and sex groupings within while the territorial, cosmopolitan group is characterized by classes and castes . . . The bonds in the small, intimate group that hold the individuals together are the sentiments, the obligations and loyalties. In the larger group the bond is territorial and commercial. In the latter there is a type of organization not to be found in the family . . .
>
> A familial society . . . is based on ethno-centrism. Patriotism is the substitute for ethnocentrism in a territorial society . . . In familial society we get solidarity; in a territorial society there is developed a sentimental attitude toward freedom . . . In our society we are guided less by sentiment and more by interest . . . In a familial society we get consensus . . . In a territorial society we get cooperation, which usually turns out to be competitive cooperation based upon individual interests. In familial society there is a moral order which means a customary and expected order . . . In the other kind of society there is a political order based not on custom but on public opinion which is in constant change and under which laws are hard to enforce."[110]

However, although Park was inclined to admire those who would take up the challenges that the *Gesellschaft* thrust upon them—he once observed that "because of the opportunity it offers, particularly to the exceptional and abnormal types of man, a great city tends to spread out and lay bare to public view in a massive manner all the human characters and traits which are ordinarily obscured and suppressed in smaller communities"[111]—several of his students took to detailing the demoralization,[112] dislocation,[113] dependency,[114] and delinquency[115] that seemed especially rampant in America's cities.[116] Some evinced a nostalgia [117] for the peace and security of the old world or small town *Gemeinschaft,* while others hoped to find a way to reconstitute the community of old inside the city of tomorrow.

It fell to the immigrant sociologist Louis Wirth to put together the negative and unpromising features of American city life and in the process give *Gemeinschaft*—in its American idealization as localized communitarianism—a renewed lease on both the sociological and the social imagination. One year before the publication of Wirth's "Urbanism as a Way of Life," Talcott Parsons had taken special note of Toennies's dichotomy, pointing out the individuating aspects of a man's social relationship if it arises under the terms of *Gesellschaft:* "The motive for entering into such a relationship is that it is the most efficient means to his end . . . All this presupposes the essential *separateness* of the parties . . . [T]he specific characteristic of *Gesellschaft* is a fusion of interests over a specific *positively defined* area. Within that area it involves a 'compromise' of interests of the parties, but it only mitigates their deeper-lying separateness, which in essentials remains untouched."[118] Wirth, who took his own specific point of departure from two essays by the German-Jewish philosopher sociologist Georg Simmel (1858–1918)—namely, "The Stranger" and "The Metropolis and Mental Life"[119]—translated the separateness on which Parsons had concentrated into social estrangement. "Characteristically," he observed, "urbanites meet one another in highly segmented roles . . . [because] the city is characterized by secondary rather than primary contacts. The contacts . . . may . . . be face to face, but they are nevertheless impersonal, superficial, transitory, and segmental."[120] Fearful of the consequences of getting to know strangers, the "reserve, . . . indifference, and . . . blasé outlook which urbanites manifest in their relationships may . . . be regarded as devices for immunizing themselves against the personal claims and expectations of others."[121] Moreover, Wirth went on to point out, "Personal disorganization, mental breakdown, suicide, delinquency, crime, corruption, and disorder might . . . under these circumstances . . . be more prevalent in the urban than in the rural community."[122] The trend toward urbanism would loose the effects of *Gesellschaft* on the entire world, he had concluded, and the city would not, indeed could not, be a haven in the heartless world to come.

Although subsequent studies modified some of Wirth's less-sanguine observations on the effects of urbanism on kinship—for example, Thomas C. Wilson has shown that "urban families are . . . as close-knit as those elsewhere . . . [and that the] bonds of kinship are equally intimate across the rural-urban continuum"[123]—other studies by the same author have thrown cold water on Wirth's and Park's hopes for a continuing rise in tolerance among generations of urbanites. Thus, Wilson observes that while "urbanism is associated with liberal racial attitudes," only the extent to which that same process promotes sustained and intimate interracial contacts will the positive attitude be translated into practices.[124] However, "urbanism increases misanthropy among whites . . . particularly because it increases the ratio of contact with subculturally alien strangers (e.g., nonwhites) to contact with strangers in general."[125] Furthermore, misanthropic and fearful whites are apt to flee: "Racial change in urban neighborhoods is typically accompanied by . . . white flight . . . [or] avoidance."[126] And the much-vaunted tolerance that attended the rural-to-urban migration did not become a part of the political outlook or social attitude of their city-bred children and grandchildren. Indeed, although the "replacement of older more prejudiced cohorts with younger less-prejudiced cohorts has contributed to society-wide reductions in prejudice in recent decades . . . , younger cohorts . . . tend to stereotype minorities more than their predecessors."[127] In 1995, nearly sixty years after Wirth had offered his observations on the positive and negative effects of urbanism, Wilson dolefully pointed out that "it is very possible that the process of prejudice reduction will reverse."[128] The Montesquieuean freedom of the city could be short-lived.

The American small town, whose wholesome character had been upheld as a model of *Gemeinschaft,* also did not go unscathed as the vast and rapid changes that overtook the post–World War II economy undermined its localized sociocultural and political autonomy. American sociologists' rural romance was brought to an end in 1958 with the publication of Arthur J. Vidich's and Joseph Bensman's path-breaking study, *Small Town in Mass Society,* whose subtitle, *Class, Power and Religion in a Rural Community,*[129] spoke to the national political economy's incursion into the lives of those who had thought they were beyond its reach and insulated from its effects. Recalling the intent of their work a decade later, the authors pointed out that their "central concern" had been with "the processes by which the small town (and indirectly all segments of American society) are continuously and increasingly drawn into the central machinery, processes and dynamics of the total society."[130] Five years after its publication, the character of the findings of Vidich's and Bensman's investigation were perceived as indicative of a great change that had taken place in America's rural communities and small towns. Such phenomena as a greater division of labor, a diversification of interest groups and associations, a transfer of local functions to state and federal agencies, a growth of both ex- and suburbanization, and the intrusion, via improved media technology, of mass societal values, fads, tastes, and innovations had, the community sociologist Roland L. Warren observed, been accompanied by a "corresponding decline in community cohesion and autonomy."[131] The *Gemeinschaft* was becoming detached from the little community.

In America's large cities, the trend toward an ever greater *Gesellschaft* has been modified by what some writers have called "the decline of the WASP"[132] and "the rise of the unmeltable ethnics."[133] Alejandro Portes's and Alex Stepick's depiction of the effects of the sociocultural transformation of Miami, a "city on the edge," as they call it,[134] resonates with what has happened or is likely to happen to other large metropolitan areas with ethnically heterogeneous populations: While "a long term trend toward integration and cultural convergence appears inevitable," they observe, "in the short to medium turn, . . . Miami will continue to be characterized by ethnic fragmentation, strife, lack of a hegemonic discourse, and the nostalgic reproduction of a foreign past."[135] New York City, in continuing its push toward ever-greater diversification and its proliferations of both traditional and innovative forms of creedal, ethnic, racial, artistic, lifestyle, and sexual preference subcommunities, "has permitted deviation from past standards which more tradition-minded groups have regarded as sacred."[136] In so doing, observe Bensman and Vidich, "the city has been seen as a source of vice, weakness and degeneracy . . . [but, at] the same time . . . , the city is attractive as a center of vice, pleasure, entertainment, culture and freedom."[137] Yet, as Hughey and Vidich point out, although there has been a resurgence of ethnicity among many of America's metropolitan residents—a consequence of the rootlessness attending the rationalization of urban life that had been anticipated only by Gustav Ratzenhofer 1842–1904),[138] whose sociological system, *except for this point,*[139] had been adapted to Chicago sociology's perspective by Albion W. Small—this new "contemporary ethnicity . . . [often] lacks specific content . . . [and] hardly suggests the sort of primordial attachments that are usually associated with traditional ethnic communities."[140] Instead, as a product of the *Gesellschaft,* the new claims on ethnicity and in behalf of multiculturalism provide "an available foundation for community for those who are unable to tolerate the impersonality, isolation, and meaninglessness of life in modern, industrial, bureaucratic society."[141] The trend first noticed by Toennies seemed to have reached its culminating point—not with the efflorescence of a democratic and enlightened civil society as so many of its advocates had hoped,[142] but rather with the emergence of existential anxiety.[143]

The Community in the Postmodern Era

Ernst Bloch (1885–1977) belonged to that body of European humanist Marxists who did not believe that a culturally diverse, socialist *Gesellschaft* would be utterly devoid of a basis for community. "The new ecumenism," he observed, "belongs to a society that is not essentially antagonistic; it belongs to a community that can grow undisturbedly."[144] He fervently believed that "socialism is the path to this; it is the finally realizable inheritance of what was meant by an inner emancipation and an outer peace."[145] However, none of these desiderata, inner emancipation, or its beneficent twin, outer peace, has yet been fully achieved. In neither the communal *Gemeinschaft*—where individuality and a sense of the personal self is suppressed by the imperatives of sociocultural solidarity—nor the urban *Gesellschaft*—where the aching isolation of the individual and the press of overwhelming bureaucratic authority produce anxiety and a desire to escape from civic freedom—has the quest for a life that provides both personal security and sociopolitical emancipation been realized.

Unlike Bloch and other European thinkers—who looked to a modern civil society in which every individual would participate in what Max Weber called "politics as a vocation,"[146] or who believed along with Marx's colleague Friedrich Engels that the "possibility of securing for every member of society, through social production, an existence which is not only fully sufficient from a material standpoint . . . , but also guarantees to them the completely unrestricted development and exercise of their physical and mental faculties . . . , now exists for the first time,"[147]—most of America's progressive intellectuals "regarded the small community as the remedy for estrangement and rootlessness, the antidote for bureaucratic collectivism, and the prescription for moral commitment to the common good."[148] But faith in a socialist panacea has declined, if it has not altogether disappeared with the disintegration of the Soviet Union and the alleged global triumph of the culture of Western capitalism;[149] while America's progressive reform movements, aiming to forge new solidarities across the older divisions of race, ethnicity, gender, class, and turf, and to found communities in such multiverse cities as San Francisco, have been thwarted. For example, an analyst of the Pacific coast scene asserts that "the negative aspect of San Francisco's celebrated social diversity is that it makes governance almost impossible and undermines the capacity to get anything done."[150] Furthermore, as Witold Rybczynski points out, although the "desire for community—or at least for a *sense* of community—is undoubtedly responsible for the success of so-called Traditional Neighborhood Development, an approach to planning suburban communities that combines smaller plots, more public spaces, and short walking distances to concentrated town centers with traditional-looking architecture . . . , a desire for local identity and old-fashioned architecture should not be confused with really wanting to return to the static communities of the past . . . It is unlikely that we will ever sacrifice our freedom and mobility (both physical and social) for the constraints implied by life in the small towns we say we admire."[151] Finally, note that when an American sociologist, who had taught at the University of Hawaii for five years (1972–1977) and been won over by "the beauty, the culture, the entire ambience" of the islands, undertook a "return to paradise" in 1994, he discovered that his native students' "sense of loss for the rural past, and for the cohesive sense of community that seemed to exist at one time" not only continued to inform the widespread nostalgia of the island state's inhabitants, but had given birth to a "local culture" movement among portions of Hawaii's youth—a movement, that is, that was also "a form of retreatism from the rapidly growing non-local culture."[152] As a mission to discover the primitive way of life, as an attempt to return to or reconstruct the little community, as a hope that full recognition and wholehearted response will be recreated in a heritage group, as a resolve to reestablish communion in the city, or as a dream of a just and humane socialist *Gemeinschaft*, the quest for community has been a vain search for an effective response to the ills and displacements of modernity and technological progress.[153]

The rise of postmodern thought has added a new dimension to this quest, best summed up in the implications of its most salient artifact and icon—*cyberspace.* A term coined in 1984 by William Gibson in *Neuromancer,* a fantasy novel, to describe a feature of society in a world dominated by computers,[154] cyberspace entails the technological advancement that separates distance from territory. It threatens to transform communication—including intimate "conversations" as well, perhaps, as the hoped-for discursive practices that Jürgen Habermas refers to in his conception of "substantive democracy," that is, a "genuine participation of citizens in processes of political will-formation"[155]—into a "consensual hallucination experienced daily by billions."[156] Cyberspace so reinforms language that such ordinary terms as "*body, meet, place,* and even *space* mean something quite different from our accustomed understanding."[157] Under the regime of cyberspace, according to Allucquère Rosanne Stone, human beings succumb to a "quiet death that comes when we have lost our presence in the discourses which shape our lives, when we no longer speak but are spoken—that is, when not we but our culture speaks through our mouths."[158]

For community, the possibility of the new age of cyberspace opens up too much opportunity for masquerade and deception and too little assurance of authenticity. As Stone reminds us in her conclusion, an elaborate meditation on the implications of Ann Rice's fictional vampire Lestat: "We are no longer unproblematically secure within the nest of our location technologies, whose function . . . is to constantly reassure us that we are without question ourselves, singular, bounded, conscious, rational; the end product of hundreds of years of societal evolution in complex dialogue with technology as Other and with gender as an othering machine."[159] The walled-in citizens of Bear Creek—the community with which I began this essay—are, thus, not only vulnerable to the ever-imaginative machinations of trespassing children, but also to the creatures who inhabit cyberspace and move effortlessly along its networked roads. Now, as Doreen Massey points out, "The global is everywhere and already, in one way or another, implicated in the local."[160] Whither community?

Is the Future of Community a Community of the Future?

Community, we have long known, is not a natural fact but, rather, a human artifact. Ever since urbanization, industrialization, and migration brought ethnically diverse strangers into contact, competition, and only grudging accommodation with one another, there has been either dream, hope, or promise of a future construction of *Gemeinschaft.* Some held that such primordial solidarities as kinship, blood, faith, ethnicity, or race would assert or reassert themselves as a "natural" basis for community formation. Others perceived the rise of non-ascriptive civic groups as a phenomenon that promised a new communal form: new friendships[161] and joint commitment to common concerns would unite otherwise disparate population segments, thereby constructing communities of interest.[162] However, while such interest groups are short-lived, or if long term, given to impersonality and bureaucratization, the primordial or "blood"-based units have all too often found it necessary to become societal rather than communal in order to achieve their aims. Thus, to give one telling example, since the end of World War II, those Indians in the western region of the United States who have not followed their brothers and sisters into the large cities have occasionally joined with their age-old enemies, the white ranchers, to oppose the federal government's Bureau of Land Management's proposals to allow strip coal mining because it would wreak havoc on both people's valuable land. One current historian of Indian life sees some communal potential in these political-economic alliances: "If Indians and non-Indians can overlook their differences and concentrate on the basics that unite them, such as the land and a shared sense of place, perhaps the next century will offer better prospects for rapport."[163] But such joint efforts, valuable as they are in terms of public interest democracy, are a far cry from the deep sentimental feelings and culturally ritualistic activities that are so often associated in ordinary people's minds with the mystique of *Gemeinschaft.*

One possible basis for community in the city and the small towns, suburbs, and exurbs drawn ever more tightly into mass and postmodern society is the global village imagery of the current environmental movement. In this regard the urban historian Sam Bass Warner Jr. has pointed out that "human and environmental issues overlap in policy because the remedies for both lie in redesigning the city so that it will be cheaper to maintain, will be more suitable for the nurture of family life, and will be more sustaining of the sociability of urban life."[164] However, two problems currently challenge this possibility. First, although the environmental movement is national, and indeed international, in scope, and draws on a broad-based ideology for its commitment, the researches of Lance de-Haven Smith have documented the fact that the "environmental movement is a coalition of people with very mundane concerns,"[165] and, moreover, that these coalitions operate at the local level with respect to very specific conditions affecting that immediate situation.[166] Interests rather than ideology or sentiment mobilize these movements. "To have an environmental movement with a philosophical ideology at its grass roots," Smith concludes, "would require a fundamental change in mass belief systems."[167] A second barrier to eco-communal development is the fact that urban and rural racial and class-based segregation practices[168] have had as one of their recently discovered effects the targeting of poor, black, and minority residential areas for waste-dumping and other forms of pollution.[169] Concerns for particularized justice in the face of such environmental discrimination are likely to divide as well as unite citizens' groups in the same general locality. Indeed, as Douglas A. Massey and Nancy A. Denton have implied, the persistence of racial segregation in the United States sets up not only a barrier to a harmonious, multi-hued national community of Americans, but also provides a source of cultural and psychic pollution of its own making: "Until we face up to the difficult task of dismantling the ghetto, the disastrous consequences of residential segregation will radiate outward to poison American society. Until we decide to end the long reign of American apartheid, we cannot hope to move forward as a people and a nation."[170]

A Less-Than-Promising Start: The New Communitarianism

Although the sociologist Amitai Etzioni has recently begun to expound a thesis about a new communitarianism, authored the first draft of "The Responsive Communitarian Platform: Rights and Responsibilities," the revised edition of which was issued on November 18, 1991, and helped to found a social movement in its behalf, its program speaks less to the older ideologies of *Gemeinschaft* than to the social and economic ills of a *Gesellschaft* society gone astray.[171] Etzioni provides a thumbnail history of the recent past that justifies his newfound commitment:

> In the fifties we had a well-established society, but it was unfair to women and minorities and a bit authoritarian. In the sixties we undermined the established society and its values. In the eighties we were told that the unbridled pursuit of self-interest was virtuous. There is now near universal agreement that the resulting world of massive street violence, the failing war against illegal drugs, unbridled greed, and so on—our well-worn list of ills—is not one we wish for our children or, for that matter, ourselves.[172]

Aside from its nostalgia for a mythologized era, the fifties[173] shorn of its authoritarianism, racism, and sexism, a "way we never were,"[174] Etzioni's communitarian organization and its agenda—a five-step program that calls consecutively for (1) shoring up the moral foundations of the family; (2) ensuring that the schools provide education in the proper values; (3) preventing the federal, state, or local governments from usurping the functions of local institutions and helping to sustain the latter by "invest[ing] more of ourselves in one another";[175] (4) embracing a national society that discourages hate crimes and book burning, and accommodates "the cuisines, music, and religious practices of the great variety of subcultures that make up America"[176] (providing, of course, that the adherents of these subcultures "subscribe to a set of overarching values: specifically the democratic process, the Constitution and its Bill of Rights, and the commitment to be respectful of one another");[177] and (5) reforming the civic order: "Individuals' rights are to be matched with social responsibilities . . . [such that] people . . . will have to dedicate more time and energy to participating in local politics and institutions . . . ," submit to drug testing, tolerate sobriety checks, and agree to the testing of their blood for the HIV virus; moreover, "aggrieved citizens [must band] together to clean up politics"[178]—are, in the words of Dean Joan W. Konner of Columbia University's School of Journalism, ". . . one part church sermon, one part reassertion of old values, one part political campaign, and one part social movement."[179] Etzioni concurs with this assessment. Indeed, to the extent that communitarianism in fact is accurately depicted by Dean Konner's statement, it fits in with older modes of reformist social action, characteristic of America since its Puritan beginnings.[180] And, despite the fact that Etzioni's exhortation that "we need to strengthen the communitarian elements in the urban and suburban centers, to provide the social bonds that sustain the moral voice," is immediately followed by a qualification—"but at the same time avoid tight networks that suppress pluralism and dissent"[181]—communitarianism's emphasis on strengthening the moral aspects of family, school, eleemosynary activities, and civic institutions echoes the "culture of discipline" that the eighteenth-century Puritans enforced in their settlements in New England.[182]

But, there is a larger problem. Current displacements of culture and economy have arisen at the same moment that consciousness of race, ethnicity, creed, gender, and sexual preference has surged. These new movements struggle to forge a different kind of community, one that focuses its attention on "events," "scenes," and "memories that flash up in moments of danger."[183] As Homi K. Bhabha points out, "These are the spaces through which minorities translate their dominant designations of difference—gender, ethnicity, class—into a solidarity that refuses both the binary politics of polarity, or the necessity of a homogeneous, unitary oppositional 'bloc.'"[184] Such a community would be different from the *Gemeinschaft* sought by Etzioni and his followers. It would, instead, resonate with what the postmodern geographer Yi-Fu Tuan calls the "protean aesthetic" that is one component of America's ideology of democracy.[185] Those who would accept it, Tuan observes, "must have an appetite for plenitude and contrarieties—for order and disorder, the grand and the comely, an overarching unity of purpose, and, within it, teeming voices that offer simultaneously division and new life."[186] Building such a community requires prior construction of a broadened culture of citizenship—and a reconceptualization of culture[187]—one suited to the twenty-first century and the contingencies of the postmodern era that it will characterize.[188]

Notes

Introduction

The epigrams heading this introduction are from Karl Mannheim, *Ideology and Utopia: An Introduction to the Sociology of Knowledge,* trans. Louis Wirth and Edward Shils (New York: Harcourt, Brace and Co., 1953), p. 188; and Tony Judt, "The Past Is Another Country: Myth and Memory in Postwar Europe," in *The Politics of Retribution in Europe: World War II and Its Aftermath,* ed. István Deák, Jan T. Gross, and Tony Judt (Princeton, N.J.: Princeton University Press, 2000), p. 315.

1. William Graham Sumner, *Folkways: A Study of the Sociological Importance of Usages, Manners, Customs, Mores, and Morals* (Boston: Ginn and Co., 1940 [1906]), p. 78.

2. Richard Hofstadter, *The Age of Reform: From Bryan to F.D.R.* (New York: Vintage Books, 1960).

3. Charles Howard Hopkins, *The Rise of the Social Gospel in American Protestantism, 1865–1915* (New Haven, Conn.: Yale University Press, 1940); Paul A. Carter, *The Decline and Revival of the Social Gospel: Social and Political Liberalism in American Protestant Churches, 1920–1940* (Hamden, Conn.: Archon Books, 1971 [1956]); and Mina Carson, *Settlement Folk: Social Thought and the American Settlement Movement, 1885–1930* (Chicago: University of Chicago Press, 1990).

4. Stanford M. Lyman, "Social Theory and Social Movements: Sociology as Sociodicy," in idem, ed., *Social Movements: Critiques, Concepts, Case Studies* (New York: New York University Press, 1995), pp. 397–435.

5. Alan Brinkley, *The Unfinished Nation: A Concise History of the American People,* 2d ed. (New York: Alfred A. Knopf, 1997), pp. 487–558, 581–632, 657–731, 803–60, 896–915, 930–49.

6. Richard Hofstadter, *The Paranoid Style in American Politics and Other Essays* (New York: Alfred A. Knopf, 1965).

7. Todd Gitlin, *The Twilight of Common Dreams: Why America Is Wracked by Culture Wars* (New York: Metropolitan Books, Henry Holt and Co., 1995).

8. Harold K. Bush Jr., *American Declarations: Rebellion and Repentance in American Cultural History* (Urbana: University of Illinois Press, 1999).

9. David Hollinger, *In the American Province: Studies in the History and Historiography of Ideas* (Baltimore: Johns Hopkins University Press, 1985), pp. 1–43, 167–75.

10. George Lundberg, *Can Science Save Us?* 2d ed. (New York: David McKay, 1961).

11. See two works by Jeffrey C. Alexander: *Theoretical Logic in Sociology, Vol. 4: The Modern Reconstruction of Classical Thought: Talcott Parsons* (Berkeley: University of

California Press, 1983); and *Twenty Lectures: Sociological Theory since World War II* (New York: Columbia University Press, 1987).

12. Quoted from Richard Hofstadter's essay, "Reflections on Violence in the United States," in Alan Brinkley, *Liberalism and Its Discontents* (Cambridge, Mass: Harvard University Press, 1998), p. 150.

13. Marshall Berman, *All That Is Solid Melts into Air: The Experience of Modernity* (New York: Penguin Books, 1988 [1982]).

14. Modris Eksteins, *Walking since Daybreak: A Story of Eastern Europe, World War II, and the Heart of Our Century* (Boston: Houghton Mifflin, 1999), pp. x–xi.

15. See Stanford M. Lyman, *Postmodernism and a Sociology of the Absurd and Other Essays on the 'Nouvelle Vague' in American Social Science* (Fayetteville: University of Arkansas Press, 1997), pp. 1–7 et passim; and Scott Lash, *Another Modernity, a Different Rationality* (Oxford, U.K.: Blackwell Publishers, Ltd., 1999), pp. 1–16, 312–46.

16. Eksteins, op. cit., p. xi.

17. See, e.g., Madan Sarup, *An Introductory Guide to Post-Structuralism and Postmodernism,* 2d ed. (Athens: University of Georgia Press, 1993), pp. 129–60.

18. Geoffrey Hawthorn, *Enlightenment and Despair: A History of Sociology* (Cambridge, U.K.: Cambridge University Press, 1976), pp. 8–27, 164–260.

19. See Robert J. Antonio, "Mapping Postmodern Social Theory," in Alan Sica, ed., *What Is Social Theory? The Philosophical Debates* (Oxford, U.K.: Blackwell Publishers, 1998), pp. 22–75.

20. See Lyman, *Postmodernism and a Sociology of the Absurd . . .*, op. cit., pp. 234–35, and Barry Smart, *Postmodernity* (London: Routledge, 1993).

21. See Pauline Marie Rosenau, *Post-Modernism and the Social Sciences: Insights, Inroads, and Intrusions* (Princeton, N.J.: Princeton University Press, 1992).

22. Alan Wolfe, "The Two Faces of Social Science," in Kai Erikson, ed., *Sociological Visions* (Lanham, Md.: Rowman and Littlefield Publishers, 1997), pp. 31–56. Quoted material from p. 51.

23. Zygmunt Bauman, "Is There a Postmodern Sociology," *Theory, Culture and Society* 5:2–3 (1998): 232. This essay is reprinted in Zygmunt Bauman, *Intimations of Postmodernity* (London: Routledge, 1992), pp. 93–113.

24. These terms are taken from J. Fekete, *Life after Postmodernism: Essays on Value and Culture* (London: Macmillan, 1988).

25. Smart, *Postmodernity* (London: Routledge, 1993), p. 65.

26. Charles Lemert, *Postmodernism Is Not What You Think* (Oxford, U.K.: Blackwell Publishers, 1997), pp. 19–53.

27. Ibid., p. 53.

28. Charles Lemert, *Social Things: An Introduction to the Sociological Life* (Lanham, Md.: Rowman and Littlefield Publishers, 1997), p. 191.

29. Jean-Francois Lyotard, *The Postmodern Explained: Correspondence, 1982–1985,* translations ed. Julian Pefanis and Morgan Thomas (Minneapolis: University of Minnesota Press, 1992), pp. 1–38.

30. Alan Sica, "Theory Then/Theory Now (or, 'The Sociology Is about to Begin,

Said the Man with the Loudspeaker'")," in Stephen P. Turner, ed., *Social Theory and Sociology: The Classics and Beyond* (Oxford, U.K.: Blackwell Publishers Ltd., 1996), pp. 256–73. Quoted material from p. 273.

31. See, e.g., the following works by Lyotard: *The Postmodern Condition: A Report on Knowledge,* trans. Geoff Bennington and Brian Massumi (Minneapolis: University of Minnesota Press, 1984); with Jean-Louis Thebaud, *Just Gaming,* trans. Wlad Godzich (Minneapolis: University of Minnesota Press, 1985); *Phenomenology,* trans. Brian Beakley (Albany: State University of New York Press, 1991); *The Differend: Phrases in Dispute,* trans. Georges Van Den Abbeele (Minneapolis: University of Minnesota Press, 1988, 1992); *The Postmodern Explained,* op. cit.; *Libidinal Economy,* trans. Iain Hamilton Grant (Bloomington: Indiana University Press, 1993); *Political Writings,* trans. Bill Readings and Kevin Paul (Minneapolis: University of Minnesota Press, 1993); *Lessons on the Analytic of the Sublime,* trans. Elizabeth Rottenberg, ed. Werner Hamacher and David E. Wellbery (Stanford, Calif.: Stanford University Press, 1994); and *Postmodern Fables,* trans. Georges Van Den Abbeele (Minneapolis: University of Minnesota Press, 1997).

32. Jean-Francois Lyotard, "Universal History and Cultural Differences," in Andrew Benjamin, ed., *The Lyotard Reader* (Oxford, U.K.: Basil Blackwell, 1989), pp. 314–23. Quoted material from p. 323.

33. Chris Jenks, *Culture* (London: Routledge, 1993), p. 137.

34. Jeffrey C. Alexander, *Fin de Siècle Social Theory: Relativism, Reduction and the Problem of Reason* (London: Verso, 1995), pp. 65–89. Quoted material from pp. 65 and 84.

35. Leslie C. Berlowitz, "Introduction," in *America in Theory,* ed. Leslie Berlowitz, Denis Donoghue, and Louis Menand (New York: Oxford University Press, 1988), p. ix.

36. See the essays collected in Homi K. Bhabha, ed., *Nation and Narration* (London: Routledge, 1990).

37. See Seymour Martin Lipset, *The First New Nation: The United States in Historical and Comparative Perspective* (New York: W. W. Norton, 1979).

38. Gunnar Myrdal, *An American Dilemma* (New York: Harper and Brothers, 1944).

39. Charles Lemert, "Dark Thoughts about the Self," in idem, ed., *Social Theory and the Politics of Identity* (Oxford, U.K.: Basil Blackwell, 1994), pp. 100–129. Quoted material from p. 107.

40. Lyman, *Postmodernism and a Sociology of the Absurd . . . ,* op. cit., pp. 83–162, 185–209.

41. Gitlin, op. cit., p. 218. For evidence of a new and more virulent racist extremism, see "Special Report: Extremism in the New Millennium," *The Intelligence Report,* Southern Poverty Law Center, Issue no. 97 (winter 2000), pp. 1–61.

42. Angela E. Oh, "Reaching toward Our Highest Aspirations: The President's Initiative on Race," in Paul M. Ong, ed., *The State of Asian America: Transforming Race Relations—A Public Policy Report* (Los Angeles: Leadership Education for Asian Pacifics and the UCLA Asian American Studies Center, 2000), pp. 475–94. Quoted material from pp. 477 and 479.

43. Yen Le Espiritu and Michael Omi, "'Who Are You Calling Asian?': Shifting

Identity Claims, Racial Classifications, and the Census," in Ong, ed., op. cit., pp. 43–102.

44. See Doobo Shim, "From Yellow Peril through Model Minority to Renewed Yellow Peril," *Journal of Communication Inquiry* 22:4 (October 1998). Reprinted in Barbara Mori, ed, *Stand! Race and Ethnicity: Contending Ideas and Opinions* (Bellevue, Calif.: Coursewise Publishing, 2000), pp. 93–106; and Robert G. Lee, "Fu Manchu Lives! Asian Pacific Americans as Permanent Aliens in American Culture," in Ong, ed., op. cit., pp. 159–87.

45. See David Yen-ho Wu, "The Construction of Chinese and Non-Chinese Identities," in Tu Wei-ming, ed., *The Living Tree: The Changing Meaning of Being Chinese Today* (Stanford, Calif.: Stanford University Press, 1991), pp. 148–66.

46. See four essays in Michael L. Krenn, ed., *Race and U.S. Foreign Policy from 1900 through World War II* (New York: Garland Publishing Co., 1998): David J. Hellwig, "Afro-American Reactions to the Japanese and the Anti-Japanese Movement, 1906–1924," pp. 175–86; John W. Dower, "Yellow, Red and Black Men," pp. 215–56; Christopher Thorne, "Racial Aspects of the Far Eastern War of 1941–1945," pp. 257–306; Richard H. Minear, "Cross-Cultural Perception and World War II: American Japanists of the 1940s and Their Images of Japan," pp. 307–32.

47. See Morrison G. Wong, "Post-1965 Asian Immigrants: Where Do They Come From, Where Are They Now, and Where Are They Going?" in Franklin Ng, ed., *The History and Immigration of Asian Americans* (New York: Garland Publishing, 1998), pp. 202–20.

48. See Franklin Ng, ed., *Asians in America: The Peoples of East, Southeast, and South Asia* (New York: Garland Publishing, 1998), 6 vols.; and Charles McClain, ed., *Asian Americans and the Law: Historical and Contemporary Perspectives* (New York: Garland Publishing, 1994), 4 vols.

49. See L. Ling-chi Wang, "Roots and the Changing Identity of the Chinese in the United States," in Tu Wei-ming, ed., op. cit., pp. 185–212.

50. See Timothy P. Fong, *The Contemporary Asian American Experience: Beyond the Model Minority* (Upper Saddle River, N.J.: Prentice Hall, 1998), pp. 233–43.

51. Andrew Gyory, *Closing the Gate: Race, Politics, and the Chinese Exclusion Act* (Chapel Hill: University of North Carolina Press, 1998).

52. For an earlier example of this argument, see Philip S. Foner and Daniel Rosenberg, eds., *Racism, Dissent, and Asian Americans from 1850 to the Present: A Documentary History* (Westport, Conn.: Greenwood Press, 1993), pp. 5–11, 165–208.

53. David Roediger, *The Wages of Whiteness: Race and the Making of the American Working Class,* rev. ed. (London: Verso, 1999).

54. Jerry Kang, "Cyber-Race," *Harvard Law Review* 113:5 (March 2000): 1130–1208. Quoted material from pp. 1138 and 1153–54.

55. On Orientalism, a term too often associated only with Edward W. Said's *Orientalism* (New York: Pantheon Books, 1978), see Bernard Lewis, *Islam and the West* (New York: Oxford University Press, 1993), pp. 99–132; and Bryan S. Turner, *Orientalism, Postmodernism and Globalism* (London: Routledge, 1994), pp. 3–76, 95–104.

56. Neil Gotanda, "Exclusion and Inclusion: Immigration and American Orientalism," in Evelyn Hu-DeHart, ed., *Across the Pacific: Asian Americans and Globalization* (Philadelphia: Temple University Press, 1999), pp. 129–51. Quoted material from p. 149.

57. Lee, op. cit., pp. 184–85.

58. Keith Tester, *The Life and Times of Post-modernity* (London: Routledge, 1993), p. 78.

59. Of course, long before the emergence of the postmodernist critique, the only occasionally recognized school of historical thought associated with such figures as Frederick Teggart, Margaret Hodgen, Robert Nisbet, and Kenneth Bock had appraised developmentalist epistemologies in the disciplines of history, sociology, and anthropology. See two works by Stanford M. Lyman, *Civilization: Contents, Discontents, Malcontents and Other Essays in Social Theory* (Fayetteville: University of Arkansas Press, 1990), pp. 76–126, 191–249; and *Postmodernism and a Sociology of the Absurd,* op. cit., pp. 43–65.

60. Dorothy Ross, "The New and Newer Histories: Social Theory and Historiography in an American Key," in Anthony Molko and Gordon S. Wood, eds., *Imagined Histories: American Historians Interpret the Past* (Princeton, N.J.: Princeton University Press, 1998), pp. 85–106. Quoted material from p. 98.

61. Tudor Parfitt, *Operation Moses: The Untold Story of the Secret Exodus of the Falasha Jews from Ethiopia* (New York: Stein and Day, 1985), pp. 6, 17, 25–26, 98. See also Louis Rapoport, *Redemption Song: The Story of Operation Moses* (San Diego, Calif.: Harcourt, Brace, Jovanovich, 1986); Claire Safran, *Secret Exodus: The Untold Story of How Operation Moses Saved the Lost Tribe of Ethiopian Jews* (New York: Prentice-Hall, 1987); and Ruth Gruber, *Rescue: The Exodus of the Ethiopian Jews* (New York: Atheneum, 1987).

62. For the concept "intrusion," see Frederick Teggart, *Theory of History* (New Haven, Conn.: Yale University Press, 1925), pp. 71–197.

63. Simcha Shtull-Traurung, "Letters from beyond the Sambatyon," in idem, ed., *Letters from beyond the Sambatyon: The Myth of the Ten Lost Tribes* (New York: Maxima New Media Ltd., 1997), p. 7.

64. "Eldad the Danite to the Jews of Spain 883," in Shtull-Traurung, ed., op. cit., pp. 18–24.

65. Ibid., pp. 25–56.

66. See Lee Eldridge Huddleston, *Origins of the American Indians: European Concepts, 1492–1729* (Austin: University of Texas Press, 1967), pp. 33–51, 69–71, 85–94, 113–14, 120–35.

67. Cf. Alan Dundes, ed., *The Flood Myth* (Berkeley: University of California Press, 1988; William Ryan and Walter Pitman, *Noah's Flood: The New Scientific Discoveries about the Event That Changed History* (New York: Simon and Schuster, Touchstone, 1998); Ronald L. Numbers, *The Creationists: The Evolution of Scientific Creationism* (New York: Alfred A. Knopf, 1992), passim; and J. Leitch Wright Jr., *The Only Land They Knew: American Indians in the Old South* (Lincoln: University of Nebraska Press, Bison Books, 1999), pp. 176–78.

68. Menasseh Ben Israel, "The Hope of Israel," in Lynn Glaser, *Indians or Jews? An Introduction* (Gilroy, Calif.: Roy V. Boswell, 1973), pp. 3–72. See Cecil Roth, *A Life of Menasseh Ben Israel: Rabbi, Printer, and Diplomat* (Philadelphia: Jewish Publication Society of America, 1934), pp. 176–290; and David S. Katz, *The Jews in the History of England, 1485–1850* (Oxford, U.K.: Clarendon Press, 1996), pp. 107–89.

69. James Adair, *Adair's History of the American Indians,* ed. S. C. Williams (New York: Promontory Press, 1930 [1775]).

70. Elias Boudinot, *A Star in the West; or, A Humble Attempt to Discover the Long Lost Ten Tribes of Israel, Preparatory to Their Return to Their Beloved City, Jerusalem* (Freeport, N.Y.: Books for Libraries Press, 1970 [1816]).

71. See Abraham J. Karp, guest curator, *Mordecai Manuel Noah/The First American Jew,* catalogue (New York: Yeshiva University Museum, 1987), pp. 55–66; Isaac Goldberg, *Major Noah: American-Jewish Pioneer* (Philadelphia: Jewish Publication Society of America, 1936), pp. 189–215; and Jonathan D. Sarna, *Jacksonian Jew: The Two Worlds of Mordecai Noah* (New York: Holmes and Meier Publishers, 1981), pp. 48, 63–70, 135–37.

72. Erich Kahler, "The Jews in Europe," trans. Alexander and Elizabeth Henderson, written in 1945, but first published in idem, *The Jews among the Nations* (New York: Frederick Ungar Publishing Co., 1967), pp. 31–94. Quoted material from p. 94.

73. See Rabbi Eliyahu Avichail, *The Tribes of Israel: The Lost and the Dispersed* (Jerusalem: Amishav, 1990). For examples of evangelical Christian responses, see Steven M. Collins, *The "Lost" Ten Tribes of Israel . . . Found!* rev. ed. (Boring, Oreg.: CPA Books, 1995); and George S. McAchran, *Lost Tribes of Israel* (West Lynn, Oreg.: M and M Publishing, 1993, 1997). For a Mormon perspective, see R. Clayton Brough, *The Lost Tribes: History, Doctrine, Prophecies, and Theories about Israel's Lost Ten Tribes* (Bountiful, Utah: Horizon Publishers, 1979, 1994).

74. Rabbi I. Harold Sharfman, *Jews on the Frontier: An Account of Jewish Pioneers and Settlers in Early America* (Malibu, Calif.: Joseph Simon/Pangloss Press, 1977), pp. 216–17.

75. See the discussion: Anthony Pagden, *The Fall of Natural Man: The American Indian and the Origins of Comparative Ethnology* (Cambridge, U.K.: Cambridge University Press, 1982); Alden T. Vaughan, *Roots of American Racism: Essays on the Colonial Experience* (New York: Oxford University Press, 1995), pp. 10, 49–57, 275 n. 69; Sacvan Bercovitch, *The Puritan Origins of the American Self* (New Haven, Conn.: Yale University Press, 1975), pp. 35–71, 136–86, 230–33.

76. See "Israel Dumps Donor Blood," *Palm Beach Post,* January 25, 1996, p. 3A; and two reports by Serge Schemann, "Ethiopians in Israel Riot over Dumping of Donated Blood," *New York Times,* January 29, 1996, p. A3; and "Israel and the Ethiopians: Welcoming Newcomers Is Not So Easy," *New York Times Week in Review,* February 4, 1996, p. 3. See also two works by William Safire, "Essay: Helping the Black Jews," *New York Times,* Op-Ed page, September 9, 1996, p. A15: and "Essay: Israel's Ethiopian Challenge," *New York Times,* Op-Ed page, July 2, 1997, p. A17. For some success stories, see Larry Derfner,"Israel's Newest Yuppies," *The Jerusalem Post,* No. 2018, July 9, 1999, p. 7.

On July 28, 1996, Israel's Navon Commission, appointed on February 13, 1996, to investigate the issue of blood donations by members of the Ethiopian community, issued a report finding flaws in the Ministry of Health's and the Blood Bank's decision-making processes and recommending the establishment of an inter-ministerial information team. See "Blood Bank: All Decisions Regarding Ethiopian Blood Made for Purely Medical Reasons," *Information Division, Israel Foreign Ministry,* March 10, 1996. URL: http://www.israel-mfa.gov.il; and "Summary of Navon Commission Report on Blood Donations by Ethiopian Immigrants," *Information Division, Israel Foreign Ministry,* July 29, 1996. URL: http://www.israel-mfa.gov.il.

77. Micha Oldenheimier, "The Next Dilemma," *Jerusalem Report* 10:6 (July 19, 1999): 33–35; "Decision Time in Ethiopia," *Jerusalem Post,* No. 2058, April 14, 2000, pp. 2, 32; Ian Fisher, "Tangling of Jewish Roots Bars Ethiopians from Israel," *New York Times,* April 19, 2000, p. A3; and "Out of Addis," *Jerusalem Post,* No. 2059, April 21, 2000, pp. 4–5.

78. James Benson, "The Call of Samaria," *Jerusalem Post,* No. 2058, April 14, 2000, pp. 16–17.

79. For various analyses of the status and situation of the Ethiopian Jews, see Louis Rapoport, *The Lost Jews: Last of the Ethiopian Falashas* (New York: Stein and Day, 1980); Simon D. Messing, *The Story of the Falashas: "Black Jews" of Ethiopia* (New York: Balshon Printing and Offset Co., 1982); Tudor Parfitt, *The Thirteenth Gate: Travels among the Lost Tribes of Israel* (Bethesda, Md.: Adler and Adler, 1987), pp. 120–48; Michael Ashkenazi and Alex Weingrod, eds., *Ethiopian Jews and Israel* (New Brunswick, N.J.: Transaction Books, 1987); Steven Kaplan, *The Beta Israel (Falasha) in Ethiopia: From Earliest Times to the Twentieth Century* (New York: New York University Press, 1992); Dr. Ruth Westheimer and Dr. Steven Kaplan, *Surviving Salvation: The Ethiopian Jewish Family in Transition* (New York: New York University Press, 1992); Teshome G. Wagaw, *For Our Soul: Ethiopian Jews in Israel* (Detroit, Mich.: Wayne State University Press, 1993); David Kessler, *The Falashas: A Short History of the Ethiopian Jews,* 3d ed., rev. (London: Frank Cass, 1996); Tudor Parfitt and Emanuela Trevisan Semi, eds., *The Beta Israel in Ethiopia and Israel: Studies on the Ethiopian Jews* (Richmond, Surrey, U.K.: Curzon Press, 1999); and Ken Blady, *Jewish Communities in Exotic Places* (Northvale, N.J.: Jason Aronson, 2000), pp. 347–402. For earlier background, see James A. Quirin, *The Evolution of the Ethiopian Jews: A History of the Beta Israel (Falasha) to 1920* (Philadelphia: University of Pennsylvania Press, 1992).

80. Hagar Salamon, *The Hyena People: Ethiopian Jews in Christian Ethiopia* (Berkeley: University of California Press, 1999), p. 124.

81. For critical discussions, see Juliet Steyn, *The Jew: Assumptions of Identity* (London: Cassell, 1999), and Laurence J. Silberstein, *The Postzionism Debates: Knowledge and Power in Israeli Culture* (New York: Routledge, 1999), esp. pp. 1–46, 165–206.

82. The bases for these critiques in fact preceded the rise of postmodernism by several decades and should be credited to the rise of scientific thought catalyzed by the Enlightenment. See e.g., Jacques Barzun, *Race: A Study in Superstition,* rev. ed. (New York: Harper Torchbooks, 1965); Elazar Barkan, *The Retreat of Scientific Racism:*

Changing Concepts of Race in Britain and the United States between the World Wars (Cambridge, U.K.: Cambridge University Press, 1992); William H. Tucker, *The Science and Politics of Racial Research* (Urbana: University of Illinois Press, 1994); Thomas F. Gossett, *Race: The History of an Idea in America,* new ed. (New York: Oxford University Press, 1997); and Ashley Montagu, *Man's Most Dangerous Myth: The Fallacy of Race,* 6th ed. (Walnut Creek, Calif.: Altamira Press, 1997).

83. See Nicholas Wade, "The Human Family Tree: 10 Adams and 18 Eves—Tracing Human History through Genetic Mutations," *New York Times,* Science Times section, May 2, 2000, pp. D1, D5.

84. Tudor Parfitt, *Journey to the Vanished City: The Search for a Lost Tribe of Israel* (Phoenix, Ariz.: Hodder and Stoughton, 1997), pp. 343–45; Nicholas Wade, "DNA Backs a Tribe's Tradition of Early Descent from the Jews," *New York Times,* May 9, 1999, pp. 1, 20; Max Amichai Heppner, "Science Ties the Lemba Closer to Mainstream Jews," *Kulanu* 6:2 (summer 1999): 1, 13; and Hillel Halkind, "An African 'Lost Tribe' Comes to TV," *Forward* 102:31, 275 (February 11, 2000), p. 11.

85. Steyn, op. cit. See also David R. Blumenthal, *The Banality of Good and Evil: Moral Lessons from the Shoah and Jewish Tradition* (Washington, D.C.: Georgetown University Press, 1999).

86. Steyn, op. cit., pp. 13–18.

87. See Peter Jackson, *Maps of Meaning: An Introduction to Cultural Geography* (London: Routledge, 1994).

88. See Patricia Yaeger, ed., *The Geography of Identity* (Ann Arbor: University of Michigan Press, 1996).

89. Geoffrey Hawthorn, Gayatri Chakravorty Spivak, Ron Aronson, and John Dunn, "The Post-modern Condition: The End of Politics?" in Gayatri Chakravorty Spivak, *The Post-Colonial Critic: Interviews, Strategies, Dialogues,* ed. Sara Harasym (New York: Routledge, 1990), pp. 17–34.

90. Charlene Spretnak, *States of Grace: The Recovery of Meaning in the Postmodern Age* (New York: Harper Collins, 1993), p. 11.

91. See Don H. Zimmerman and Melvin Pollner, "The Everyday World as Phenomenon," in Jack D. Douglas, ed., *Understanding Everyday Life: Toward the Reconstruction of Sociological Knowledge* (Chicago: Aldine Publishing Co., 1970), pp. 80–103.

92. See two works by Stanford M. Lyman and Marvin B. Scott: *A Sociology of the Absurd* (New York: Appleton-Century-Crofts, 1970); 2d ed. (Dix Hills, N.Y.: General Hall, 1989); and *The Drama of Social Reality* (New York: Oxford University Press, 1975).

93. See Steven Galt, "Who Is the Political Actor? An Existential-Phenomenological Approach," in Kevin Thompson and Lester Embree, eds., *Phenomenology of the Political* (Dordrecht, The Netherlands: Kluwer Academic Publishers, 2000), pp. 11–28.

94. See Marvin B. Scott and Stanford M. Lyman, *The Revolt of the Students* (Columbus, Ohio: Charles Merrill Publishing Co., 1970).

95. Lyman and Scott, *The Drama of Social Reality,* op. cit., pp. 101–62.

96. Stanford M. Lyman, "The Drama in the Routine: A Prolegomenon to a

Praxiological Sociology," *Social Theory* 8:2 (fall 1990): 217–23; reprinted in idem, *Postmodernism and a Sociology of the Absurd . . .*, op. cit., pp. 286–94, 383–85.

97. See Robert D. Benford and Scott A. Hunt, "Dramaturgy and Social Movements: The Social Construction and Communication of Power," in Stanford M. Lyman, ed., *Social Movements: Critiques, Concepts, Case Studies* (New York: New York University Press, 1995), pp. 84–112; and Daniel Cefai, "Making Sense of Politics in Public Spaces: The Phenomenology of Political Experiences and Activities," in Lester Embree, ed., *Schutzian Social Science* (Dordrecht, The Netherlands: Kluwer Academic Publishers, 1999), pp. 135–58.

98. Edward W. Soja, *Thirdspace: Journeys to Los Angeles and Other Real-and-Imagined Places* (Cambridge, Mass.: Blackwell's Publishing Co., 1996).

99. Herbert Blumer, "Moulding of Mass Behavior through the Motion Picture," *Publications of the American Sociological Society* 29 (August 1935): 115–27.

100. Beverly Merrill Kelley with John J. Pitney, Craig R. Smith, and Herbert E. Gooch III, *Reelpolitik: Political Ideologies in '30s and '40s Films* (Westport, Conn.: Praeger Publishers, 1998), p. 2.

101. Lyman, *Postmodernism and a Sociology of the Absurd,* op. cit., pp. 230–33.

102. See Steve Vineberg, "'American Beauty': No Joy in the Gilded Suburbs," *Chronicle of Higher Education* 46:10 (October 29, 1999): B10.

103. Alfred Schutz, *The Phenomenology of the Social World,* trans. George Walsh and Frederick Lehnert (Evanston, Ill.: Northwestern University Press, 1967), pp. 139–214.

104. Sigmund Freud, *The Future of an Illusion,* trans. W.D. Robson-Scott (Garden City, N.Y.: Doubleday, Anchor Books, 1957), p. 99.

105. See David J. Skal, *Screams of Reason: Mad Science and Modern Culture* (New York: W. W. Norton, 1998), p. 317.

106. Maurice R. Stein, *The Eclipse of Community: An Interpretation of American Studies* (Princeton, N.J.: Princeton University Press, 1960).

107. Ibid., p. 329.

108. J. Hector St. John de Crèvecoeur, *Letters from an American Farmer* (New York: E. P. Dutton, 1957 [1782]), pp. 35–82.

109. Israel Zangwill, *The Melting Pot: Drama in Four Acts,* new and rev. ed. (New York: Macmillan, 1922 [1909]), esp. pp. 184–85.

110. Horace Kallen, *Culture and Democracy in the United States: Studies in the Group Psychology of the American Peoples* (New York: Boni and Liveright, 1924; reprint, New York: Arno Press and the *New York Times,* 1970).

111. Randolph S. Bourne, *War and the Intellectuals: Collected Essays,* 1915–1919, ed. Carl Resek (New York: Harper Torchbooks, 1964), pp. 107–33.

112. Michael W. Hughey and Arthur J. Vidich, "Ethnicity and Community in America," in idem, eds., *The Ethnic Quest for Community: Searching for Roots in the Lonely Crowd,* Research in Community Sociology, vol. 3 (Greenwich, Conn.: JAI Press, 1993), pp. 3–14. Quoted material from p. 7.

113. Gian Biagio Conte, *The Rhetoric of Imitation: Genre and Poetic Memory in Virgil*

and Other Latin Poets, trans. Charles Segal (Ithaca, N.Y.: Cornell University Press, 1986), pp. 23–24.

114. Henrik de Man, *Vermassung und Kulturverfall: Eine Diagnose unserer Zeit,* p. 136, a book published in Bern in 1951. The English translation is taken from Wolf Lepenies, *Melancholy and Society,* trans. Jeremy Gaines and Doris Jones (Cambridge, Mass.: Harvard University Press, 1992), p. 183.

115. See Frank E. Manuel and Fritzie P. Manuel, *Utopian Thought in the Western World* (Cambridge, Mass.: Belknap Press of Harvard University Press, 1979).

116. Jean-Francois Lyotard, *The Postmodern Condition: A Report on Knowledge,* op. cit., p. xxiv.

117. Georg Simmel, *The Conflict in Modern Culture and Other Essays,* trans. Peter Etzkorn (New York: Teacher's College Press, 1968), pp. 11–46.

Chapter One. Gunnar Myrdal's *An American Dilemma* after a Half Century: Critics and Anticritics

1. The first paragraph of this introduction is adapted from the first page of an earlier essay of mine, "Gunnar Myrdal's *An American Dilemma,*" published as chapter 4 of my book, *The Black American in Sociological Thought: A Failure of Perspective* (New York: G. P. Putnam's Sons, 1972), p. 99. In that essay (pp. 99–120) I offered a critique of Myrdal's study, making the point that the Swedish scholar had not moved sufficiently far from the conceptual frameworks of the American social scientists whom he criticizes, that his mechanistic model of cumulative causation has much in common with the evolutionary functionalist approaches that he repudiates, and that his thesis about the American Creed fails to heed the possibility that the average white American might find no difficulty in maintaining the contradictory ethos of racism alongside his or her commitment to the Creed.

2. Gunnar Myrdal, with the assistance of Richard Sterner and Arnold Rose, *An American Dilemma: The Negro Problem and Modern Democracy* (New York: Harper and Brothers, 1944), p. xlvi.

3. Ibid., pp. xlvii–xlviii.

4. Ibid., p. liii.

5. Ibid., p. liv.

6. Ibid., p. lv.

7. Loc. cit.

8. Richard Swedberg, "Introduction to the Transaction Edition," in Gunnar Myrdal, *The Political Element in the Development of Economic Theory,* trans. Paul Streeter (New Brunswick, N.J.: Transaction Publishers, 1990), pp. vii–xxxvii. The first edition was published in London by Routledge and Kegan Paul, Ltd., in 1953.

9. Gunnar Myrdal, "Gunnar Myrdal's *An American Dilemma*—Has It Been Resolved?" *Worldview* (December 1972). Reprinted in Gunnar Myrdal, *Against the Stream: Critical Essays on Economics* (New York: Vintage, 1975), pp. 293–307.

10. Sissela Bok, "Foreword," *An American Dilemma Revisited: Race Relations in a*

Changing World, ed. Obie Clayton Jr. (New York: Russell Sage Foundation, 1996), pp. xi–xxii.

11. For two differing accounts of the Carnegie sponsorship, see John H. Stanfield, *Philanthropy and Jim Crow in American Social Science* (Westport, Conn.: Greenwood Press, 1985), pp. 139–84; and Walter A. Jackson, *Gunnar Myrdal and America's Conscience: Social Engineering and Racial Liberalism, 1938–1987* (Chapel Hill: University of North Carolina Press, 1990), pp. 10–35.

12. See Herbert Aptheker, with an "Introduction" by Doxey A. Wilkerson, *The Negro People in America: A Critique of Gunnar Myrdal's* "An American Dilemma" (New York: International Publishers, 1946).

13. Stephen Graubard, "An American Dilemma Revisited," in Clayton Jr., ed., op. cit., p. 2.

14. Ralph Bunche, *The Political Status of the Negro in the Age of FDR,* ed. Dewey W. Grantham (Chicago: University of Chicago Press, 1973), pp. 77–78, 212, 254, 311–12, 419, 421, 489, 492, 564, 598, 604–5; Brian Urquhart, *Ralph Bunche: An American Life* (New York: W. W. Norton, 1993), pp. 58–59; Myrdal, *An American Dilemma,* op. cit., pp. 796–97, 831–36, 1405–6.

15. Myrdal, *An American Dilemma,* op. cit., pp. 1035–64.

16. Ibid., pp. 88n, 1031–34, 1048–49, 1053–54.

17. Ibid., pp. 662, 690–91, 1049–51.

18. Ibid., pp. 1388–89 n. 2, 1051–52.

19. Ibid., pp. 1053–54, fn. d.

20. Ibid., pp. 670, 674, 691, 1378, 1384–86.

21. Ibid., p. 1057, fn. a.

22. Ibid., p. 1055.

23. Ibid., p. 1057.

24. Ibid., p. 1064.

25. Loc. cit.

26. Gerald David Jaynes and Robin M. Williams, "Summary and Conclusions," *A Common Destiny: Blacks and American Society,* a report by the Committee on the Status of Black Americans, Commission on Behavioral and Social Sciences and Education, National Research Council (Washington, D.C.: National Academy Press, 1989), p. 4.

27. Reynolds Farley, *The New American Reality: Who We Are, How We Got Here, Where We Are Going* (New York: Russell Sage Foundation, 1996), p. 266.

28. Douglas S. Massey and Nancy A. Denton, *American Apartheid: Segregation and the Making of the Underclass* (Cambridge, Mass.: Harvard University Press, 1993).

29. Farley, op. cit., p. 266.

30. Myrdal, *An American Dilemma,* op. cit., p. 1015.

31. Ibid., p. 1021.

32. Steven A. Holmes, "Scholar Takes on His Toughest Study of Race," *New York Times,* September 28, 1997, pp. 1, 16.

33. See, e.g., George M. Fredrickson, "America's Caste System: Will It Change?" *New York Review of Books* 44 (October 23, 1997): 68–75; Orlando Patterson, *The Ordeal*

of Integration: Progress and Resentment in America's "Racial" Crisis (Washington, D.C.: Civitas/Counterpoint, 1997), esp. pp. 147–204; Nathan Glazer, *We Are All Multiculturalists Now* (Cambridge, Mass.: Harvard University Press, 1997); and Anthony K. Appiah, "The Multiculturalist Misunderstanding," *New York Review of Books* 44 (October 9, 1997): 30–36; John Higham, ed., *Civil Rights and Social Wrongs: Black-White Relations since World War II* (University Park: Pennsylvania State University Press, 1997); and Arthur M. Melzer, Jerry Weinberger, and M. Richard Zinman, eds., *Multiculturalism and American Democracy* (Lawrence: University Press of Kansas, 1998).

34. Celeste Michelle Condit and John Louis Lucaites, *Crafting Equality: America's Anglo-African Word* (Chicago: University of Chicago Press, 1993), esp. pp. 188–232. See also the discussion in Richard Harvey Brown, *Toward a Democratic Science: Scientific Narration and Civic Communication* (New Haven, Conn.: Yale University Press, 1998), esp. pp. 214–26.

35. David W. Southern, op. cit., pp. 127–54, 225–60.

36. Robert C. Smith, *Racism in the Post–Civil Rights Era: Now You See It, Now You Don't* (Albany: State University of New York Press, 1995).

37. See, e.g., David R. Goldfield, *Black, White, and Southern: Race Relations and Southern Culture, 1940 to the Present* (Baton Rouge: Louisiana State University Press, 1990), pp. 3, 7, 13, 29, 119. See also Bertram D. Doyle, *The Etiquette of Race Relations: A Study in Social Control* (New York: Schocken Books, 1971 [1937]).

38. Bunche, op. cit., passim; Urquhart, op. cit., pp. 81–91.

39. Robert R. Edgar, "Prologue," in idem, ed., *An African American in South Africa: The Travel Notes of Ralph J. Bunche, 28 September 1937–1 January 1938* (Athens: Ohio University Press, 1992), p. 23. For Raper's contributions to the race question, see Arthur F. Raper, *Preface to Peasantry: A Tale of Two Black Belt Counties* (New York: Atheneum, 1968 [1936]).

40. See Stanfield, op. cit., pp. 119–38; Richard Robbins, *Sidelines Activist: Charles S. Johnson and the Struggle for Civil Rights* (Jackson: University Press of Mississippi, 1996). For Johnson's own contributions to the understanding of the race question, see Charles S. Johnson and Associates, *To Stem This Tide: A Survey of Racial Tensions in the United States* (New York: AMS Press, 1969 [1943]); *Backgrounds to Patterns of Negro Segregation* (New York: Thomas Y. Crowell, Apollo, 1970 [1943]); *Bitter Canaan: The Story of the Negro Republic* (New Brunswick, N.J.: Transaction Books, 1987).

41. Robbins, op. cit., pp. 207–8 n. 17.

42. Stanfield, op. cit., pp. 170–71.

43. Doxey A. Wilkerson, "Introduction" in Aptheker, op. cit., p. 10.

44. Aptheker, op. cit., p. 66.

45. Oliver Cromwell Cox, *Caste, Class and Race: A Study in Social Dynamics* (New York: Monthly Review Press, 1959), pp. 509–38. Quoted material is from pp. 509 and 538. For discussions of Cox's life and works, see Butler A. Jones, "The Tradition of Sociology Teaching in Black Colleges: The Unheralded Professionals," in James E. Blackwell and Morris Janowitz, eds., *Black Sociologists: Historical and Contemporary Perspectives* (Chicago: University of Chicago Press, 1974), pp. 155–63; and Herbert M.

Hunter and Sameer Y. Abraham, "Introduction: The Life and Career of Oliver C. Cox," in idem, eds., *Race, Class and World System: The Sociology of Oliver C. Cox* (New York: Monthly Review Press, 1987), pp. xvii–1.

46. See Cedric J. Robinson, *Black Marxism: The Making of the Black Radical Tradition* (London: Zed Books, 1983).

47. At a meeting of "a group of representative southern Negroes" in Durham, North Carolina, on October 20, 1942, when World War II was raging, the assembled body urged immediate abolition of the poll tax, abolition of the white primary, "abolition of all forms of discriminatory practices, evasions of the law, and intimidations of citizens seeking to exercise their right of franchise"; discontinuance of exclusion of Negroes from juries; enforcement of civil rights protecting Negroes from police beatings and other abuses; hiring of Negro policemen; enforcement of truly equal separate facilities where the latter have the force of law; enforcement of laws forbidding lynching; appointment of qualified Negroes to positions of social planning and administration; lifting of employment restrictions on Negroes in industry, service, agriculture, and education; industrial training and other education for Negroes; opening opportunities for Negroes in the armed services; improved health and welfare benefits; and a recognition that the "correction of these problems is not only a moral matter but a practical necessity in winning the war and winning the peace."

On April 8, 1943, a "Statement of [the] Conference of White Southerners on Race Relations" acknowledged the truths contained in the Negroes' statement but asserted that "The solution of these problems can be found only in men of both races who are known to be men of determined good will. The ultimate solution will be found in evolutionary methods and not in ill-founded revolutionary movements which promise immediate solutions."

Both statements are found in Johnson, *To Stem This Tide,* op. cit., pp. 131–42.

48. J. Edgar Hoover, "Memorandum to Special Agent Ridgely," October 11, 1919, in William L. Van Deburg ed., *Modern Black Nationalism from Marcus Garvey to Louis Farrakhan* (New York: New York University Press, 1997), p. 33.

For a comprehensive report on the governmental surveillance of African American protests in the 1920s, see Theodore Kornweibel Jr., *Seeing Red: Federal Campaigns against Black Militancy, 1919–1925* (Bloomington: Indiana University Press, 1998).

49. See Howard W. Odum, *Race and Rumors of Race: The American South in the Early Forties* (Baltimore: Johns Hopkins University Press, 1997 [1943]), pp. 142–55.

50. Robert E. Park, "Racial Ideologies," in William Fielding Ogburn, ed., *American Society in Wartime* (Chicago: University of Chicago Press, 1943), pp. 165–84.

51. Patrick S. Washburn, *A Question of Sedition: The Federal Government's Investigation of the Black Press during World War II* (New York: Oxford University Press, 1986), p. 171.

52. Robert A. Hill, comp. and ed., *The FBI's RACON: Racial Conditions in the United States during World War II* (Boston: Northeastern University Press, 1995), p. 75.

53. Athan G. Theoharis and John Stuart Cox, *The Boss: J. Edgar Hoover and the Great American Inquisition* (Philadelphia: Temple University Press, 1998), p. 302n.

54. Clayborne Carson, David J. Garrow, Gerald Gill, Vincent Harding, and Darlene Clark Hine, eds., *The Eyes on the Prize Civil Rights Reader: Documents, Speeches, and First-Hand Accounts from the Black Freedom Struggle, 1954–1990* (New York: Viking, 1991), pp. 500–590; and Kenneth O'Reilly, *"Racial Matters": The FBI's Secret File on Black America, 1960–1972* (New York: Free Press, 1989); and Ward Churchill and Jim Vander Wall, *Agents of Repression: The FBI's Secret Wars against the Black Panther Party and the American Indian Movement* (Boston: South End Press, 1990), pp. 1–102, 353–88.

55. Kenneth O'Reilly, *Black Americans: The FBI Files,* ed. David Gallen (New York: Carroll and Graf Publishers, 1994), pp. 83–129, 130–38, 382–423.

56. David J. Garrow, *The FBI and Martin Luther King, Jr.* (New York: Penguin Books, 1981). For a comprehensive account, see the two published volumes of an as-yet-unfinished trilogy by Taylor Branch: *Parting the Waters: America in the King Years, 1954–1963* (New York: Simon and Schuster, 1988); and *Pillar of Fire: America in the King Years, 1963–1965* (New York: Simon and Schuster, 1998). Four volumes of *The Papers of Martin Luther King,* ed. Clayborne Carson (Berkeley: University of California Press, 1992, 1994, 1997, 2000) have been published. On the FBI's surveillance of King and other civil rights leaders, see Theoharis and Cox, op. cit., pp. 354–78, 411 et passim; Athan Theoharis, ed., *From the Secret Files of J. Edgar Hoover* (Chicago: Ivan R. Dee, 1991), pp. 93–130; Curt Gentry, *J. Edgar Hoover: The Man and the Secrets*(New York: W. W. Norton, 1991), pp. 441–42, 483–85, 501–10, 527–28, 561–86, 606–7; Richard Gid Powers, *G-Men: Hoover's FBI in American Popular Culture* (Carbondale: Southern Illinois University Press, 1983), pp. 265–80; Gerald D. McKnight, *The Last Crusade: Martin Luther King, the FBI, and the Poor People's Campaign* (Boulder, Colo.: Westview Press, 1998).

57. Elijah Muhammad, *Message to the Black Man in America* (Chicago: Muhammad Mosque of Islam, No. 2, 1965); Claude Andrew Clegg III, *An Original Man: The Life and Times of Elijah Muhammad*(New York: St. Martin's Press, 1997); Karl Evanzz, *The Messenger: The Rise and Fall of Elyah Muhammad* (New York: Pantheon, 1999). On the nation of Islam, see E. U. Essien-Udom, *Black Nationalism: A Search for Identity in America* (Chicago: University of Chicago Press, 1962); and C. Eric Lincoln, *The Black Muslims in America,* 3d ed. (Grand Rapids, Mich.: Eerdmans Publishing Co., 1994).

58. *The Autobiography of Malcolm X,* with the assistance of Alex Haley (New York: Grove Press, 1965); Clayton Carson, *Malcolm X: The FBI File* (New York: Carroll and Graf, 1991). On Malcolm X's assassination, see Peter Goldman, *The Death and Life of Malcolm X,* 2d ed. (Urbana: University of Illinois Press, 1979); Karl Evanzz, *The Judas Factor: The Plot to Kill Malcolm X* (New York: Thunder's Mouth Press, 1992).

59. Adam Fairclough, *Race and Democracy: The Civil Rights Struggle in Louisiana, 1915–1972* (Athens: University of Georgia Press, 1995), p. 81. See also Murray Friedman, "The White Liberal's Retreat," in Alan F. Westin, ed., *Freedom Now! The Civil Rights Struggle in America* (New York: Basic Books, 1964), p. 320–28.

60. There is a vast literature on the civil rights movement. Some representative works are: John Egerton, *Speak Now against the Day: The Generation before the Civil*

Rights Movement in the South (New York: Alfred A. Knopf, 1994); Aldon D. Morris, *The Origins of the Civil Rights Movement: Black Communities Organizing for Change* (New York: Free Press, 1984); Charles W. Eagles, ed., *The Civil Rights Movement in America* (Jackson: University Press of Mississippi, 1986); Larry Hampton and Steve Fayer with Sarah Flynn, *Voices of Freedom: An Oral History of the Civil Rights Movement from the 1950s through the 1980s* (New York: Bantam Books, 1990); Fred Powledge, *Free at Last? The Civil Rights Movement and the People Who Made It* (Boston: Little, Brown and Co., 1991); Glen T. Eskew, *But for Birmingham: The Local and National Movement in the Civil Rights Struggle* (Chapel Hill: University of North Carolina Press, 1997); Juan Williams, *Eyes on the Prize: America's Civil Rights Years, 1954–1965* (New York: Viking, 1987); Carson, et al., eds., *The Eyes on the Prize Reader,* op. cit., pp. 1–499, 591–728; Sally Belfrage, *Freedom Summer* (Greenwich, Conn.: Fawcett, 1968); Elizabeth Sutherland, ed., *Letters from Mississippi* (New York: Signet, 1966); Joanne Grant, ed., *Black Protest: 350 Years of History, Documents, and Analyses* (New York: Fawcett Columbine, 1996), pp. 237–482.

61. See Donald B. King and Charles W. Quick, ed., *Legal Aspects of the Civil Rights Movement* (Detroit, Mich.: Wayne State University Press, 1965); Albert P. Blaustein and Robert L. Zangrando, eds., *Civil Rights and the American Negro: A Documentary History* (New York: Washington Square Press, 1968), pp. 355–656; Merl E. Reed, *Seedtime for the Modern Civil Rights Movement: The President's Committee on Fair Employment Practice, 1941–1946* (Baton Rouge: Louisiana State University Press, 1991); Foster Rhea Dulles, *The Civil Rights Commission: 1957–1965* (East Lansing: Michigan State University Press, 1968); Robert D. Loevy, ed., *The Civil Rights Act of 1964: The Passage of the Law That Ended Racial Segregation* (Albany: State University of New York Press, 1997); Hugh Davis Graham, *The Civil Rights Era: Origins and Development of National Policy* (New York: Oxford University Press, 1990).

62. John Dittmer, *Local People: The Struggle for Civil Rights in Mississippi* (Urbana: University of Illinois Press, 1994), p. 83. See also Charles M. Payne, *I've Got the Light of Freedom: The Organizing Tradition and the Mississippi Freedom Struggle* (Berkeley: University of California Press, 1995), and two review essays—Michael W. Hughey, "The Rise and Fall of a People's Movement," pp. 451–58, and Robert Washington, "Reclaiming the Civil Rights Movement," pp. 459–73, both in *International Journal of Politics, Culture, and Society* 9:3 (spring 1996).

63. "Judge Sebe Dale's Charge to the Pearl River County Grand Jury (Poplarville *Democrat,* Nov. 5, 1959) . . . ," Appendix B in Howard Smead, *Blood Justice: The Lynching of Mack Charles Parker* (New York: Oxford University Press, 1986), pp. 208–12. Quotation from p. 210.

64. Myrdal, *An American Dilemma,* op. cit., p. 587.

65. Smead, op. cit., pp. 3–23.

66. Stephen J. Whitfield, *A Death in the Delta: The Story of Emmett Till* (New York: Free Press, 1988).

67. Herman Talmadge, *You and Segregation* (Birmingham, Ala.: Vulcan Press, 1966), p. 42. Quoted in Whitfield, op. cit., p. 9.

68. Myrdal, *An American Dilemma,* op. cit., p. 587.

69. Ibid., op. cit., p. 587–88.

70. By contrast, the activities undertaken by the liberal-minded Columbia-educated sociologist at the University of North Carolina, Howard W. Odum (1884–1954), in behalf of the Southern Negro in the 1930s yielded "few tangible results to show for his decade's service in interracial activities." Daniel Joseph Singal, *The War Within: From Victorian to Modernist Thought in the South, 1919–1945* (Chapel Hill: University of North Carolina Press, 1982), p. 151.

71. Whitfield, op. cit., p. 134.

72. Rhoda Lois Blumberg, *Civil Rights: The 1960s Freedom Struggle,* rev. ed. (Boston: Twayne Publishers, 1991), p. 7.

73. Nicolaus Mills, *Like a Holy Crusade: Mississippi 1964—The Turning of the Civil Rights Movement in America* (Chicago: Ivan R. Dee, 1992). See also William M. Van Deburg, *New Day in Babylon: The Black Power Movement and American Culture, 1965–1975* (Chicago: University of Chicago Press, 1992); Clayborne Carson, *In Struggle: SNCC and the Black Awakening of the 1960s* (Cambridge, Mass.: Harvard University Press, 1995); and David Chappell, *Inside Agitators: White Southerners in the Civil Rights Movement* (Baltimore: Johns Hopkins University Press, 1994).

74. For the assassination of Medgar Evers by Byron de la Beckwith—who, only after three trials, two ending in mistrials, was convicted of the murder in 1994, see Adam Nossiter, *Of Long Memory: Mississippi and the Murder of Medgar Evers* (Reading, Mass.: Addison-Wesley Publishing Co., 1994); and Maryanne Vollers, *Ghosts of Mississippi: The Murder of Medgar Evers, the Trials of Byron de la Beckwith, and the Haunting of the New South* (Boston: Little, Brown and Co., 1995). For de la Beckwith's connection to the Christian Identity Movement, see Reed Massengill, *Portrait of a Racist: The Man Who Killed Medgar Evers?* (New York: St. Martin's Press, 1994), pp. 4–11, 56–62, 91–98, 123–24, 197–98, 250–51, 278–312. For the Christian Identity Movement and its origins in British Israelitism and its affiliation with the Aryan Nation, see O. Michael Friedman, *Origins of the British Israelites: The Lost Tribes* (San Francisco: Mellen Research University Press, 1993); Michael Barkun, *Religion and the Racist Right: The Origins of the Christian Identity Movement,* rev. ed. (Chapel Hill: University of North Carolina Press, 1997); James Ridgeway, *Blood in the Face: The Ku Klux Klan, Aryan Nations, Nazi Skinheads, and the Rise of a New White Culture* (New York: Thunder's Mouth Press, 1991); Morris Dees with James Corcoran, *Gathering Storm: America's Militia Threat* (New York: Harper Collins, 1996); and two works by James A. Aho, *The Politics of Righteousness: Idaho Christian Patriotism* (Seattle: University of Washington Press, 1990); and *This Thing of Darkness: A Sociology of the Enemy* (Seattle: University of Washington Press, 1994). For the effects of Evers's murder on American popular culture, see Willie Morris, *The Ghosts of Medgar Evers: A Tale of Murder, Mississippi, and Hollywood* (New York: Random House, 1998).

75. For the origins and usages of this term, see David Goodman Croly and George Wakeman, *Miscegenation: The Theory of the Blending of the Races Applied to the American White and Negro* (Upper Saddle River, N.J.: Literature Press/Gregg Press,

1970 [1864]); Forrest G . Wood, *Black Scare: The Racist Response to Emancipation and Reconstruction* (Berkeley: University of California Press, 1968), pp. 53–79; Ashley Montagu, "Appendix B: The Term 'Miscegenation,'" *Man's Most Dangerous Myth: The Fallacy of Race,* 5th ed. (New York: Oxford University Press, 1974), pp. 445–47. For Myrdal's discussion, see *An American Dilemma,* op. cit., pp. 105–6, 113, 123–27, 135, 586–87, 607, 696–98, 1197, 1203–12.

76. Myrdal, *An American Dilemma,* op. cit., pp. 60–67.

77. *Loving vs. Virginia,* 388 U.S. 1 (1967).

78. For an analysis of the constitutionality of the several states' miscegenation statutes, see Andrew D. Weinberger, "A Reappraisal of the Constitutionality of 'Miscegenation' Statutes," Appendix G in Montagu, op. cit., 4th ed. (Cleveland, Ohio: World Publishing Co., Meridian Books, 1965), pp. 402–24.

79. Paul Spickard, *Mixed Blood: Intermarriage and Ethnic Identity in Twentieth-Century America* (Madison: University of Wisconsin Press, 1989), pp. 3–22, 233–373.

80. See three works by Edward Byron Reuter, *The Mulatto in the United States* (New York: Negro Universities Press, 1969 [1918]); *Race Mixture: Studies in Intermarriage and Race Mixture* (New York: Negro Universities Press, 1969 [1931]); with an introduction and revision by Jitsuichi Masuoka, *The American Race Problem* (New York: Thomas Y. Crowell, 1970), pp. 124–37. See also Edwin R. Embree, *Brown Americans: The Story of a Tenth of the Nation* (Fairfield, N.J.: Augustus M. Kelley, 1977 [1943]).

81. Naomi Zack, *Race and Mixed Race* (Philadelphia: Temple University Press, 1993), p. 36.

82. Ibid.

83. F. James Davis, *Who Is Black? One Nation's Definition* (University Park: Pennsylvania State University Press, 1991).

84. Virginia R. Dominguez, *White by Definition: Social Classification in Creole Louisiana* (New Brunswick, N.J.: Rutgers University Press, 1986), pp. 149–81. See also William Faulkner Rushton, *The Cajuns: From Acadia to Louisiana* (New York: Farrar, Straus, Giroux, 1979); Carl A. Brasseaux, *The Founding of New Acadia: The Beginnings of Acadian Life in Louisiana, 1765–1803* (Baton Rouge: Louisiana State University Press, 1987); and Carl A. Brasseaux, Keith P. Fontenot, and Claude F. Oubre, *Creoles of Color in the Bayou Country* (Jackson: University Press of Mississippi, 1994).

85. Stanford M. Lyman, "The Race Question and Liberalism: Casuistries in American Constitutional Law," *International Journal of Politics, Culture, and Society* 5:2 (winter 1991): 183–247; Ian F. Haney Lopez, *White by Law: The Legal Construction of Race* (New York: New York University Press, 1996); Rogers M. Smith, *Civic Ideals: Conflicting Visions of Citizenship in U.S. History* (New Haven, Conn.: Yale University Press, 1997).

86. Thus, Gilbert Haven, Methodist Bishop of Massachusetts, predicted with alloyed enthusiasm at the end of the Civil War that "the daughters of those haughty Southerners, who have shrank from their touch as leprous, shall gratefully accept the offers of the sons of their fathers' slaves"; while Moncure Daniel Conway, a Southern

abolitionist who had fled to England during the Civil War, asserted that "the mixture of the blacks and whites is good; . . . the person so produced is, under ordinarily favourable circumstances, healthy, handsome, and intelligent . . . I believe that such a combination would evolve a more complete character than the unmitigated Anglo-Saxon." George M. Fredrickson, *The Black Image in the White Mind: The Debate on Afro-American Character and Destiny, 1817–1914* (New York: Harper and Row, 1971), pp. 121–22. In the post–Civil War era, the former codirector of the Confederacy's Nitre Bureau, Joseph Le Conte (1823–1901) proposed the cross-breeding of the Freedmen and -women with marginal elements among the whites so that "civilization . . . will no longer be Anglo-Saxon, or Teutonic, or European, or Aryan, or Caucasian, but human . . . The final civilization will thus be coextensive with human nature, with the earth surface, and with the life of humanity." Joseph Le Conte, *The Race Problem in the South* (New York: D. Appleton, 1892; Miami: Mnemosyne Publishing Co., 1969), pp. 374–75. In the twentieth century, Israel Zangwill (1864–1926), most famous for his advocacy of widespread interethnic and interracial marriage in his melodrama, *The Melting Pot,* would later repudiate his progressive attitude toward Negro-white marriages on both aesthetic and cultural grounds. See Israel Zangwill, *The Melting Pot: Drama in Four Acts,* new and rev. ed. (New York: Macmillan, 1922 [1909]), pp. 204–7. See also Stanford M. Lyman, *Postmodernism and a Sociology of the Absurd and Other Essays on the "Nouvelle Vague" in American Social Science* (Fayetteville: University of Arkansas Press, 1997), pp. 185–209.

87. See two works by Lester F. Ward, *Pure Sociology: A Treatise on the Origin and Spontaneous Development of Society,* 2d ed. (New York: Macmillan, 1907; reprint, New York: Augustus M. Kelley, 1970), pp. 205–20, 240–357, 358–60, 364–416, 544–75; and *Applied Sociology: A Treatise on the Conscious Improvement of Society, by Society* (Boston: Ginn and Co., 1906), pp. 37–49, 97–223, 326–39. See also Arthur J. Vidich and Stanford M. Lyman, *American Sociology: Worldly Rejections of Religion and Their Directions* (New Haven, Conn.: Yale University Press, 1985), pp. 20–35.

88. Norman Podhoretz, "My Negro Problem—And Ours," *Commentary* 35 (February 1963): 93–101. Reprinted in Bernard E. Segal, ed., *Race and Ethnic Relations: Selected Readings* (New York: Thomas Y. Crowell, 1966), pp. 239–50.

89. Ibid., p. 248.

90. Cf. Myrdal's discussion of this popular form of pseudo-reasoning as basic to the Southern whites' discourse on race in *An American Dilemma,* op. cit., pp. 53–60.

91. Podhoretz, op. cit., p. 250.

92. Ibid., p. 249.

93. Ibid., p. 250.

94. Loc. cit.

95. Judith Miller, "Think Tank: Banishing Racial Strife on the Wings of Love," *New York Times,* Arts and Ideas section, May 23, 1998, p. A17.

96. Norman Mailer, *The White Negro* (San Francisco: City Lights, 1957). In an essay by Gayle Wald, "'A Most Disagreeable Mirror': Reflections on White Identity in *Black Like Me,*" in *Passing and the Fictions of Identity,* ed. Elaine K. Ginsberg (Durham, N.C.:

Duke University Press, 1996), pp. 151–77, at p. 163, Professor Wald writes: "In the tradition of white hipsterism exemplified by Mailer's "White Negro" essay, passing for black has served as a mode through which white men in particular have symbolized their alienation from cultural norms and their pleasurable embrace of marginality and radicalism. By adopting black radical chic as a mode of self-conscious unorthodoxy, white liberals have attempted to indicate their solidarity with the struggles of marginalized African Americans, as well as their belief in basic principles of racial equality . . . Here the marginality ascribed to black identity is associated not only with freedom and autonomy—precisely those qualities that would seem to be conferred by white status—but also with a disruptive power, an ability to interfere, shock, terrorize, to play with ideas of centrality and marginality." In *Bulworth,* it seems to me, the eponymous senator is a veritable paragon of Wald's characterization of a "white Negro."

In one sense, *Bulworth* is an unsuccessful foray into "racial cross-dressing," wherein its eponymous hero occupies what Marjorie Garber calls the "space of desire," interpreted, in a racial context, by Michael Rogin, *Blackface, White Noise: Jewish Immigrants in the Hollywood Melting Pot* (Berkeley: University of California Press, 1996), p. 32, as "calling into question the repressive division between man and woman, aristocrat and commoner, white and black."

97. Quoted in Mailer, op. cit., p. A17.

98. See Stanford M. Lyman, "Race, Sex and Servitude: Images of Black Americans in Movies," *International Journal of Politics, Culture, and Society* 4:1 (fall 1990): 49–77. Reprinted in Stanford M. Lyman, *Color, Culture, Civilization: Race and Minority Issues in American Society* (Urbana: University of Illinois Press, 1994), pp. 183–216.

99. See Donald Bogle, *Toms, Coons, Mulattoes, Mammies, and Bucks: An Interpretive History of Blacks in American Films,* 3d ed. (New York: Continuum, 1996), pp. 145, 182, 194, 201, 212–18, 366.

100. William E. Cross, *Shades of Black: Diversity in African-American Identity* (Philadelphia: Temple University Press, 1991), pp. 41, 157–87, 220–23. Quotation from p. 159.

101. Miller, op. cit., p. 217.

102. Loc. cit.

103. Jody David Armour, *Negrophobia and Reasonable Racism: The Hidden Costs of Being Black in America* (New York: New York University Press, 1997). On the mystique of the tragic mulatto, see Freda Scott Giles, "From Melodrama to the Movies: The Tragic Mulatto as a Character Type," in Naomi Zack, *American Mixed Race: The Culture of Microdiversity* (Lanham, Md.: Rowman and Littlefield Publishers, 1995), pp. 63–78.

104. Rainier Spencer, "Race and Mixed Race: A Personal Tour," in William S. Penn, ed., *As We Are Now: Mixblood Essays on Race and Identity* (Berkeley: University of California Press, 1997), pp. 126–39.

105. A self- and group identifying term employed by an association of students at the University of California, Berkeley, whose mixed ancestry includes at least one Asian forebear.

106. A term once used by the multiracial, multiethnic supporters of Jesse Jackson's campaigns for public office, as well as a general term of reference for mixed-race groups. Jon Michael Spencer, *The New Colored People: The Mixed Race Movement in America* (New York: New York University Press, 1997), pp. 15–49.

107. Naomi Zack, *Race and Mixed Race,* op. cit.

108. Joel Williamson, *New People: Miscegenation and Mulattos in the United States* (New York: Free Press, 1980).

109. See G. Reginald Daniel, "Beyond Black and White: The New Multiracial Consciousness," in Maria P. P. Root, ed., *Racially Mixed People in America* (Newbury Park, Calif.: Sage Publications, 1992), pp. 333–41.

110. For various usages of this term, see Geoffrey Fox, *The Hispanic Nation: Culture, Politics and the Construction of Identity* (Tucson: University of Arizona Press, 1996), p. 2; Brewton Berry, *Almost White: A Study of Certain Racial Hybrids in the Eastern Untied States* (New York: Macmillan, 1963), pp. 40–51. See also Stanford M. Lyman, "The Spectrum of Color," *Social Research* 31 (autumn 1964): 364–73; Carl Gutierrez-Jones, *Rethinking the Borderlands: Between Chicano Culture and Legal Discourse* (Berkeley: University of California Press, 1995), pp. 57–75.

111. Karen I. Blu, *The Lumbee Problem: The Making of an American Indian People* (Cambridge, U.K.: Cambridge University Press, 1980); Gerald M. Sider, *Lumbee Indian Histories: Race, Ethnicity, and Indian Identity in the Southern United States* (Cambridge, U.K.: Cambridge University Press, 1993).

112. David Steven Cohen, *The Ramapo Mountain People* (New Brunswick, N.J.: Rutgers University Press, 1974).

113. Kingsley Davis, "Intermarriage in Caste Societies," *American Anthropologist* 43 (July–September 1941): 388–95.

114. Elaine K. Ginsberg, ed., *Passing and the Fictions of Identity* (Durham, N.C.: Duke University Press, 1996).

115. G. Reginald Daniel, "Passers and Pluralists: Subverting the Racial Divide," in Root, ed., op. cit., pp. 91–107. See also W. McKee Evans, *To Die Game: The Story of the Lowry Band, Indian Guerrillas of Reconstruction* (Baton Rouge: Louisiana State University Press, 1971).

116. Berry, op. cit., James T. Wooten, "Carolina Mestizos Seeking Ethnic Identity as Indians," *New York Times,* August 3, 1972, p. 35; and "Indians and Blacks Seized in Carolina," *New York Times,* April 18, 1973, p. 42.

117. "Multiracial Checkoff Is a Vote for Accuracy," editorial, *San Francisco Chronicle,* June 8, 1997, p. A10.

118. John Michael Spencer, op. cit., p. 20.

119. Stanford M. Lyman, *Postmodernism and a Sociology of the Absurd,* op. cit., pp. 1–8, 83–105, 185–264.

120. John Dollard, *Caste and Class in a Southern Town* (Madison: University of Wisconsin Press, 1988 [1937]), pp. 134–87, 267–433.

121. John P. Pittman, "Malcolm X: Masculinist Practice and Queer Theory," in Naomi Zack, ed., *Race/Sex: Their Sameness, Difference, and Interplay* (New York: Routledge, 1997), pp. 205–18. Quotation from p. 213.

122. Donna J. Haraway, *Modest-Witness @ Second-Millennium: Femaleman Meets Oncomouse: Feminism and Technoscience* (New York: Routledge, 1997), pp. 213–66.

123. Cf. Cecile Ann Lawrence, "Racelessness," in Zack, ed., *American Mixed Race,* op. cit., pp. 25–38.

124. Haraway, op. cit., pp. 263–64.

125. Ibid., p. 264.

126. Ibid., p. 262.

127. Loc. cit.

128. Loc cit.

129. Michael Omi and Howard Winant, *Racial Formation in the United States from the 1960s to the 1990s,* 2d ed. (New York: Routledge, 1994), p. 60.

130. Ibid., p. 98.

131. Joel Williamson, *New People: Miscegenation and Mulattoes in the United States,* op. cit., p. 195.

132. Cyntha L. Nakashima, "An Invisible Monster: The Creation and Denial of Mixed-Race People in America," in Root, op. cit., pp. 162–78. Quotation from p. 177.

133. *Report of the National Advisory Commission on Civil Disorders* (New York: Bantam Books, 1968), p. 35.

134. Ibid., pp. 35–108. See also Gerald Horne, *Fire This Time: The Watts Uprising and the 1960s* (Charlottesville: University Press of Virginia, 1995).

135. See Myrdal, *An American Dilemma,* op. cit., pp. 1021–24.

136. Lyndon B. Johnson, An Address, delivered at the Inaugural Centennial Convocation, January 6, 1963. Published as "Introduction" in Arnold Rose, ed., *Assuring Freedom to the Free: A Century of Emancipation in the USA* (Detroit, Mich.: Wayne State University Press, 1964), pp. 10–15. Quotation from p. 11.

137. The following quotations are taken from "Appendix C: Excerpts from President Lyndon B. Johnson's Address to the Nation on Civil Disorders, July 27, 1967," in *Report of the National Advisory Commission on Civil Disorders,* op. cit., pp. 538–41.

138. *Report of the National Advisory Commission on Civil Disorders,* op. cit., p. 407.

139. Urban America, Inc., and the Urban Coalition, *One Year Later: An Assessment of the Nation's Response to the Crisis Described by the National Advisory Commission on Civil Disorders* (New York: Frederick A. Praeger, 1969).

140. Ibid., p. 116.

141. Arnold Rose, *The Negro's Morale: Group Identification and Protest* (Minneapolis: University of Minnesota Press, 1949), p. 144.

142. Urban America, Inc., and the Urban Coalition, op. cit., p. 116.

143. Gunnar Myrdal, "Toward a Better America," an address given to student audiences in the United States, in idem, *Against the Stream: Critical Essays on Economics,* op. cit., pp. 266–92. Quotation from p. 283.

144. Ibid., p. 283.

145. Ibid., p. 284.

146. Loc. cit.

147. Ibid., p. 284

148. Ibid., pp. 287–91.

149. Ibid., p. 289.
150. Ibid., pp. 291–92.
151. Ibid., p. 292.
152. Ibid., p. 291.
153. Ibid., p. 284.
154. Ibid., p. 292.
155. Gunnar Myrdal, "The Worldwide Emancipation of Underdeveloped Nations," in Arnold Rose, ed., *Assuring Freedom to the Free,* op. cit., pp. 97–118. Quotation from pp. 117–18.
156. See Stephen Jay Gould, *Ontogeny and Phylogeny* (Cambridge, Mass.: Belknap Press of Harvard University Press, 1977).
157. Myrdal, "The Worldwide Emancipation of Underdeveloped Nations," op. cit., pp. 7–100.
158. Ibid., p. 99.
159. Ibid., p. 100.
160. Ibid., p. 99.
161. Gunnar Myrdal, "Gunnar Myrdal's *An American Dilemma*—Has It Been Resolved?" *Worldview* (December 1972). The following draws on the republication of this essay in Myrdal, *Against the Stream,* op. cit., pp. 293–307. Quotation from p. 293.
162. Loc. cit.
163. James Baldwin, Nathan Glazer, Sidney Hook, Gunnar Myrdal, and Norman Podhoretz, "Liberalism and the Negro: A Round-Table Discussion," *Commentary* 37 (March 1964): 25–42. Reprinted in Segal, ed., op, cit., pp. 459–92. Hereafter cited as Round-Table.
164. Myrdal, *An American Dilemma,* op. cit., pp. 28–29, 50–54, 67, 310, 620, 667, 1389.
165. Ibid., p. 1078.
166. Round-Table, op. cit., p. 469.
167. Round-Table, op. cit., p. 475.
168. Round-Table, op. cit., p. 469.
169. Loc. cit.
170. Loc. cit.
171. See, e.g., Alan B. Anderson and George W. Pickering, *Confronting the Color Line: The Broken Promise of the Civil Rights Movement in Chicago* (Athens: University of Georgia Press, 1986); J. Brian Sheehan, *The Boston School Integration Dispute: Social Change and Legal Maneuvers* (New York: Columbia University Press, 1984); and Ronald P. Formisano, *Boston against Busing: Race, Class and Ethnicity in the 1960s and 1970s* (Chapel Hill: University of North Carolina Press, 1991).

Talcott Parsons attempted to combine Myrdal's thesis with his own form of evolutionary functionalism, defining and describing a process of "inclusion" that eventually—if nothing interfered to halt its progress—would admit black Americans to "full citizenship" in the United States. The process proceeded in stages, the final one of which, Parsons believed, was at hand, provided that America would leave off of its war in Vietnam, extend to blacks the benefits for the poor begun in the New Deal, the students on America's college campuses would cease their disruptive and disorderly rebellions, and the African Americans would give up their nationalistic and particularistic excesses. Then, and only then, Parsons seemed to be arguing, could the inclusion of the Negro in accordance with Myrdal's beliefs about the American Creed proceed along their inevitable course. See Talcott Parsons, "Full Citizenship for the Negro American? A Sociological Problem," *Daedalus* 94:4 (fall 1965): 1009–54. For a critique, see Stanford M. Lyman, *The Black American in Sociological Thought,* op. cit., pp. 145–70.

172. Fred R. Harris, "Preface to the 1988 Edition," *The Kerner Report: The 1968 Report of the National Advisory Commission on Civil Disorders* (New York: Pantheon Books, 1988), pp. ix–xi. Quotation from p. x.

173. Ibid., p. xi.

174. Loc. cit. Harris proved to be all too prescient on the matter of affirmative action. For case studies, see James E. Jones, "The Rise and Fall of Affirmative Action," in Hill and Jones Jr., op. cit., pp. 345–69; and Lydia Chavez, *The Color Bind: California's Battle to End Affirmative Action* (Berkeley: University of California Press, 1998). In defense of affirmative action, see, e.g., Michel Rosenfeld, *Affirmative Action and Justice: A Philosophical Constitutional Inquiry* (New Haven, Conn.: Yale University Press, 1991); Ronald J. Fiscus, *The Constitutional Logic of Affirmative Action,* ed. Stephen L. Wasby (Durham, N.C.: Duke University Press, 1992); Barbara R. Bergman, *In Defense of Affirmative Action* (New York: Basic Books, 1996); and Orlando Patterson, *The Ordeal of Integration; Progress and Resentment in America's Racial Crisis* (Washington, D.C.: Civitas/Counterpoint, 1997), pp. 147–70; William G. Bowen and Derek Bok, *The Shape of the River: Long-Term Consequences of Considering Race in College and University Admissions* (Princeton, N.J.: Princeton University Press, 1998).

175. Fred R. Harris and Roger W. Wilkins, eds., *Quiet Riots: Race and Poverty in the United States: The Kerner Report Twenty Years Later* (New York: Pantheon Books, 1988), p. xi.

176. Ibid., p. 184.

177. Gary Orfield, "Separate Societies: Have the Kerner Warnings Come True?" in ibid., pp. 100–122, quotation from p. 122.

178. See Gary Orfield, "School Desegregation after Two Generations: Race, Schools, and Opportunity in Urban Society," in Hill and Jones Jr., op. cit., pp. 234–62. In 1984, Jennifer L. Hochschild had described what she called a "new American dilemma" arising out of the nation's inability thus far to sort out the paradoxes entailed in pursuing diversity, freedom, liberalism, and democracy in public education. See Jennifer L. Hochschild, *The New American Dilemma: Liberal Democracy and School Desegregation* (New Haven, Conn.: Yale University Press, 1984).

179. Reynolds Farley, *Blacks and Whites: Narrowing the Gap?* (Cambridge, Mass.: Harvard University Press, 1984); Reynolds Farley and Walter R. Allen, *The Color Line and the Quality of Life in America* (New York: Oxford University Press, 1987), esp. pp. 103–59; Reynolds Farley, *The New American Reality,* op. cit., pp. 208–71; and, in general, Reynolds Farley, "The Common Destiny of Blacks and Whites: Observations

about the Social and Economic Status of the Races," in Hill and Jones Jr., op. cit., pp. 197–233.

180. See among the many works on the racist practices of America's labor unions by Herbert Hill: "Labor Unions and the Negro," *Commentary* 28 (December 1959): 479–88; "Black Labor in White America," in Joan Grant, ed., op. cit., pp. 510–15; "The Racial Practices of Organized Labor: The Age of Gompers and After," in Arthur M. Ross and Herbert Hill, eds., *Employment, Race, and Poverty: A Critical Study of the Disadvantaged Status of Negro Workers from 1865 to 1965* (New York: Harcourt, Brace and World, 1967), pp. 365–402; "Race, Ethnicity and Organized Labor: The Opposition to Affirmative Action," *New Politics*, n.s., 1:2 (winter 1987): 31–82; "Reply," *New Politics*, n.s., 1:3 (summer 1987): 61–71; *Black Labor and the American Legal System: Race, Work, and the Law* (Madison: University of Wisconsin Press, 1985); "Myth-Making as Labor History: Herbert Gutman and the United Mine Workers of America," *International Journal of Politics, Culture, and Society* 2:3 (spring 1989): 132–200; "The Problem of Race in American Labor History," paper presented at the 61st annual meeting of the Southern Historical Association, New Orleans, La., November 9, 1995; "Black Workers, Organized Labor and Title VII of the 1964 Civil Rights Act: Legislative History and Litigation Record," in Hill and Jones Jr., op. cit., pp. 263–344.

181. Harris and Wilkins, op. cit., p. 180. The term *underclass* has sparked a vociferous debate. See Michael B. Katz, ed., *The "Underclass" Debate: Views from History* (Princeton, N.J.: Princeton University Press, 1993).

182. Harris and Wilkins, op. cit., pp. 172–84.

183. Haki R. Madhubuti, "Missing Movement, Missing Fathers: The Culture of Short Lives and Low Expectations," in idem, ed., *Why L.A. Happened: Implications of the '92 Los Angeles Rebellion* (Chicago: Third World Press, 1993), pp. 95–104. Quotation from p. 104.

184. Andrew Hacker, *Two Nations: Black and White, Separate, Hostile, Unequal*, Expanded and updated ed. (New York: Ballantine Books, 1995), pp. 238–39.

185. David K. Shipler, *A Country of Strangers: Blacks and Whites in America* (New York: Alfred A. Knopf, 1997).

186. Ibid., p. 389.

187. Obie Clayton Jr., ed., *An American Dilemma Revisited*, op. cit.

188. Robert A. Dentler, "The Political Situation and Power Prospects of African Americans in Gunnar Myrdal's Era and Today," in Clayton Jr., op. cit., pp. 25–44. Quotation from p. 44.

189. Reynolds Farley, "Black-White Residential Segregation: The Views of Myrdal in the 1940s and Trends of the 1980s," in Clayton Jr., op. cit., pp. 45–76. Quotation from p. 74.

190. Ronald F. Ferguson, "Shifting Challenges: Fifty Years of Economic Change toward Black-White Earnings Equality," in Clayton Jr., op. cit., pp. 76–111. Quotation from p. 105.

191. William Darity, "The Undesirables, America's Underclass in the Managerial

Age: Beyond the Myrdal Theory of Racial Inequality," in Clayton Jr., op. cit., pp. 112–37. Quotation from p. 131.

192. John Sibley Butler, "Myrdal Revisited: The Negro in Business, the Professions, Public Service, and Other White-Collar Occupations," in Clayton Jr., op. cit., pp. 138–68. Quotation from pp. 164–65.

193. Walter R. Allen and Joseph O. Jewell, "The Miseducation of Black America: Black Education since *An American Dilemma*," in Clayton Jr., op. cit., pp. 169–90. Quotation from p. 189.

194. William Rodormor, "The Minority Report," *California Monthly* 108: 6 (June 1998): p. 13.

195. Obie Clayton Jr., "The Church and Social Change: Accommodation, Moderation, or Protest," in Clayton Jr., op. cit., pp. 191–208. Quotation from p. 206.

196. Susan Welch, Michael W.. Combs, Lee Sigelman, Timothy Bledsoe, "Justice for All: Still an American Dilemma," in Clayton Jr., op. cit., pp. 209–25. Quotation from p. 224.

197. Samuel Walker, "'A Strange Atmosphere of Consistent Illegality': Myrdal on 'The Police and Other Public Contacts,'" in Clayton Jr., op. cit., pp. 226–46. Quotation from p. 242.

198. Cassia C. Spohn, "Courts, Sentences, and Prisons," in Clayton Jr., op. cit., pp. 247–68. Quotation from p. 261. For further evidence of the lack of progress on this issue, see Katheryn K. Russell, *The Color of Crime: Racial Hoaxes, White Fear, Black Protectionism, Police Harassment, and Other Macroagressions* (New York: New York University Press, 1998).

199. Antonio McDaniel, "The Dynamic Racial Composition of the United States," in Clayton Jr., op. cit., pp. 269–87. Quotation from p. 283.

200. Doris Wilkinson, "Gender and Social Inequality: The Prevailing Significance of Race," in Clayton Jr., op. cit., pp. 288–300. Quotation from p. 299.

201. Walter A. Jackson, *Gunnar Myrdal and America's Conscience: Social Engineering and Racial Liberalism, 1938–1987* (Chapel Hill: University of North Carolina Press, 1990), p. 51.

202. Michael W. Hughey, "Americanism and Its Discontents: Protestantism, Nativism, and Political Heresy in America," *International Journal of Politics, Culture, and Society* 5:4 (summer 1992): 533–53. Quotation from p. 534.

203. Loc. cit

204. See two works by Max Weber, *The Protestant Ethic and the Spirit of Capitalism,* trans. Talcott Parsons (New York: Charles Scribner's Sons, 1930), pp. 113–54, 200 n. 23, 217 n. 1; and *The Sociology of Religion,* trans. Ephraim Fischoff (Boston: Beacon Press, 1963), pp. 92–94. See also the discussion of Arminianism and of the race question in Seymour Martin Lipset, *American Exceptionalism: A Double-Edged Sword* (New York: W. W. Norton, 1996), pp. 60–76, 113–50.

205. Sidney E. Ahlstrom, *A Religious History of the American People* (New Haven, Conn.: Yale University Press, 1972), p. 404 n. 1.

206. Timothy L. Smith, *Revivalism and Social Reform in Mid-Nineteenth Century*

America (New York: Abingdon Press, 1957), pp. 88–89. Quoted in Seymour Martin Lipset, *The First New Nation: The United States in Historical and Comparative Perspective* (New York: W. W. Norton, 1979), p. 161.

207. Ernst Troeltsch, *The Social Teachings of the Christian Churches,* trans. Olive Wyon (New York: Harper Torchbooks, 1960 [1911]), II, pp. 635–36.

208. Lipset, *The First New Nation,* op. cit., p. 164. Emphasis supplied.

209. Loc. cit.

210. For the idea of U.S. civil religion, see Robert N. Bellah, "Civil Religion in America," and "American Civil Religion in the 1970s," in *American Civil Religion,* ed. Donald G. Jones and Russell E. Richey (San Francisco: Mellen Research University Press, 1990), pp. 21–44, 255–72. For further discussions, see Robert N. Bellah, *The Broken Covenant: American Civil Religion in Time of Trial* (New York: Seabury Press, Crossroad, 1975). For a critique of Bellah's thesis, see Michael W. Hughey, *Civil Religion and Moral Order; Theoretical and Historical Dimensions* (Westport, Conn.: Greenwood Press, 1983), pp. 157–70.

211. Quoted in Jackson, op. cit., p. 150.

212. Myrdal, *The Political Element in the Development of Economic Theory,* op. cit., p. 46.

213. Myrdal, *An American Dilemma,* op. cit., pp. 1–25. Not all scholars put such faith in Christian universalism. To take one outstanding example, historian Forrest G. Wood writes: "Christianity, in the five centuries since its message was first carried to the peoples of the New World—and, in particular, to the natives and the transplanted Africans of English North America and the United States—has been fundamentally racist in its ideology, organization, and practice." *The Arrogance of Faith: Christianity and Race in America from the Colonial Era to the Twentieth Century* (New York: Alfred A. Knopf, 1990), p. xviii.

214. Myrdal, "Toward a Better America," op. cit., p. 291.

215. Ibid., p. 266.

216. "Text of the Supreme Court Opinions, May 17, 1954" and "Appendix to Appellant's Briefs," both in Kenneth B. Clark, *Prejudice and Your Child* (Middletown, Conn.: Wesleyan University Press, 1988), pp. 156–84.

217. Kenneth B. Clark, "Racial Progress and Retreat: A Personal Memoir," in Hill and Jones Jr., op. cit., pp. 3–18.

218. John H. Stanfield, *Philanthropy and Jim Crow in American Social Science,* op. cit., pp. 170–71.

219. Doxey A. Wilkerson, "Introduction," in Herbert Aptheker, *The Negro People in America: A Critique of Gunnar Myrdal's* An American Dilemma, op. cit., pp. 7–16.

220. Joel Williamson, *The Crucible of Race: Black-White Relations in the American South since Emancipation* (New York: Oxford University Press, 1984), pp. 248–49.

221. Berman E. Johnson,, *The Dream Deferred: A Survey of Black America, 1840–1896* (Dubuque, Iowa: Kendall/Hunt Publishing Co., 1993), p. 142.

222. Charles E. Silberman, *Crisis in Black and White* (New York: Random House, 1964), p. 10.

223. Myrdal, *The Political Element in the Development of Economic Theory,* op. cit., pp. 44–49.

224. Hughey, op. cit., pp. 164–67. See also Adam B. Seligman, *The Idea of Civil Society* (Princeton, N.J.: Princeton University Press, 1992), pp. 1–144.

225. See Stanford M. Lyman, "Race Relations as Social Process: Sociology's Resistance to a Civil Rights Orientation," in Hill and Jones Jr., eds., op. cit., pp. 370–401.

226. Georg Simmel, "The Problem of Religion Today (1911)," in *Essays on Religion,* ed. and trans. Horst Jürgen Helle in collaboration with Ludwig Nieder (New Haven, Conn.: Yale University Press, 1997), pp. 7–19; and *Schopenhauer and Nietzsche,* trans. Helmut Loiskandl, Deena Weinstein, and Michael Weinstein (Amherst: University of Massachusetts Press, 1986), pp. 4–5, 10, 118, 138–44, 150–51, 168.

227. Troeltsch, op. cit., II, pp. 819–20.

228. Weber, *The Sociology of Religion,* op. cit., pp. 100–101.

229. Herbert Hill, "The Racial Practices of Organized Labor: The Age of Gompers and After," in Ross and Hill, eds., op. cit., pp. 365–402; Horace R. Cayton and George S. Mitchell, *Black Workers and the New Unions* (Chapel Hill: University of North Carolina Press, 1939); Ray Marshall, *The Negro and Organized Labor* (New York: John Wiley and Sons, 1965); William B. Gould, *Black Workers in White Unions: Job Discrimination in the United States* (Ithaca, N.Y.: Cornell University Press, 1977); and, in general, Herbert Hill, "The Problem of Race in American Labor History." Paper presented at the annual meeting of the Southern Historical Association, New Orleans, La., November 9, 1995.

230. See two works by Alexander Saxton, *The Indispensable Enemy: Labor and the Anti-Chinese Movement in California* (Berkeley: University of California Press, 1971); and *The Rise and Fall of the White Republic: Class Politics and Mass Culture in Nineteenth-Century America* (London: Verso, 1990). See also two works by Noel Ignatiev, *How the Irish Became White* ((New York: Routledge, 1995); and "Immigrants and Whites," in Noel Ignatiev and John Garvey, eds., *Race Traitor* (New York: Routledge, 1996), pp. 15–23; and Theodore W. Allen, *The Invention of the White Race, Vol. I: Racial Oppression and Social Control; Vol. II: The Origin of Racial Oppression in Anglo-America* (London: Verso, 1994; 1997); and David R. Roediger, *The Wages of Whiteness: Race and the Making of the American Working Class* (London: Verso, 1991), esp. pp. 95–184.

231. James Ridgeway, op. cit.; Sara Diamond, *Roads to Dominion: Right-Wing Movements and Political Power in the United States* (New York: Guilford Press, 1995), pp. 66–91, 140–60, 257–73, 307–12; Lyman Tower Sargent, ed., *Extremism in America: A Reader* (New York: New York University Press, 1995), pp. 115–97, 359–66; Kenneth S. Stern, *A Force upon the Plain: The American Militia Movement and the Politics of Hate* (New York: Simon and Schuster, 1996); Morris Dees with James Corcoran and the Klanwatch/Militia Task Force, *False Patriots: The Threat of Antigovernment Extremists* (Montgomery, Ala.: Southern Poverty Law Center, 1996).

232. Hendrik Hertzberg and Henry Louis Gates Jr., "Comment: The African-American Century: A reality that is more complicated, and more heroic, than the myth," *New Yorker* 72:10 (April 29–May 6, 1996): 9–10. Quotation from p. 10.

233. This term and its meaning are matters of considerable controversy. See three works by William Julius Wilson, *The Declining Significance of Race: Blacks and*

Changing American Institutions, 2d ed. (Chicago: University of Chicago Press, 1980); *The Truly Disadvantaged: The Inner City, the Underclass, and Public Policy* (Chicago: University of Chicago Press, 1987); and *When Work Disappears: The World of the New Urban Poor* (New York: Alfred A. Knopf, 1996). A critique of Wilson's argument will be found in Robert C. Smith, *Racism in the Post–Civil Rights Era: Now You See It, Now You Don't* (Albany: State University of New York Press, 1995), pp. 105–44. See also Michael B. Katz, ed., *The "Underclass" Debate: Views from History,* op. cit.

234. Hertzberg and Gates Jr., op. cit., p. 10. On June 29, 1998, the Center for Disease Control in the United States reported that "although African Americans make up 13 percent of the United States population . . . , they account for about 57 percent of all new infections with human immunodeficiency virus, which causes AIDS . . . And while the death rate from AIDS is dropping overall, the disease remains the leading cause of death among black people aged 25 to 44." Sheryl Gay Stolberg, "Eyes Shut, Black America Is Being Ravaged by AIDS," *New York Times* 147:51,203 (June 29, 1998), pp. A1, A12. Quotation from p. A1.

235. Among many works written in opposition to affirmative action, see Robert K. Fullinwider, *The Reverse Discrimination Controversy: A Moral and Legal Analysis* (Totowa, N.J.: Rowman and Littlefield, 1980); Charles Murray, *Losing Ground: American Social Policy, 1950–1980* (New York: Basic Books, 1984), pp. 13, 43, 85, 91–94, 106, 221–23; Clint Bolick, *Changing Course: Civil Rights at the Crossroads* (New Brunswick, N.J.: Transaction Books, 1988); Shelby Steele, *The Content of Our Character: A New Vision of Race in America* (New York: St. Martin's Press, 1990), pp. 111–26; Frederick R. Lynch, *Invisible Victims: White Males and the Crisis of Affirmative Action* (New York: Praeger, 1991); Herman Belz, *Equality Transformed: A Quarter-Century of Affirmative Action* (New Brunswick, N.J.: Transaction Books, 1991); Russell Nieli, ed., *Racial Preference and Racial Justice: The New Affirmative Action Controversy* (Washington, D.C.: Ethics and Policy Center, 1991); Richard A. Epstein, *Forbidden Grounds: The Case against Employment Discrimination Laws* (Cambridge, Mass.: Harvard University Press, 1992); Carl Cohen, *Naked Racial Preference: The Case against Affirmative Action* (Lanham, Md.: Madison Books, 1995); and Terry Eastland, *Ending Affirmative Action: The Case for Colorblind Justice* (New York: Basic Books, 1996).

For the several varieties of defense of affirmative action, see, inter alia, John E. Fleming, Gerald R. Gill, and David H. Swinton, *The Case for Affirmative Action for Blacks in Higher Education* (Washington, D.C.: Howard University Press, 1978); Herman Schwartz, "Affirmative Action," in Leslie W. Dunbar, ed., *Minority Report: What Has Happened to Blacks, Hispanics, American Indians, and Other Minorities in the Eighties* (New York: Pantheon Books, 1984), pp. 58–74; Herbert Hill, "Race, Ethnicity and Organized Labor: The Opposition to Affirmative Action," op. cit., pp. 31–82; and "Discussion: Race, Ethnicity and Organized Labor" with thirteen discussants and a reply by Hill, *New Politics,* n.s., 1:3 (summer 1987): 22–71; Michel Rosenfeld, *Affirmative Action and Justice: A Philosophical and Constitutional Inquiry,* op. cit.; Ronald J. Fiscus, *The Constitutional Logic of Affirmative Action,* ed. Stephen L. Wasby, op. cit.; James E. Jones Jr., "The Rise and Fall of Affirmative Action," in Hill and Jones Jr., op. cit., pp. 345–69; Stephen Steinberg, *Turning Back: The Retreat from Racial Justice in American Thought and Policy* (Boston: Beacon Press, 1995), pp. 164–78; Barbara R. Bergman, *In Defense of Affirmative Action,* op. cit.; Leslie G. Carr, *"Color-Blind" Racism* (Thousand Oaks, Calif.: Sage Publications, 1997), pp. 86–170; Orlando Patterson, *The Ordeal of Integration: Progress and Resentment in America's "Racial" Crisis,* op. cit., pp. 147–70; David Roediger, "White Workers, New Democrats, and Affirmative Action," in Wahneema Lubiano, ed., *The House That Race Built: Black Americans, U.S. Terrain* (New York: Pantheon, 1997), pp. 48–65; Walter Feinberg, *On Higher Ground: Education and the Case for Affirmative Action* (New York: Teachers College Press, 1998); Jacqueline Jones, *American Work: Four Centuries of Black and White Labor* (New York: W. W. Norton, 1998), pp. 301–94; and Bowen and Bok, op. cit.

See also Alan H. Goldman, *Justice and Reverse Discrimination* (Princeton, N.J.: Princeton University Press, 1979); Paul Burstein, *Discrimination, Jobs, and Politics: The Struggle for Equal Employment Opportunity in the United States since the New Deal* (Chicago: University of Chicago Press, 1985); Richard Jenkins and John Solomos, eds., *Racism and Equal Opportunities in the 1980s* (Cambridge, U.K.: Cambridge University Press, 1987); Kathanne W. Greene, *Affirmative Action and Principles of Justice* (New York: Greenwood Press, 1989); Stephanie L. Witt, *The Pursuit of Race and Gender Equity in American Academe* (New York: Praeger, 1990); Stephen M. Cahn, ed., *Affirmative Action and the University: A Philosophical Inquiry* (Philadelphia: Temple University Press, 1993); Nicolaus Mills, ed., *Debating Affirmative Action: Race, Gender, Ethnicity, and the Politics of Inclusion* (New York: Delta-Dell Pub. Co., 1994); John Edwards, *When Race Counts: The Morality of Racial Preference in Britain and America* (London: Routledge, 1995); John David Skrentny, *The Ironies of Affirmative Action: Politics, Culture, and Justice in America* (Chicago: University of Chicago Press, 1996); Richard D. Kahlenberg, *The Remedy: Class, Race, and Affirmative Action* (New York: Basic Books, 1996); George E. Curry, ed., *The Affirmative Action Debate* (Reading, Mass.: Addison-Wesley Pub. Co., 1996); Darien A. McWhirter, *The End of Affirmative Action: Where Do We Go from Here?* (New York: Birch Lane Press, Carol Pub. Co., 1996); and Lydia Chavez, *The Color Bind: California's Battle to End Affirmative Action,* op. cit.

236. The mainstream opposition to multiculturalism finds its voice in Arthur M. Schlesinger Jr., *The Disuniting of America: Reflections on a Multicultural Society,* rev. ed. (New York: W. W. Norton, 1998). However, scholarly studies and philosophical ruminations have thrown considerable light on this as-yet-inchoate development. See, e.g., Charles P. Henry, *Culture and African American Politics* (Bloomington: Indiana University Press, 1990); Philip Perlmutter, *Divided We Fall: A History of Ethnic, Religious, and Racial Prejudice* (Ames: Iowa State University Press, 1992), pp. 228–335; Becky W. Thompson and Sangeeta Tyagi, eds., *Beyond a Dream Deferred: Multicultural Education and the Politics of Excellence* (Minneapolis: University of Minnesota Press, 1993); Elizabeth Higginbotham, "Sociology and the Multicultural Curriculum: The Challenges of the 1990's and Beyond," *Race, Sex and Class: An Interdisciplinary Journal* 1:1 (fall 1993): 13–24; two works by David Theo Goldberg: *Racist Culture: Philosophy*

and the Politics of Meaning (Oxford, U.K.: Blackwell, 1993); and idem, ed., *Multiculturalism: A Critical Reader* (Oxford, U.K.: Blackwell, 1994); "Multiculturalism and Diversity," *National Forum: The Phi Kappa Phi Journal* 74:1 (winter 1994): 3–45; Richard Bernstein, *Dictatorship of Virtue: Multiculturalism and the Battle for America's Future* (New York: Alfred A. Knopf, 1994); David A. Hollinger, *Postethnic America: Beyond Multiculturalism* (New York: Basic Books, 1995); Joel S. Kahn, *Culture, Multiculture, Postculture* (London: Sage, 1995); Will Kymlicka, *Multicultural Citizenship: A Liberal Theory of Minority Rights* (Oxford, U.K.: Clarendon Press, 1995); Arthur Asa Berger, *Cultural Criticism: A Primer of Key Concepts* (Thousand Oaks, Calif.: Sage, 1995), pp. 135–73; William E. Connolly, *The Ethos of Pluralization* (Minneapolis: University of Minnesota Press, 1995); Stuart Hall and Paul duGay, eds., *Questions of Cultural Identity* (London: Sage, 1996); Robert John Ackermann, *Heterogeneities: Race, Gender, Class, Nation and State* (Amherst: University of Massachusetts Press, 1996); Lucius T. Outlaw Jr., *On Race and Philosophy* (New York: Routledge, 1996); Nathan Glazer, *We Are All Multiculturalists Now,* op. cit.; Joseph Tilden Rhea, *Race Pride and the American Identity* (Cambridge, Mass.: Harvard University Press, 1997); John J. Miller, *The Unmaking of Americans: How Multiculturalism Has Undermined America's Assimilation Ethic* (New York: Free Press, 1997); Arthur M. Melzer, et al., eds., *Multiculturalism and American Democracy,* op. cit.

237. See Stanford M. Lyman, *Postmodernism and a Sociology of the Absurd and Other Essays on the "Nouvelle Vague" in American Social Science,* op. cit., pp. 83–105, 185–209.

238. Herbert Hill ("Black Workers, Organized Labor, and Title VII . . . ," op. cit., p. 329) writes: "Race supplanted class as an organizing principle of American politics in the postreform period that began after judicial enforcement of the civil rights legislation enacted in the 1960s, and given the white hostility to black advancement, racism became the decisive factor in determining the politics of the nation. Paradoxically, the coalition formed in the period of Franklin D. Roosevelt's New Deal was shattered by its last major victory; the adoption of the Civil Rights Act of 1964."

239. Charles Lemert (*Postmodernism Is Not What You Think* [Malden, Mass.: Blackwell Publishers, 1997], p. 128) writes: "It is obvious that the destabilizing of the modern world is associated with a curious but undeniable, energizing of identity as the topic of widespread political interest." Robert G. Dunn (*Identity Crisis: A Social Critique of Postmodernity* [Minneapolis: University of Minnesota Press, 1998], p. 149) observes: "The formation of new global relationships and a heightened sense of global interdependency, rapidly changing structures of production and consumption, major changes in the structure and social composition of labor markets, the collective impact of the new social movements—all contributed to and reflected the destabilization of modern forms of culture and identity and the concomitant rise of new groupings and movements. Earlier models of order . . . became increasingly ineffective."

240. Krishan Kuman, *From Post-Industrial to Post-Modern Society: New Theories of the Contemporary World* (Malden, Mass.: Blackwell Publishers, 1995), p. 122.

241. Myrdal, "An American Dilemma—Has It Been Resolved?" op. cit., p. 301.

242. Sissela Bok, "Foreword," op. cit., p. xvi.

243. Ibid., p. xvii.

244. Quoted in Nat Hentoff, *Living the Bill of Rights: How to be an Authentic American* (New York: Harper Collins, 1998), p. 90.

245. *Brown vs. Board of Education* 347 U.S. 483 (1954).

246. Clark reprinted the entire decision, including the footnote, in his book, *Prejudice and Your Child,* 2d ed., op. cit., pp. 158–65. The criticism did not cease, however. In 1983, in "School Desegregation: The Social Science Role," *American Psychologist* 38 (1983): 869–77, H. B. Gerard criticized the usage made of Clark's work and urged a more conservative application of social science to public policy. Clark caused a reply, Stewart W. Cook, "Desegregation: A Reply to Gerard," to be reprinted as Appendix 6, pp. 236–72, of the Wesleyan University Press edition of *Prejudice and Your Child.*

247. Kenneth B. Clark, "The Role of the Social Sciences in Desegregation," presidential address to the Society for the Psychological Study of Social Issues, Chicago, September 5, 1960. Reprinted as Appendix 5 in Clark, *Prejudice and Your Child,* 2d ed., op. cit., pp. 207–35.

248. Ibid., pp. 207–8.

249. Kenneth B. Clark, *Dark Ghetto: Dilemmas of Social Power* (New York: Harper and Row, 1965), p. 203.

250. Gunnar Myrdal, "Foreword," in ibid., pp. x–xi.

251. Kenneth B. Clark, *Pathos of Power* (New York: Harper and Row, 1974), p. 127.

252. Ibid., pp. 127–28.

253. Ibid., p. 128.

254. Kenneth B. Clark, "Introduction: The Dilemma of Power," in Talcott Parsons and Kenneth B. Clark, eds., *The Negro American* (Boston: Houghton Mifflin, 1966)), pp. xi–xviii. Quotation from p. xviii.

255. Ibid., p. xi.

256. Kenneth B. Clark, "The Civil Rights Movement: Momentum and Organization," in ibid., pp. 595–625.

257. Ibid., p. 623.

258. "Liberalism and the Negro: A Round-Table Discussion," in Segal, op. cit., p. 486. Emphasis in original.

259. Kenneth B. Clark, "Racial Progress and Retreat: A Personal Memoir," in Hill and Jones Jr., eds., op. cit., pp. 3–18. Quotation from pp. 15–18.

260. Ibid., p. 17.

261. Ibid., p. 18.

262. Quoted from Benjamin Disraeli, *Sybil; or, The Two Nations,* 1845, in Andrew Hacker, *Two Nations: Black and White, Separate, Hostile, Unequal,* expanded and updated ed. (New York: Ballantine Books, 1995), p. ix.

263. Ibid., pp. 249–62.

264. Ibid., pp. 207–22.

265. Ibid., p. 222.

266. Ibid., p. 241.

267. Alexis de Tocqueville, *Democracy in America,* ed. J. P. Mayer and Max Lerner, trans. George Lawrence (New York: Harper and Row, 1966).

268. See George Wilson Pierson, *Tocqueville and Beaumont in America* (New York: Oxford University Press, 1938).

269. For varying interpretations of Tocqueville's observations, see: Max Lerner, *Tocqueville and American Civilization* (New Brunswick, N.J.: Transaction Publishers, 1994 [1966]); two works by Seymour Drescher, *Dilemmas of Democracy: Tocqueville and Modernization* (Pittsburgh: University of Pittsburgh Press, 1968); and idem, ed. and trans., *Tocqueville and Beaumont on Social Reform* (New York: Harper Torchbooks, 1968); Doris S. Goldstein, *Trial and Faith: Religion and Politics in Tocqueville's Thought* (New York: Elsevier Scientific Publishing Co., 1975); John Stone and Stephen Mennell, eds., *Alexis de Tocqueville on Democracy, Revolution, and Society: Selected Writings* (Chicago: University of Chicago Press, 1980); Whitney Pope in collaboration with Lucetta Pope, *Alexis de Tocqueville, His Social and Political Theory* (Beverly Hills, Calif.: Sage Publications, 1986); and Roger Boesche, *The Strange Liberalism of Alexis de Tocqueville* (Ithaca, N.Y.: Cornell University Press, 1987).

270. Hacker, op. cit., p. 243.

271. Alexis de Tocqueville, "Report on Abolition" (1839); and "On the Emancipation of the Slaves," a series published in *Le Siecle,* October 22 and December 14, 1843, in Drescher, ed., op. cit., pp. 98–136 and 137–73.

272. See the two letters from Alexis de Tocqueville to Arthur de Gobineau, November 17, 1853, and December 20, 1853, in *Alexis de Tocqueville: Selected Letters on Politics and Society,* ed. Roger Boesche and trans. James Toupin and Roger Boesche (Berkeley: University of California Press, 1985), pp. 297–301, 302–5.

273. Alexis de Tocqueville, *Writings on Empire and Slavery,* trans. and ed. Jennifer Pitts (Baltimore: Johns Hopkins University Press, 2001). See Alexis de Tocqueville, *"Colonialism in Algeria,"* in Stone and Mennell, eds., op. cit., pp. 345–47; Goldstein, op. cit., pp. 110–17; and Boesche, *The Strange Liberalism . . . ,* op. cit., pp. 215–18.

274. Hacker, op, cit., p. 243.

275. Gustave de Beaumont, "Note on the Social and Political Condition of the Negro Slaves and of Free People of Color," Appendix A, in idem, *Marie or Slavery in the United States: A Novel of Jacksonian America, translated from the French by Barbara Chapman* (Stanford, Calif.: Stanford University Press, 1958 [1835]), pp. 189–215.

276. Ibid., Appendix I, pp. 226–31. Quotation from pp. 230–31.

277. Hacker, op. cit., p. 245.

278. Loc. cit.

279. See three works by Nathan Glazer, *Affirmative Discrimination: Ethnic Inequality and Public Policy* (New York: Basic Books, 1975); *Ethnic Dilemmas, 1964–1982* (Cambridge Mass.: Harvard University Press, 1983), pp. 159–229; and "The Affirmative Action Stalemate," *The Public Interest* 90 (winter 1988): 99–114.

280. Glazer, *Ethnic Dilemmas,* op. cit., pp. 97–156.

281. Nathan Glazer, "Is 'Integration' Possible in New York's Schools?" *Commentary* 30:3 (September 1960): 185–93. Reprinted in Hubert H. Humphrey, ed., *School*

Desegregation: Documents and Commentaries (New York: Thomas Y. Crowell Co., 1964), pp. 185–98.

282. See two recent works by Nathan Glazer: *We Are All Multiculturalists Now,* op. cit.; and "In Defense of Preference," *New Republic* (April 6, 1998): 18–19, 24–25.

283. Richard Rorty, *Achieving Our Country: Leftist Thought in Twentieth-Century America,* The William Massey Sr. Lectures in the History of American Civilization (Cambridge, Mass.: Harvard University Press, 1998), p. 100.

284. See James Traub, "Nathan Glazer Changes His Mind, Again," *New York Times Magazine,* June 28, 1998, pp. 23–25.

285. Nathan Glazer, "American Epic: Then and Now," *The Public Interest* 130 (winter 1998): 3–20.

286. Oscar Handlin, *The Uprooted,* 2d ed., enlarged (Boston: Little Brown and Co., An Atlantic Monthly Press Book, 1973), p. 3. Glazer gives this example in "American Epic . . . ," op. cit., p. 18.

287. See Thomas J. LaBelle and Christopher R. Ward, *Multiculturalism and Education: Diversity and Its Impact on Schools and Society* (Albany: State University of New York Press, 1994).

288. Glazer, "America Epic," op. cit., p. 19.

289. Ibid., p. 20.

290. Loc. cit.

291. Glazer, *We Are All Multiculturalists Now,* op. cit., pp. 116–17.

292. Ibid., pp. 120–21.

293. Ibid., p. 121.

294. Robert Post and Michael Rogin, eds., "Race and Representation: Affirmative Action," Special Issue, *Representations* 55 (summer 1996): 1–186. See also Chavez, op. cit.

295. See three articles that appeared in *Asian Week* 19:38 (May 14–20, 1998): Leland Y. Lee, "Bilingual-Ed Needs Reform—Not Prop. 227," p. 5; Bill Wong, "How Prop. 227 May Hurt Families: Communication Doesn't Always Improve When English Does," p. 6; and Emil Guillermo, "Prop. 227 Is Bad—But It's Not Racist," p. 7.

296. Patricia Healy, "Berkeley Struggles to Stay Diverse in Post-Affirmative Action Era: It Sees 52 Percent Drop in Black and Hispanic Freshmen in First Class Admitted under Proposition 209," *Chronicle of Higher Education* 44:38 (May 29, 1998): A31–A33.

297. *Hopwood vs. Texas* 78 F, 3d 932 (1996); McWhirter, op. cit., pp. 127–29; James Traub, "Testing Texas," *New Republic,* April 6, 1998, pp. 20–21; Douglas Lederman, "Texas Regents to Appeal 'Hopwood' Ruling," *Chronicle of Higher Education* 44:38 (May 29, 1998): p. A36.

298. See the "Special Section on Affirmative Action," *Telos* 106 (winter 1996): 139–64, as well as the book reviews, pp. 165–94. See also two essays on affirmative action that appeared in *New Politics,* n.s., 5:3 (summer 1995): Barry Finger, "Racism and Affirmative Action," pp. 23–30; and Leith Mullings, "Racism Remains Pervasive," pp. 31–34; and, in a later issue of *New Politics* n.s., 6:4 (winter 1998): Reginald Wilson, "Affirmative Action and the Left," pp. 35–38.

299. See two works by Stanford M. Lyman, "Asians, Blacks, Hispanics, Amerinds: Confronting Vestiges of Slavery," in Vincent Parrillo, ed., *Rethinking Today's Minorities* (New York: Greenwood Press, 1991), pp. 63–86; and *Postmodernism and a Sociology of the Absurd*, op. cit., pp. 83–209; and Stanford M. Lyman and Arthur J. Vidich, *Social Order and the Public Philosophy: An Analysis and Interpretation of the Work of Herbert Blumer* (Fayetteville: University of Arkansas Press, 1988), pp. 55–94, esp. pp. 76–91.

300. See two works by Stephen L. Carter, *Reflections of an Affirmative Action Baby* (New York: Basic Books, 1991); and *The Dissent of the Governed: A Meditation on Law, Religion, and Loyalty.* The William E. Massey Sr. Lectures in the History of American Civilization 1995 (Cambridge, Mass.: Harvard University Press, 1998), pp. 17, 22–24, 67–69, 122–26.

301. Glenn C. Loury, "How to Amend Affirmative Action," *The Public Interest* 127 (spring 1997): 33–43.

302. See the following works by Thomas Sowell: *Say's Law: An Historical Analysis* (Princeton, N.J.: Princeton University Press, 1972); *Black Education: Myths and Tragedies* (New York: David McKay Co., 1972); *Classical Economics Reconsidered* (Princeton, N.J.: Princeton University Press, 1974); *Race and Economics* (New York: David McKay Co., 1975); ed. with the assistance of Lynn D. Collins, *Essays and Data on American Ethnic Groups* (Washington, D.C.: Urban Institute, 1978); *Knowledge and Decisions* (New York: Basic Books, 1980); *Markets and Minorities* (New York: Basic Books, 1981); *Pink and Brown People and Other Controversial Essays* (Stanford, Calif.: Hoover Institution Press, 1981); *Ethnic America: A History* (New York: Basic Books, 1981); *The Economics and Politics of Race: An International Perspective* (New York: William Morrow and Co., 1983); *Civil Rights: Rhetoric or Reality?* (New York: William Morrow and Co., 1984); *Marxism: Philosophy and Economics* (New York: William Morrow and Co., 1985); *Compassion Versus Guilt and Other Essays* (New York: William Morrow and Co., 1987); *A Conflict of Visions: Ideological Origins of Political Struggles* (New York: William Morrow and Co., 1987); *Judicial Activism Reconsidered* (Stanford, Calif.: Hoover Institution, 1989); *Preferential Policies: An International Perspective* (New York: William Morrow and Co., 1990); *Inside American Education: The Decline, the Deception, the Dogmas* (New York: Free Press, 1993); *Race and Culture: A World View* (New York: Basic Books, 1994); *The Vision of the Anointed: Self-Congratulation as a Basis for Social Policy* (New York: Basic Books, 1995); *Migrations and Cultures: A World View* (New York: Basic Books, 1996); *Late-Talking Children* (New York: Basic Books, 1997); *Conquests and Cultures: An International History* (New York: Basic Books, 1998).

303. Cf. Nathan Glazer and Daniel P. Moynihan, *Beyond the Melting Pot: The Negroes, Puerto Ricans, Jews, Italians, and Irish of New York City,* 2d ed. (Cambridge, Mass.: M.I.T. Press, 1970), pp. xi–xxvi, xliii–lvii, 24–85, 299–315.

304. "Liberalism and the Negro: A Round-Table Discussion," in Segal, op. cit., p. 466.

305. Loc. cit. For a historical account that shows that the enforcement of civil rights was far more difficult than Glazer's remarks suggest, see Hugh Davis Graham, *The Civil Rights Era: Origins and Development of National Policy, 1960–1972,* op. cit., pp. 27–204, 420–76.

306. Glazer, "In Defense of Preference," op. cit., p. 19.

307. "Liberalism and the Negro: A Round-Table Discussion," in Segal, op. cit., p. 467.

308. Loc. cit.

309. Glazer, "In Defense of Preference," op. cit., p. 19.

310. Loc. cit.

311. Ibid., p. 24.

312. Traub, "Nathan Glazer Changes His Mind, Again," op. cit.

313. Glazer, "In Defense of Preference," op. cit., p. 25.

314. Stephan Thernstrom and Abigail Thernstrom (*America in Black and White: One Nation Indivisible* [New York: Simon and Schuster, 1997], pp. 16–17) point out: "As two authors for whom the 1960s were formative years, we remain committed to race neutral policies. Not simply because they are morally right; in a society already deeply divided along lines of race, we see divisive race-conscious programs as dangerous."

315. Abigail Thernstrom, "The Drive for Racially Inclusive Schools," in Harold Orlans and June O'Neill, eds., *Affirmative Action Revisited,* a special issue of *The Annals of the American Academy of Political and Social Science* 523 (September 1992): 131–43.

316. Thernstrom and Thernstrom, op. cit., pp. 13, 52, 496–97, 527. For the analyses and position of Derrick Bell, see the following: *Race, Racism and American Law,* 2d ed. (Boston: Little Brown and Co., 1980); *Faces at the Bottom of the Well: The Permanence of Racism* (New York: Basic Books, 1992); "Remembrances of Racism Past: Getting beyond the Civil Rights Decline," in Hill and Jones Jr., op. cit., pp. 73–82; *Confronting Authority: Reflections of an Ardent Protester* (Boston: Beacon Press, 1994); *Gospel Choirs: Psalms of Survival in an Alien Land Called Home* (New York: Basic Books, 1996); and "The Strange Career of Randall Kennedy," *New Politics,* n.s., 7:1 (summer 1998): 55–68.

317. See Joseph G. Conti and Brad Stetson, *Challenging the Civil Rights Establishment: Profiles of a New Black Vanguard* (Westport, Conn.: Praeger Publishers, 1993), pp. 193–226.

318. Quoted in Thernstrom and Thernstrom, op. cit., p. 540.

319. Ibid., p. 396.

320. Loc. cit.

321. Traub, op. cit., p. 25. For Wolfe's position, based on his survey of the social attitudes of white middle-class Americans, see Alan Wolfe, *One Nation, After All: What Middle-Class Americans Really Think about God, Country, Family, Racism, Welfare, Immigration, Homosexuality, Work, the Right, the Left, and Each Other* (New York: Viking, Penguin, 1998).

322. Abigail Thernstrom and Stephen Thernstrom, "The Prescience of Myrdal," *The Public Interest* 128 (summer 1997): 36–54.

323. Stephen Steinberg, "Up from Slavery: The Myth of Black Progress," *New Politics,* n.s., 7:1 (summer 1998): 69–81. Quotation from p. 75.

324. "Liberalism and the Negro: A Round-Table Discussion," op. cit., p. 469.

325. Steinberg, "Up from Slavery," op. cit., p. 70, singles out Carl N. Degler's "The Negro in America—Where Myrdal Went Wrong," *New York Times Magazine,* December 7, 1969, pp. 64ff., for asserting, "Myrdal's optimism is the greatest weakness in his book." Steinberg, who has developed a powerful critique of conservative

perspectives on the race and ethnic issues in America,—[see, e.g., *The Ethnic Myth: Race, Ethnicity, and Class in America,* updated ed. (Boston: Beacon Press, 1989); *Turning Back: The Retreat from Racial Justice in American Thought and Policy* (Boston: Beacon Press, 1995); "Race and Radicalism in the 1960s," *New Politics,* n.s., 5:3 (summer 1995): 41–54; and "Science and Politics in the Work of William Julius Wilson," *New Politics* 6:2 (winter 1997): 72–83]—believes that "by idealizing human nature and American democracy, Myrdal failed to grasp the depth of American racism, or to anticipate the decades of political struggle that lay ahead." Steinberg also criticizes Myrdal's failure to see that black insurgency, rather than the positive operation of the American Creed on white people's consciences, would be crucial for the extension of civil rights, and for regarding "the Negro masses as irredeemably passive . . . [while he] looked to political elites and the labor movement as instruments of social change." In 1972, it should be noted, Myrdal ["An American Dilemma—Has It Been Resolved," op. cit., p. 299] insisted "I did see the Negro rebellion . . . I even foresaw that the Negro rebellion would have its start in the South," but he conceded that "I saw the [Negro] church as rather passive . . . , and did not foresee the active role it would come to play in the Negro rebellion." For a sensitive study of the role that certain black youths played in the civil rights movement, see David Halberstam, *The Children* (New York: Random House, 1998). Halberstam reports (p. 721) that in 1955 he carried "a copy of Gunnar Myrdal's *An American Dilemma,* the most important and influential book I had read at the time and probably have read since . . . to Jackson, Mississippi, ready to be a heroic reporter."

326. Steinberg, "Up from Slavery," op. cit., p. 75.

327. Ibid., pp. 75–77.

328. Thernstrom, "The Prescience of Myrdal," op. cit., p. 53.

329. Stephen Thernstrom, "Farewell to Preferences?" *The Public Interest* 130 (winter 1998): 34–49. Quotation from p. 49.

330. Myrdal, *An American Dilemma,* op. cit., pp. 1021–22.

331. Abigail Thernstrom and Stephan Thernstrom, "The Prescience of Myrdal," op. cit., p. 34.

332. Stephan Thernstrom and Abigail Thernstrom, *America in Black and White,* op. cit., p. 544.

333. Stephan Thernstrom, "Farewell to Preferences?" op. cit., p. 49.

334. Myrdal, "Toward a Better America," op. cit., p. 290.

335. See Lawrence D. Bobo, "The Color Line, the Dilemma, and the Dream: Race Relations in America at the Close of the Twentieth Century," in John Higham, ed., *Civil Rights and Social Wrongs: Black-White Relations since World War II,* op. cit., pp. 31–58.

336. For an illuminating breakdown of the several meanings of "success" and their relationship to the "American Dream," see Jennifer L. Hochschild, *Facing Up to the American Dream: Race, Class, and the Soul of the Nation* (Princeton, N.J.: Princeton University Press, 1995), pp. 157–260.

337. Cf. Charles R. Lawrence III, "Race and Affirmative Action: A Critical Race

Perspective," in David Kairys, ed., *The Politics of Law: A Progressive Critique,* 3d ed. (New York: Basic Book, 1998), pp. 312–27.

338. W. Arthur Lewis, *Racial Conflict and Economic Development.* The W. E. B. DuBois Lectures, 1982 (Cambridge, Mass.: Harvard University Press, 1985), p. 121.

339. Loc. cit.

340. Bart Landry, "The Enduring Dilemma of Race in America," in Alan Wolfe, ed., *America at Century's End* (Berkeley: University of California Press, 1991), pp. 185–207. Quotation from p. 207.

341. Loc. cit.

342. John Higham, "Coda: Three Reconstructions," in Higham, ed., op. cit., pp. 179–89.

343. Ibid., p. 186.

344. Loc. cit.

345. Ibid., pp. 188–89.

346. Ibid., p. 189.

347. Loc. cit.

348. Bruce Ackerman, *The Future of the Liberal Revolution* (New Haven, Conn.: Yale University Press, 1992), p. 123.

349. Loc. cit.

350. Ernst B. Haas, *Nationalism, Liberalism, and Progress: The Rise and Decline of Nationalism* (Ithaca, N.Y.: Cornell University Press, 1997), I, p. 352.

351. Loc. cit.

352. Ackerman, op. cit., p. 22.

Chapter Two. The "Yellow Peril" Mystique: Origins and Vicissitudes of a Racist Discourse

1. The original measurement of societal distance was devised by the U.S.C. sociologist Emory Bogardus. See his "Social Distance: A Measuring Stick," *Survey Graphic Number* 56:3 (May 1, 1926): 169–70, 206, 208, 210, wherein he asserted: "Race prejudice is measurable in terms of social distance, and racial goodwill expands to the degree that social distance shrinks" (p. 210).

2. Paul Spickard, "Who Is an American? Teaching about Ethnic and Racial Hierarchy," *Immigration and Ethnic Newsletter* 31:1 (May 1999): 1, 8–9. Quoted statement from p. 1.

3. Ibid., p. 8.

4. In 1920, Emory Bogardus found it necessary to observe in a book whose purpose was "To Help win the War for Democracy" (emphasis in original): "The Japanese in Our Country, with certain exceptions, are an un-American portion of our population." Emory Bogardus, *Essentials of Americanization,* rev. ed. (Los Angeles: Jesse Ray Miller, University of Southern California Press, 1920), pp. 9, 25.

5. Calvin Sims, "Koreans See Dark Scenario in U.S. Precaution," *New York Times,* December 26, 1999, p. 8. See also Calvin Sims, "North and South Koreans Meet on Mountain Path," *New York Times,* February 15, 2000, p. A3.

6. James Sterngold, "Coalition Fears an Asian Bias in Nuclear Case," *New York Times,* December 13, 1999, pp. A1, A26. On December 10, Dr. Lee was arrested and charged with fifty-nine counts of mishandling atomic and nuclear data—including, reportedly, allegations that he not only had transferred and copied secret documents but also altered three of them, removing or hiding their classified markings, and that he had made tape copies of others in 1993, 1994, and 1997. In September 2000, fifty-eight of these counts were dropped. Dr. Lee pleaded guilty to one count and was released. (Matthew Purdy, "The Making of a Suspect: The Case of Wen Ho Lee," *New York Times,* February 4, 2001, pp. 1, 18–19; and Matthew Purdy with James Sterngold, "The Prosecution Unravels: The Case of Wen Ho Lee," *New York Times,* February 5, 2001, pp. A1, A15. He had not been accused of giving secret information to an unauthorized person or to a foreign power. James Risen, "Tight Curbs on Use of Nuclear Secrets in Scientist's Trial," *New York Times,* December 8, 1999, p. A9.) Before Lee's indictment some journalists suggested that there was little evidence to support a charge of espionage against the Taiwan-born scientist who is a naturalized American citizen. (See Lars-Erik Nelson, "China Spy Plot: Less Than What Meets the Eye," *New York Daily News,* May 5, 1999; Steven Aftergood, "How Not to Combat Chinese Espionage," *Los Angeles Times,* July 4, 1999; Peter Grier, "China Spy Case: Real or Imagined?" *Christian Science Monitor,* August 26, 1999; Bob Drogin, "Chinese Spy Case Produces Heavy Fallout, Little Else," *Los Angeles Times,* September 20, 1999; Robert Schmidt, "Crash Landing," URL:http://wenholee.org/brillo.htm, November, 1999; Vernon Loeb and Walter Pincus, "New Spy Data Suggests Scientist Is Innocent," *San Jose Mercury News,* November 19, 1999; Robert Scheer, "Commentary," *Los Angeles Times,* November 23, 1999.) Frank Wu, "Task Force Reports Findings: What It Means for API Lab Scientists," and Janet Dong, "API Lab Employees File Suit, *Asian Week* 21:22 (January 27–February 2, 2000): 11–13.

Friends and supporters of Dr. Lee and a coalition of Asian American civil rights groups had formed a defense fund and encouraged the formation of support groups for the accused scientist. (William J. Broad, "Friends Rally Support for Los Alamos Scientist," *New York Times,* December 21, 1999, p. D1; "Asian American Scientist Files Bias Complaint," *New York Times,* December 24, 1999, p. A14; James Sterngold, "For Asian Americans a New Political Resolve," *New York Times,* September 22, 1999, pp. A1, A21.) On December 20, 1999, Dr. Lee and his family filed suit against the FBI and the Justice and Energy Departments, charging them with violating provisions of the Privacy Act of 1974. (Neil A. Lewis, "Imprisoned Scientist Sues U.S. Agencies," *New York Times,* December 21, 1999, p. A23; "Family of Dr. Lee Announces Filing . . . ," URL:http://www.wenholee.org/media122099.htm; James Sterngold, "Two Sides Clash over Bail for Indicted Atom Scientist," *New York Times,* December 28, 1999, p. A16; James Sterngold, "Atom Scientist Is Denied Bail, But Possibility Is Held Out," *New York Times,* December 30, 1999, p. A19, "Wen Ho Lee Attorneys Say 'Mishandled Information' Was Available in Public Domain," *Pacific Citizen* 130:9 [March 3–7, 2000]: 1, 8.)

7. Quoted in Bill Mesler, "The Spy Who Wasn't," *Nation* 269:5 (October 9/6, 1999): 13.

8. Cf. His remarks quoted on William J. Broad, "Spies vs. Sweatt: The Debate over China's Nuclear Advance," *New York Times,* September 7, 1999, pp. A1, A14–15.

9. Lars-Erik Nelson, "Washington: The Yellow Peril," *New York Review of Books* 46:12 (July 15, 1999): 10.

10. Paul D. Moore, "China's Subtle Spying," Op-Ed essay, *New York Times,* September 2, 1999, p. A21. On December 24, 1999, a federal judge announced that he would review Dr. Lee's lawyers' request for bail for their client. Lee had not been charged with espionage. "Judge to Hear Request to Release Nuclear Scientist Awaiting Trial," *New York Times,* December 25, 1999, p . A13. Bail was denied.

11. Thus, Lieutenant General J. L. DeWitt, commander of the Western Defense Command and Fourth Army, included in his justification for the forced evacuation of a persons of Japanese descent from the Pacific coast of the United States the allegation that "more than 115, 000 persons of Japanese ancestry *resided along the coast and were significantly concentrated near* many highly sensitive installations essential to the war effort." U.S. Army, Western Defense Command and Fourth Army, *Final Report: Japanese Evacuation from the West Coast, 1942* (Washington, D.C.: Government Printing Office, 1943), p. vii.

12. Fox Butterfield and Joseph Kahn, "Chinese Intellectuals in U.S. Say Spying Case Unfairly Casts Doubts on Their Loyalties," *New York Times,* May 16, 1999, p. 26.

13. Meihong Xu and Larry Engelmann, *Daughter of China: A True Story of Love and Betrayal* (New York: John Wiley and Sons, 1999).

14. "Illegal Chinese Immigrants Posing as Japanese," *Pacific Citizen* 129:9 (August 27–September 2, 1999): 5.

15. Somini Sengupta, "Women Keep Garment Jobs by Sending Babies to China," *New York Times,* September 14, 1999, pp. A1, A21.

16. See Yasuko I. Takezawa, *Breaking the Silence: Redress and Japanese American Ethnicity* (Ithaca, N.Y.: Cornell University Press, 1995), pp. 98–103, 170–72.

17. Qian Xuesen's career in the United States and in China is discussed in *Report of the Select Committee on U.S. National Security and Military/Commercial Concerns with the People's Republic of China.* House of Representatives. 105th Congress. 2d Session. Report 105–851. Declassified May 25, 1999, in part, pursuant to House Resolution 5, as amended, 106th Congress, 1st session. Kenneth deGraffenreid, ed. (Washington, D.C.: Regnery Publishing, 1999), pp. 165–67. His situation is mentioned in Butterfield and Kahn, op. cit., p. 26.

18. Quoted in David E. Sanger, "50 Years Made China Change. But Not the Fear of It," *New York Times,* October 3, 1999, p. 4.

19. See Ling Chi Wang, "China Spy Scandal Taps Reservoir of Racism." URL:http://www.minorities-jb.com/asian/news/spying3c.html; and Helen Zia, "Presumed Guilt @ Los Alamos: Questions Mainstream Reporters (Who Should Know Better) Should Be Asking Themselves," URL:http://www.minorities-jb.com/asian/news/zia3b.html

20. Butterfield and Kahn, op. cit., p. 26. The arrest of Wen Ho Lee appears to be

an instance of "racial profiling," or selective prosecution, in that former CIA director John M. Deutch had committed the same "crime"—placing large volumes of classified materials on his home computer—but was neither fully investigated nor charged. See James Risen, "C.I.A. Inquiry of Its Ex-Director Was Stalled at Top, Report Says: Case Involved Handling of Secret Computer Files," *New York Times,* February 1, 2000, pp. A1, A16; and "Security Lapses; Don't Let Deutch off Hook—Incident Bears Comparison to Los Alamos Case," Editorial, *Sun-Sentinel, South Florida,* February 25, 2000, p. 22A. See also Associated Press, "Energy Probe Finds Racial Profiling in Wake of Wen Ho Lee Case," *Pacific Citizen* 130:4 (January 28–February 3, 2000): 1, 6; George M. Ong, "On Behalf of Wen Ho Lee," Letter to the editor, *Asian Week* 21:19 (January 6–12, 2000): 4; and L. Ling-chi Wang, "A Request to Feinstein," *Asian Week* 21:21 (January 20–January 26, 2000): 6.

21. Max Weber, "Critical Studies in the Logic of the Cultural Sciences: A Critique of Eduard Meyer's Methodological Views," in idem, *The Methodology of the Social Sciences,* trans. and ed. Edward A. Shils and Henry A. Finch (New York: Free Press, 1949), pp. 113–88, esp. pp. 182–85. See also the discussion of the usefulness of this analogy in Seymour Martin Lipset, *The First New Nation: The United States in Historical and Comparative Perspective* (New York: W. W. Norton, 1979), pp. 6–9.

22. See two works by Edward Said, *Orientalism* (New York: Pantheon, 1978); and *Culture and Imperialism* (New York: Alfred A, Knopf, 1993).

23. Bryan S. Turner, *Orientalism, Postmodernism and Globalism* (London: Routledge, 1994), pp. 101–2. See also the critique of Said's thesis in Bernard Lewis, *Islam and the West* (New York: Oxford University Press, 1993), pp. 99–132.

24. See Harold Garfinkel, "Respecification: evidence for locally produced, naturally accountable phenomena of order, logic, reason, meaning, method, etc. in and as of the essential haecceity of immortal ordinary society (I)-an announcement of studies," in *Ethnomethodology and the Human Sciences,* ed. Graham Button (New York: Cambridge University Press, 1993), pp. 10–19.

25. Turner, op. cit., p. 21.

26. Cf. Lena Jayussi, "Values and moral judgement: communicative praxis as a moral order," in Button, ed., op, cit., p. 227–51, esp. pp. 243–49.

27. Herbert Blumer, "The Nature of Race Prejudice," *Social Process in Hawaii* 5 (June 1939): 11–20. Reprinted in Stanford M. Lyman and Arthur J. Vidich, *Social Order and the Public Philosophy: An Analysis and Interpretation of the Work of Herbert Blumer* (Fayetteville: University of Arkansas Press, 1988), pp. 183–95. Quoted material from p. 185.

28. Herbert Blumer, "Race Prejudice as a Sense of Group Position," *Pacific Sociological Review* 1 (spring 1958): 3–7. Reprinted in Lyman and Vidich, op. cit., pp. 196–207.

29. Blumer, "The Nature of Race Prejudice," in Lyman and Vidich, op. cit., p. 190.

30. Richard Austin Thomas, *The Yellow Peril, 1890–1924* (New York: Arno Press, 1979), pp. 1–3. See also William F. Wu, *The Yellow Peril: Chinese Americans in American Fiction, 1850–1940* (Hamden, Conn.: Archon Books, 1982).

31. Jonathan D. Spence, *The Chan's Great Continent: China in Western Minds* (New York: W. W. Norton, 1998), pp. 81–100.

32. Ibid., p. 99.

33. Richard Austin Thompson, *The Yellow Peril, 1890–1924* (New York: Arno Press, 1978), pp. 1–6.

34. Wolfram Eberhard, *A History of China,* rev. and enlarged ed. (Berkeley: University of California Press, 1969), p. 230.

35. Richard Austin Thompson, op. cit., pp. 2–3.

36. Ibid., p. 3.

37. Arthur deGobineau, "Events in Asia (1880–1881)," in Michael D. Biddiss, ed., *Gobineau: Selected Political Writings* (New York: Harper and Row, 1970), p. 242.

38. Victor Purcell, *The Boxer Uprising: A Background Study* (Cambridge, U.K.: Cambridge University Press, 1963), p. 90.

39. Thompson, op. cit., pp. 2–3. A slightly different description of the painting will be found in Gary Y. Okihiro, *Margins and Mainstreams: Asians in American History and Culture* (Seattle: University of Washington Press, 1994), pp. 118–19.

40. Purcell, op. cit., pp. 263–71.

41. Limin Chu, *The Images of China and the Chinese in the Overland Monthly, 1868–1875, 1883–1935,* Ph.D. diss., Duke University, 1965 (Ann Arbor: University Microfilms, 1966), pp. 307–23.

42. William B. Farwell, *The Chinese at Home and Abroad—Together with The Report of the Special Committee of the Board of Supervisors of San Francisco on the Condition of the Chinese Quarter of that City* (San Francisco: A. L. Bancroft and Co., 1885; reprint, San Francisco: R and E Research Associates, 1970), pp. 104–11.

43. H[arry] H[ubbell] Kane, *Opium-Smoking in America and China: A Study of Its Prevalence, and Effects, Immediate and Remote, on the Individual and the Nation* (New York: G. P. Putnam's Sons, 1882; reprint, New York: Arno Press, 1976), pp. 1–19, 32–45.

44. John Berda Gardner, *The Image of the Chinese in the United States, 1885–1915,* Ph.D. diss., University of Pennsylvania, 1961 (Ann Arbor: University Microfilms, 1970), pp. 25–27.

45. Frank Shay, reporter, *Chinese Immigration: The Social, Moral, and Political Effect of Chinese Immigration. Testimony Taken before a Committee of the Senate of the State of California* (Sacramento, Calif.: State Printing Office, 1876; reprint, San Francisco: R and E Research Associates, 1970), pp. 44, 47, 60–63, 89, 100, 116, 124, 132, 152.

46. California Legislature, "Chinese Immigrants Are Harming California," Memorial to Congress, 1877. Reprinted in William Dudley, ed., *Asian Americans: Opposing Viewpoints* (San Diego: Greenhaven Press, 1997), pp. 36–45, esp. pp. 40–43. Chinese students were first excluded from California's public schools, then segregated in San Francisco's "Oriental" school. See Charles M. Wollenberg, "'Yellow Peril' in the Schools (I)," in *The Asian American Educational Experience: A Source Book for Teachers and Students,* ed. Don T. Nakanishi and Tina Yamano Nishida (New York: Routledge, 1995), pp. 3–12.

47. Roger Daniels, *Concentration Camps: North America-Japanese in the United*

States and Canada during World War II (Malabar, Fla.: Robert E. Krieger Pub. Co., 1981), pp. 1–41. See also Gray Brechin, *Imperial San Francisco: Urban Power, Earthly Ruin* (Berkeley: University of California Press, 1999), pp. 156–70.

48. Robert Wolters, *A Short and True History of the Taking of California and Oregon by the Chinese in the Year A.D. 1899* (San Francisco: A. L. Bancroft, 1882).

49. Jacobus tenBroek, Edward N. Barnhart, and Floyd W. Matson, *Prejudice, War and the Constitution* (Berkeley: University of California Press, 1954), p. 19.

50. Chu, op. cit., p. 307.

51. H. J. West, *The Chinese Invasion* (San Francisco: Bacon and Co., 1873), p. 5. Quoted in tenBroek, Barnhart, and Matson, op. cit., p. 19.

52. Atwell Whitney, *Almond-Eyed* (San Francisco: A. L. Bancroft, 1878). The plot of this novel is summarized in tenBroek, Barnhart, and Matson, op. cit., p. 18.

53. Pierton W. Dooner, *Last Days of the Republic* (San Francisco: Alta California Publishing House, 1880), pp. 257–58.

54. Jeffery M. Dorwart, *The Pigtail War: American Involvement in the Sino-Japanese War, 1894–1895* (Amherst: University of Massachusetts Press, 1975), pp. 91–113; Chester Holcombe, *The Real Chinese Question* (New York: Young People's Missionary Movement, 1909 [1900]), pp. 115.147; Chu, op. cit., pp. 237–47.

55. Cited in tenBroek, Barnhart, and Matson, op. cit., p. 19.

56. Austin Lewis, quoted from Joan London, *Jack London and His Times* (Garden City, N.Y.: Doubleday, 1939), p. 191, in Clarice Stasz, *American Dreamers: Charmian and Jack London* (New York: St. Martin's Press, 1988), p. 75.

57. Stasz, op. cit., p. 159.

58. Jack London, "The Yellow Peril," in *Revolution and Other Essays* (New York: Macmillan, 1910), pp. 282–83. Quoted in Richard Hofstadter, *Social Darwinism in American Thought* (Boston: Beacon Press, 1967 [1944]), p. 189.

59. Jack London, "The Unparalleled Invasion," in *Moon-Face and Other Stories* (New York: Macmillan, 1904, 1919), pp. 71 ff. Quoted in tenBroek, Barnhart, and Matson, op. cit., pp. 19–20.

60. See, e.g., Samuel Gompers and Hermann Gudstadt, "Some Reasons for Chinese Exclusion. Meat vs. Rice. American Manhood against Asiatic Coolieism. Which Shall Survive?" Originally published by the American Federation of Labor. (Washington, D.C.: Government Printing Office, 1902), pp. 3–30.

61. Garder, op. cit., p. 89.

62. Oto E. Mundo, *The Recovered Continent: A Tale of the Chinese Invasion* (Columbus, Ohio: Harper, Osgood, 1898).

63. Ibid., p. 194. Quoted in William F. Wu, *The Yellow Peril: Chinese Americans in American Fiction, 1850–1940* (Hamden, Conn.: Archon Books, 1982), p. 38.

64. Carl Crow, *Four Hundred Million Customers: The Experiences—Some Happy, Some Sad—of an American in China, and What They Taught Him* (New York: Halcyon House, 1937).

65. Chu, op. cit., pp. 307–23. Quotation from p. 307.

66. Ibid., p. 10.

67. Ibid., pp. 309–10.

68. Dooner, op. cit., p. 245.

69. Ibid., pp. 251–52.

70. Chu, op. cit., pp. 311–12.

71. See, e.g., Sucheng Chan, ed., *Entry Denied: Exclusion and the Chinese Community in America, 1882–1943* (Philadelphia: Temple University Press, 1991).

72. Adah F. Battele, "The Sacking of Grubbville," *Overland Monthly*, 2d series, 20 (December 1892): 573–77.

73. William W. Crane, "The Year 1899," *Overland Monthly*, 2d series, 11 (June 1893): 579–89.

74. Chu, op. cit., p. 314.

75. Chu, op. cit., pp. 314–18; Wu, op. cit., pp. 43–44.

76. Alexander Saxton, *The Rise and Fall of the White Republic: Class Politics and Mass Culture in Nineteenth-Century America* (London: Verso, 1990).

77. In 1903, W. E. B. DuBois wrote, "The Problem of the twentieth century is the problem of the color-line,—the relation of the darker to the lighter races of men in Asia and Africa, in America and the islands of the sea." W. E. B. DuBois, "The Souls of Black Folk," in *Writings: The Suppression of the African Slave Trade; The Souls of Black Folk; Dusk of Dawn; Essays and Articles,* text selection and notes by Nathan Huggins (New York: Literary Classics of the United States, 1986), p. 372.

78. Maurice Muret, *The Twilight of the White Races,* trans. Mrs. Touzalin (New York: Charles Scribner's Sons, 1926), p. 256.

79. Ibid., p. 257.

80. See Hsi-sheng Ch'i, *Warlord Politics in China, 1916–1928* (Stanford, Calif.: Stanford University Press, 1976).

81. Muret, op. cit., p. 257.

82. Stuart Creighton Miller, *The Unwelcome Immigrant: The American Image of the Chinese, 1785–1882* (Berkeley: University of California Press, 1969); Arthur Bonner, *Alas! What Brought Thee Hither? The Chinese in New York, 1800–1950* (Teaneck, N.J.: Fairleigh Dickinson University and Cranbury, N.J.: Associated University Presses, 1997); John Kuo Wei Tchen, *New York before Chinatown: Orientalism and the Shaping of American Culture, 1776–1882* (Baltimore: Johns Hopkins University Press, 1999).

83. Thomas Nast, artist, "Every Dog (No Distinction of Color) Has His Day," *Harper's Weekly*, February 8, 1879. Reprinted in Bonner, op. cit., p. 50; and in Philip Choy, Lorraine Dong, and Marlon K. Hom, *The Coming Man: Nineteenth-Century American Perceptions of the Chinese* (Seattle: University of Washington Press, 1994), p. 118.

84. Thomas Nast, artist, "The Chinese Question," *Harper's Weekly*, February 18, 1871. Reprinted in Choy, Dong, and Hom, op. cit., p. 119.

85. Thomas Nast, artist, "Uncle Sam's Thanksgiving Dinner," *Harper's Weekly*, November 20, 1869, p. 745. Reprinted in Choy, Dong, and Hom, op. cit., p. 120.

86. Thomas Nast, artist, "'The Nigger Must Go,' and 'The Chinese Must Go,'" *Harper's Weekly*, September 18, 1879. Reprinted in Choy, Dong, and Hom, op. cit., p. 117.

87. Felix Regamey, "Pennsylvania—War of Races in the City of Brotherly Love—Colored Washerwomen Berating Chinese Laundrymen," *Frank Leslie's Illustrated Newspaper*, September 25, 1869, p. 32. Reprinted in Choy, Dong, and Hom, op. cit., p. 122.

88. G. F. Keller, illustrator, "The Ship of State Glided Noiselessly to Her Doom," frontispiece; "The Governor of California," between pp. 48–49; "Chinese Mandarins in Washington," between pp. 96–97; "The War of the Races," between pp. 160–61; "The Beginning of the End," between pp. 208–9, in Dooner, op. cit. These drawings are reprinted in Choy, Dong, and Hom, op. cit., pp. 128–32.

89. Choy, Dong, and Hom, op. cit., pp. 76, 81, 88–90, 104–11, 127, 134–35, 151. Recently, works examining the actual role of Chinese women in the periods of both free immigration and exclusion have thrown new light and greater importance on a hitherto neglected area of Chinese American history and social organization. See among many: Huping Ling, "Chinese Merchant Wives in the United States," pp. 79–92; Yem Siu Fong, "Expressing Self: The Development of Personal Autonomy in Second-Generation Chinese Women," pp. 93–102; Marjorie Lee, "On Contradiction: The Second Generation," pp. 93–110, in Munson A. Kwok et al., *Origins and Destinations: Forty-one Essays on Chinese America* (Los Angeles: Chinese Historical Society of Southern California and UCLA Asian American Studies Center, 1994); Benson Tong, *Unsubmissive Women: Chinese Prostitutes in Nineteenth-Century San Francisco* (Norman: University of Oklahoma Press, 1994); two works by Judy Yung, *Unbound Feet: A Social History of Chinese Women in San Francisco* (Berkeley: University of California Press, 1995); and *Unbound Voices: A Documentary History of Chinese Women in San Francisco* (Berkeley: University of California Press, 1999); Huping Ling, *Surviving on the Gold Mountain: A History of Chinese American Women and Their Lives* (Albany: State University of New York Press, 1998); and George Anthony Peffer, *If They Don't Bring Their Women Here: Chinese Female Immigration before Exclusion* (Urbana: University of Illinois Press, 1999).

90. Robert G. Lee, *Orientals: Asian Americans in Popular Culture* (Philadelphia: Temple University Press, 1999), pp. 35–36.

91. John Kuo Wei Tchen, "Quimbo Appo's Fear of Fenians: Chinese-Irish-Anglo Relations in New York City," in Ronald H. Bayor and Timothy J. Meagher, eds., *The New York Irish* (Baltimore: Johns Hopkins University Press, 1996), pp. 125–52.

92. *The WASP,* November 7, 1885, p. 3. Quoted in Philip P. Choy, Lorraine Dong, and Marlon K. Hom, op. cit., p. 125.

93. J. B. Arkhaus, artist, "The 'Fourth' of the Future," *The WASP,* n.d., pp. 8–9. Pictured in Choy, Dong, and Hom, op. cit., p. 133. Quoted description by Choy, Dong, and Hom will be found on p. 124.

94. G. F. Keller, artist, "A Statue for Our Harbor," *The WASP,* November 11, 1881, p. 320. Reprinted in Choy, Dong, and Hom, op. cit., p. 136.

95. Lee, op. cit., pp. 89, 68–69.

96. For a lengthy defense of Harte and a study of the literary usages to which "Plain Language from Truthful James" was put, see William Purviance Fenn, *Ah Sin and His*

Brethren in American Literature, a monograph delivered before the Convocation of the College of Chinese Studies, June 1933. (Peiping [Beijing]: College of Chinese Studies cooperating with California College in China, 1933), esp. pp. 45–128. Fenn (1903–1993), born in New Rochelle, New York, followed his father, Rev. Courtney H. Fenn, author of a report on the Boxer rebellion, and compiler of the first Bible concordance in Chinese and a Chinese-English dictionary, into the ministry, rising to the position of general secretary of the United Board for Christian Higher Education in Asia. At the time of his delivery of *Ah Sin and His Brethren in American Literature,* he was professor and head of the Department of Foreign Languages, University of Nanking. See Obituary, "William P. Fenn, 90, Protestant Missionary," *New York Times,* April 25, 1993, p. 21. See also Jonathan Spence, *The Chan's Great Continent: China in Western Minds,* op. cit., pp. 123–37.

97. Francis Bret Harte, "Plain Language from Truthful James," *Table Mountain,* 1870. Reprinted in Fenn, op. cit., pp. ix–x. The poem was inserted in the *Congressional Record* in 1879. E. P. Hutchinson, *Legislative History of American Immigration Policy, 1798–1865* (Philadelphia: University of Pennsylvania Press, 1981), p. 73.

98. Jonathan G. Utley, "American Views of China, 1900–1915: The Unwelcome But Inevitable Awakening," in Jonathan Goldstein, Jerry Israel, and Hilary Conroy, eds., *America Views China: American Images of China Then and Now* (Bethlehem, Penn.: Lehigh University Press, 1991), pp. 114–31, esp. pp. 114–16.

99. Robert Bogdan, *Freak Show: Presenting Human Oddities for Amusement and Profit* (Chicago: University of Chicago Press, 1990), pp. 65, 98–99.

100. Utley, op. cit., p. 116.

101. See Cay Van Ash and Elizabeth Sax Rohmer, *Master of Villainy: A Biography of Sax Rohmer* (London: Tom Stacey, 1972).

102. Robert McClellan, *The Heathen Chinee: Study of American Attitudes toward China, 1890–1905* (Columbus: Ohio State University Press, 1971), p. 253. For Japan-U.S. conceptions of one another before the Meiji period, see Peter Duus, *The Japanese Discovery of America: A Brief History with Documents* (Boston: Bedford Books, 1997).

103. Robert F. Heizer and Alan F. Almquist, *The Other Californians: Prejudice and Discrimination under Spain, Mexico, and the United States to 1920* (Berkeley: University of California Press, 1971), p. 178. The treatment of Japanese students, who, in 1905, were ordered into the "Oriental" school reserved for Chinese, created an international crisis. See Charles Wollenberg, "'Yellow Peril' in the Schools (II)," in Nakanishi and Nishida, op. cit., pp. 13–29.

104. Disputed anthropological theories about the "race" to which Japanese belonged entered into American law in the U.S. Supreme Court's decision that the immigrants from Japan were not "Caucasians" and, therefore, not white. Thus, until 1952, the *Issei,* i.e., the immigrant generation, were classified as aliens ineligible for United States citizenship. See "Naturalization Cases," in the Consulate-General of Japan, comp., *Documental History of Law Cases Affecting Japanese in the UnitedStates, 1916–1924, Vol. I: Naturalization Cases and Cases Affecting Constitutional and Treaty Rights* (San Francisco: The Consulate-General of Japan, 1925; reprint, New York: Arno Press, 1978), pp. 1–214.

See also Dr. Moritoshi Fukuda, S.J.D., *Legal Problems of Japanese Americans: Their History and Development in the United States* (Tokyo: Keio Tsushin Co., 1980), p. 3–94.

105. See e.g., the critical but ambiguous analysis of the question, "Is Japan Militant?" given by James A. B. Scherer, *The Japanese Crisis* (New York: Frederick A. Stokes Co., 1916), pp. 41–66.

106. Editorial, *Organized Labor,* March 17, 1900. Quoted in tenBroek, Barnhart, and Matson, op. cit., p. 24, and in Heizer and Almquist, op. cit., pp. 178–79.

107. Editorial, *Organized Labor,* March 11, 1905. Quoted in tenBroek, Barnhart, and Matson, op. cit., p. 26.

108. Editorial, *San Francisco Chronicle,* November 14, 1906. Quoted in tenBroek, Barnhart, and Matson, op. cit., p. 341 n. 78.

109. Earl Miner, *The Japanese Tradition in British and American Literature* (Princeton, N.J.: Princeton University Press, 1958, 1966), p. 276.

110. Robert E. Park, "Behind Our Masks," *Survey Graphic* 56:3 (May 1, 1926): 135–39. Park's essay was illustrated with photographs of Japanese Noh masks provided by Irene Lewisohn.

111. Roger Daniels, *The Politics of Prejudice: The Anti-Japanese Movement in California and the Struggle for Japanese Exclusion,* University of California Publications in History, vol. 71 (Berkeley: University of California Press, 1962), pp. 65–78.

112. See the essays collected in Peter Duus, Ramon H. Myers, and Mark R. Peattie, eds., *The Japanese Informal Empire in China, 1895–1937* (Princeton, N.J.: Princeton University Press, 1989); Ramon H. Myers and Mark R. Peattie, eds., *The Japanese Colonial Empire, 1895–1945* (Princeton, N.J.: Princeton University Press, 1984); and in Peter Duus, Ramon H. Myers, and Mark R. Peattie, eds., *The Japanese Wartime Empire, 1931–1945* (Princeton, N.J.: Princeton University Press, 1996), and a Japanese scholar's defense of Japan's arms in Asia and the Pacific: Seiji G. Ishida, *The International Position of Japan as a Great Power,* Studies in History, Economics and Public Law, vol. 24:3 (New York: Columbia University Press, 1905; reprint, New York: AMS Press, 1968). See also two works by Hilary Conroy: *The Japanese Frontier in Hawaii, 1868–1898,* University of California Publications in History, vol. 46 (Berkeley: University of California Press,1953); and *The Japanese Seizure of Korea, 1868–1910: A Study of Realism and Idealism in International Relations* (Philadelphia: University of Pennsylvania Press, 1960); and Toyokichi Iyenaga, "Japan in South Manchuria," an address delivered at Clark University on November 23, 1911, in George H. Blakeslee, ed., *Japan and Japanese-American Relations: Clark University Addresses* (New York: G. E. Stechert and Co., 1912), pp. 249–74.

113. See Alex Ladenson, "The Background of the Hawaiian-Japanese Labor Convention of 1886," *Pacific Historical Review* 9:4 (December 1940): 389–400. Reprinted in Dennis M. Ogawa with the assistance of Glen Grant, ed., *Kodomo no tame ni: For the Sake of the Children* (Honolulu: University Press of Hawaii, 1978), pp. 13–19; Yukiko Kimura, *Issei: Japanese Immigrants in Hawaii* (Honolulu: University Press of Hawaii, 1988), pp. 3–130; Franklin Odo and Kazuko Sinoto, *A Pictorial History of the Japanese in Hawaii, 1885–1924* (Honolulu: Bishop Museum Press, 1985), pp. 20–125,

152–203; Ronald Takaki, *Pau Hana: Plantation Life and Labor in Hawaii, 1835–1920* (Honolulu: University Press of Hawaii, 1983); and Dr. James H. Okakata, Chrmn., Publication Committee, ed., *A History of Japanese in Hawaii* (Honolulu: United Japanese Society of Hawaii, 1971), pp. 69–197.

114. Yamato Ichihashi, *Japanese Immigration: Its Status in California* (San Francisco: R and E Research Associates, 1970 [1915]), pp. 21–64; T. Iyenaga and Kenoski Sato, *Japan and the California Problem* (New York: G. P. Putnam's Sons, 1921), pp. 33–197; Tasuku Harada, *The Japanese Problem in California: Answers (by Representative Americans) to Questionnaire* (San Francisco: Privately Printed, 1922; reprint, San Francisco: R and E Research Associates, 1971); Jean Pajus, *The Real Japanese California* (Berkeley: James J. Gillick Co., 1937; reprint, San Francisco: R and E Research Associates, 1971); and Roger Daniels, *Asian America: Chinese and Japanese in the United States since 1850* (Seattle: University of Washington Press, 1988), pp. 100–185.

115. Yamato Ichihashi, *Japanese in the United States: A Critical Study of the Problems of the Japanese Immigrants and Their Children* (Stanford, Calif.: Stanford University Press, 1932; reprint, New York: Arno Press and the *New York Times*, 1969).

116. Robert E. Park, "Racial Assimilation in Secondary Groups with Particular Reference to the Negro," *Publication of the American Sociological Society* 8 (1913): 66–83; also in *American Journal of Sociology* 13 (March 1914): 606–19. Reprinted in Robert E. Park, *Race and Culture: The Collected Papers of Robert Ezra Park,* ed. Everett Cherrington Hughes et al. (Glencoe, Ill.: Free Press, 1950), vol. 1, pp. 204–20. Quoted material, p. 209.

117. Cabinet resolution of Dececember 30, 1903, *Nihon Gaiko Bunsho* 36/I, no. 50. Quoted in Ian Nish, *The Origins of the Russo-Japanese War* (London: Longman Group Ltd., 1985, 1996), p. 201.

118. Moritoshi Fukuda, op. cit., p. 33.

119. See Thomas A. Bailey, *Theodore Roosevelt and the Japanese-American Crisis: An Account of the International Complications Arising from the Race Problem on the Pacific Coast* (Gloucester, Mass.: Peter Smith, 1964 [1934]).

120. *Harper's Weekly,* November 1906. Quoted in Frank F. Chuman, *The Bamboo People: The Law and Japanese-Americans* (Del Mar, Calif.: Publisher's Inc., 1976), p. 348 n. 8.

121. Eugene Anschel, *Homer Lea, Sun Yat-sen, and the Chinese Revolution* (New York: Praeger, 1984). See also Marius B. Jansen, *The Japanese and Sun Yat-sen* (Cambridge, Mass.: Harvard University Press, 1954); and Carl Glick, *Double Ten: Captain O'Banion's Story of the Chinese Revolution* (London: Whittlesey House-McGraw-Hill Book Co., 1945).

122. Homer Lea, *The Valor of Ignorance* (New York: Harper and Brothers, 1942 [1909]), p. 69.

123. Ibid., p. 81.

124. Ibid., p. 81–82.

125. Ibid., p. 69.

126. Ibid., p. 111. Lea reprinted the Anglo-Japanese pact in an appendix, pp. 221–22.

127. Ibid., p. 87.
128. Loc. cit.
129. Ibid., p. 88.
130. Loc. cit.
131. Ibid., p. 91.
132. Ibid., p. 88.
133. Ibid., pp. 142–42.
134. Ibid., p. 248.
135. Ibid., p. 173.
136. Ibid., p. 220.
137. Ibid., p. 178.
138. Ibid., p. 179.
139. Ibid., pp. 178–220.
140. Toyokichi Iyenaga, ed., *Japan's Real Attitude toward America: A Reply to Mr. George Bronson Rea's "Japan's Place in the Sun—The Menace to America"* (New York: G. P. Putnam's Sons, 1916).
141. Ibid., p. 17.
142. Ibid., p. 26.
143. Loc. cit.
144. Loc. cit.
145. Ibid., p. 27.
146. Ibid., p. 12.
147. Ibid., p. 13.
148. Ibid., p. 27.
149. The Hon. Iichiro Tokutomi, *Japanese-American Relations,* trans. Sukeshige Yanagiwara (New York: Macmillan, 1922), p. 139.
150. Ibid., p. 143.
151. K. K. Kawakami, *Japan in World Politics* (New York: Macmillan, 1917), p. xv.
152. This idea had some supporters in the United States. See the discussion and the sources cited in Stanford M. Lyman, "Background to Internment: Bishop Yoshiaki Fukuda's Mission of Justice in America," in Rev. Yoshiaki Fukuda, *My Six Years of Internment: An* Issei's *Struggle for Justice* (San Francisco: Konko Church of San Francisco and the Research Information Center of the Konko Churches of America, 1990), pp. 85–99, esp. pp. 90–93 and p. 98 nn. 43–49.
153. K. K. Kawakami, *The Real Japanese Question* (New York: Macmillan, 1921), p. 234. See also K. K. Kawakami, *Japan and World Peace* (New York: Macmillan, 1919), pp. 63–71.
154. His Excellency Tsuyoshi Inukai, Prime Minister of Japan, "Introduction," K. K. Kawakami, *Japan Speaks on the Sino-Japanese Crisis* (New York: Macmillan, 1932), p. xii.
155. Ibid., p. 138.
156. Ibid., p. 111. Ironically, the Japanese occupation of Manchuria and Shanghai would prove to be a lifeline for thousands of East European Jews, who, with the help of a Japanese consul, a Japanese Protestant minister, and a few Japanese military officers,

escaped the Holocaust. See Martin Tokayer and Mary Swartz, *The Fugu Plan: The Untold Story of the Japanese and the Jews in World War II* (New York: Weatherhill, Inc., 1996) [1979]); Yukiko Sugihara, *Visas for Life,* trans. Hiroki Sugihara, ed. Lani Silver and Eric Saul (San Francisco: Small World Productions, 1993); Hillel Levine, *In Search of Sugihara: The Elusive Japanese Diplomat Who Risked His Life to Rescue 10,000 Jews from the Holocaust* (New York: Free Press, 1996); Abraham Kotsuji, *From Tokyo to Jerusalem* (New York: Bernard Geis-Random House, 1964); David Kranzler, *Japanese, Nazis and Jews: The Jewish Refugee Community of Shanghai, 1938–1945* (New York: Yeshiva University Press, 1976); and two books by Ben-Ami Shillony, *Politics and Culture in Wartime Japan* (Oxford, U.K.: Clarendon Press, 1981); and *The Jews and the Japanese: The Successful Outsiders* (Rutland, Vt.: Charles E. Tuttle, 1991). For Jewish memoirs of the Shanghai experience, see Rena Krasno, *Strangers Always: A Jewish Family in Wartime Shanghai* (Berkeley: Pacific View Press, 1992); Ernest G. Heppner, *Shanghai Refuge: A Memoir of the World War II Jewish Ghetto* (Lincoln: University of Nebraska Press, 1993); Evelyn Pike Rubin, *Ghetto Shanghai* (New York: Shengold Publishers, 1993); and James R. Ross, *Escape to Shanghai: A Jewish Community in China* (New York: Free Press, 1994). See also Solly Gaynor, *Light One Candle: A Survivor's Tale from Lithuania to Jerusalem* (New York: Kodansha International, 1995), pp. 33–50, 346–49.

157. K. K. Kawakami, *Manchouko: Child of Conflict* (New York: Macmillan, 1933), p. v.

158. I have here borrowed anti-Chinese phrases from Donald Keene, *Appreciations of Japanese Culture* (Tokyo: Kodansha International, 1981 [1971]), p. 273.

159. Japanese as well as white defenders of the *Issei* and their American-born offspring attempted to refute the accusations against them, but as the 1942 incarceration of all persons of Japanese descent living along the Pacific coast would show, their writings and speeches would have little effect on either policy or public opinion. For examples, see "Asia, Japan: Consular Reports," in Department of Commerce and Labor, *Special Consular Reports: Emigration to the United States,* 58th Congress, House of Representatives, Vol. XXX: Document No. 732 (Washington, D.C.: Government Printing Office, 1904), pp. 192–97; Herbert B. Johnson, D.D., *Discrimination against the Japanese in California: A Review of the Real Situation* (Berkeley: Courier Publishing Co., 1907; reprint, San Francisco; R and E Research Associates, 1971); The Japanese Association of the Pacific Northwest, *Japanese Immigration: An Exposition of Its Real Status* (Seattle: JAPN, publishers, 1907; reprint, San Francisco: R and E Research Associates, 1972); Kiichi Kanzaki, *California and the Japanese* (San Francisco: n.p., 1921; reprint, San Francisco: R and E Research Associates, 1971); H. A. Millis, *The Japanese Problem in the United States: An Investigation for the Commission on Relations with Japan Appointed by the Federal Council of the Churches of Christ* (New York: Macmillan, 1915); Allan A. Hunter, *Out of the Far East* (New York: Friendship Press, 1934; reprint, San Francisco: R and E Research Associates, 1972).

160. For an outstanding example of a missionary's life-long attempt to improve intercultural understanding and prevent war with Japan, see five books by Sidney Lewis Gulick (1860–1945): *The White Peril in the Far East: An Interpretation of the Significance*

of the Russo-Japanese War (New York: Fleming H. Revell, 1905); *The American Japanese Problem: A Study of the Racial Relations of the East and the West* (New York: Charles Scribner's Sons, 1914; reprint, Newark, N.J.: Jerome S. Ozer, 1971); *Working Women of Japan* (New York: Missionary Education Movement of the United States and Canada, 1915); *American Democracy and Asiatic Citizenship* (New York: Charles Scribner's Sons, 1918); *The East and the West: A Study of Their Psychic and Cultural Characteristics* (Rutland, Vt.: Charles E. Tuttle, 1963). For a biography of Gulick, see Sandra C. Taylor, *Advocate of Understanding: Sidney Gulick and the Search for Peace with Japan* (Kent, Ohio: Kent State University Press, 1984).

161. Jesse Frederick Steiner, *The Japanese Invasion: A Study in the Psychology of Inter-Racial Contacts* (Chicago: A. C. McClurg, 1917; reprint, New York: Arno Press, 1978).

162. Ibid., pp. 68–92.

163. Quoted in tenBroek, Barnhart, and Matson, op. cit., p. 35. On Ross, see Arthur J. Vidich and Stanford M. Lyman, *American Sociology: Worldly Rejections of Religion and Their Directions* (New Haven, Conn.: Yale University Press, 1985), pp. 151–67; and Sean H. McMahon, *Social Control and Public Intellect: The Legacy of Edward A. Ross* (New Brunswick, N.J.: Transaction Publishers, 1999), pp. 13–25, 107–36.

164. Jesse Frederick Steiner, "Some Factors Involved in Minimizing Race Friction on the Pacific Coast," *Annals of the American Academy of Political and Social Science* 93 (January 1921): 116–20.

165. Steiner, *The Japanese Invasion,* op. cit., p. 193. Twenty-five years after *The Japanese Invasion* was published, Steiner, who had become a professor of sociology at the University of Washington in Seattle, testified before the House of Representatives hearings on national defense migration, opposing the military's plan for the mass evacuation along the Pacific coast but proposing that the *Nisei* be treated in accordance with their educational experiences—the American-born, American-educated, and "thoroughly Americanized" to be let alone; the *Kibei,* i.e., those *Nisei* who had received some of their education in Japan, to be subjected to evacuation and surveillance together with the *Issei,* now dubbed "enemy aliens," and those *Nisei* who had not applied for renunciation of their dual citizenship status in Japan. "Testimony of J. F. Steiner, Professor, Department of Sociology, University of Washington, Seattle, Washington," *House of Representatives, Select Committee Investigating National Defense Migration,* March 2, 1942 (Washington, D.C.: Government Printing Office, 1942; reprint, New York: Arno Press, 1978), pp. 11557–64. Needless to say, neither Congress nor the military made such fine distinctions, preferring to remove all persons of Japanese descent from what was now deemed an area in danger of Japanese invasion, sabotage, and espionage and regarding the American Japanese as "Japs." See *Final Report: Japanese Evacuation From the West Coast, 1942* (Washington, D.C.: Government Printing Office, 1943).

166. John S. Chambers, "The Japanese Invasion," *Annals of the American Academy of Political and Social Science* 93 (January 1921): 23–29. Quoted material on p. 25.

167. Andrew W. Lind, *An Island Community: Ecological Succession in Hawaii* (New York: Greenwood Press, 1968 [1938]), pp. 210–44.

168. Gary Y. Okihiro, *Cane Fires: The Anti-Japanese Movement in Hawaii, 1865–1945* (Philadelphia: Temple University Press, 1991), pp. 86–87. The fear had been voiced as early as 1902 when the *Second Report of the U.S. Commissioner of Labor on Hawaii* stated, "At present a *laissez faire* policy [on immigration to Hawaii] is being pursued, which—so far as present tendencies indicate—will result in a few years in making the islands practically Japanese . . . [T]hey readily adopt Occidental habits, but they do not amalgamate with Caucasians and are intensely alien in their sympathies, religion, and customs." Quoted in Andrew W. Lind, *Hawaii's Japanese: An Experiment in Democracy* (Princeton, N.J.: Princeton University Press, 1946), pp. 12–13. And, it would be reiterated in 1927 in W. A. Kinney's *Hawaii's Capacity for Self-Government All but Destroyed* (Salt Lake City, Utah: Frank L. Jensen, publisher, 1927), p. 188: "The Asiatics have come to Hawaii, not as immigrants . . . but more by way of invasion and adventure—the Japanese, particularly, came with the set purpose of returning again to Japan, and are now staying on . . . largely with thoughts of ultimate aggression, . . . and . . . they are receiving direct encouragement from the government of Japan."

169. See Yamato Ichihashi, *The Washington Conference and After: A Historical Survey* (Stanford, Calif.: Stanford University Press, 1928.)

170. Warren Jefferson Davis, *Japan: The Air Menace of the Pacific* (Boston: Christopher Publishing Co., 1928; reprint, New York: Arno Press, 1970), pp. 48–75.

171. Ibid., p. 155.

172. Ibid., p. 130.

173. Ibid., p. 154.

174. Loc. cit.

175. Hector C. Bywater, *The Great Pacific War* (New York: St. Martin's Press, 1991 [1924]). For a biography of Bywater, see William H. Honan, *Visions of Infamy: The Untold Story of How Journalist Hector C. Bywater Devised the Plans That Led to Pearl Harbor* (New York: St. Martin's Press, 1991).

176. William H. Honan, "Introduction," in Bywater, op. cit., pp. iv–vi.

177. Ibid., p. 321.

178. Ibid., p. xi.

179. John E. Orchard, "The Japanese Dilemma," in Joseph Barnes, ed., *Empire in the East* (Freeport: Books for Libraries Press, 1970 [1934]), p. 39.

180. Carl Crow, *Japan and America: A Contrast* (New York: Robert M. McBride, 1916), p. 312.

181. Robert C. Kiste, "United States," in K. R. Howe, Robert C. Kiste, and Brij V. Val, eds., *Tides of History: The Pacific Islands in the Twentieth Century* (Honolulu: University of Hawaii Press, 1994), pp. 227–57, esp. pp. 239–49.

182. James H. Okahata, op. cit., pp. 257–62.

183. Bob Kumamoto, "The Search for Spies: America Counterintelligence and the Japanese American Community, 1931–1942," *Amerasia Journal* 6:2 (fall 1979): 45–75. See also Peter Irons, *Justice at War: The Story of the Japanese American Internment Cases* (New York: Oxford University Press, 1983), pp. 19–24; Roger Daniels, *Asian America: Chinese and Japanese in the United States since 1850* (Seattle: University of Washington

Press, 1988), pp. 199–224; Mitchell T. Maki, Harry H. L. Kitano, and S. Megan Berthold, *Achieving the Impossible Dream: How Japanese Americans Obtained Redress* (Urbana: University of Illinois Press, 1999), pp. 25–35.

184. See two books by Gordon W. Prange: *At Dawn We Slept: The Untold Story of Pearl Harbor* ((New York: Penguin Books, 1991 [1981]); idem with Donald M. Goldstein and Katherine V. Dillon, *December 7, 1941: The Day the Japanese Attacked Pearl Harbor* (New York: McGraw-Hill Book Co., 1988).

185. Gary Y. Okihiro, *Storied Lives: Japanese American Students and World War II* (Seattle: University of Washington Press, 1999), p. 25.

186. See J. Garner Anthony, *Hawaii under Army Rule* (Honolulu: University Press of Hawaii, 1975 [1955]); Roger Daniels, *The Decision to Relocate the Japanese Americans* (Philadelphia: J. B. Lippincott Co., 1975); and Paul Frederick Clark, *Those Other Camps: An Oral History Analysis of Japanese Alien Enemy Internment during World War II,* M.A. thesis, California State University, Fullerton, 1980 (Ann Arbor: UMI Dissertation Services, 1980). Sometime during the 1930s, William Crane, a journalist who had worked for the *Wall Street Journal* but joined the Communist Party of the United States in 1932 and, later, would become an underground agent doing clandestine work for the Soviets, conducted a survey of the West Coast's Chinese and Japanese populations, taught English to a Japanese immigrant who was also a spy, and acted as co-publisher of a Japanese newspaper in Los Angeles. See John Earl Haynes and Harvey Klehr, *Venona: Decoding Soviet Espionage in America* (New Haven, Conn.: Yale University Press, 1999), p. 227.

187. Fears of a Japanese cooptation of African Americans had led the FBI to focus on the Nation of Islam leader, Elijah Mohammed. Their investigations revealed that Satohata Takahashi, an agent of Japan's Black Dragon Society, had sought to win over the Muslim sect's followers to the Japanese cause. See Karl Evanzz, *The Messenger: The Rise and Fall of Elijah Mohammed* (New York: Pantheon Books, 1999), pp. 105–11, 121–49.

188. U.S. Army Western Defense Command and Fourth Army, *Final Report . . . ,* op. cit., p. 34.

189. See the essays published in "Commemorative Issue: Japanese American Internment," *Amerasia Journal* 19:1 (winter 1993): v–viii, 1–162. A hitherto under-investigated feature of Japanese life—one that would indicate the progress of acculturation—sports, has recently been given extensive coverage. (See the special holiday issue of the national publication of the Japanese American Citizens League devoted entirely to "Community Ties through Sports," *Pacific Citizen* 29:23 [December 1999]: 6–110.)

190. Executive Order 9066. 3 C.F.R. 1092–93. February 19, 1942. Reprinted in Nobuya Tsuchida, *American Justice: Japanese American Evacuation and Redress Cases* (Minneapolis: Asian/Pacific American Learning Resource Center, University of Minnesota, 1988), p. 29.

191. *Hirabayashi vs. U.S.,* 320 U.S. 81 (1943); *Yasui vs. U.S.,* 320 U.S. 115 (1943); *Korematsu vs. U.S.,* 323 U.S. 214 (1944); *Ex Parte Endo,* 323 U.S. 283 (1944).

192. Michi Nishiura Weglyn, *Years of Infamy: The Untold Story of America's*

Concentration Camps, updated ed. (Seattle: University of Washington Press, 1996); and Audrie Girdner and Anne Loftis, *The Great Betrayal: The Evacuation of the Japanese-Americans during World War II* (London: Macmillan, 1969).

193. Donald E. Collins, *Native American Aliens: Disloyalty and the Renunciation of Citizenship by Japanese Americans during World War II* (Westport, Conn.: Greenwood Press, 1985); and R. Scott Corbett, *Quiet Passages: The Exchange of Civilians between the United States and Japan during the Second World War* (Kent, Ohio: Kent State University Press, 1987).

194. See two works by C. Harvey Gardiner, *The Japanese and Peru, 1873–1973* (Albuquerque: University of New Mexico Press, 1975); and *Pawns in a Triangle of Hate: The Peruvian Japanese and the United States* (Seattle: University of Washington Press, 1981). See also John K. Emmerson, *The Japanese Thread: A Life in the U.S. Foreign Service* (New York: Holt, Rinehart, and Winston, 1978), pp. 1–53, 125–49; and John K. Emmerson and Harrison M. Holland, *The Eagle and the Rising Sun: America and Japan in the Twentieth Century* (Reading, Mass.: Addison-Wesley Publishing Co., 1988), pp. 41–57. For the Peruvian Japanese in the American courts, see two articles by Edward N. Barnhart, "Japanese Internees from Peru," *Pacific Historical Review* 31:2 (May 1962): 169–78; and "Citizenship and Political Tests in Latin American Republics in World War II," *Hispanic American Historical Review* 42:3 (August 1962): 297–332. See also Corbett, op. cit., pp. 139–66.

195. Orville C. Shirey, *Americans: The Story of the 442nd Combat Team* (Washington, D.C.: Infantry Journal Press, 1946).

196. Thomas D. Murphy, *Ambassadors in Arms: The Story of Hawaii's 100th Battalion* (Honolulu: University of Hawaii Press, 1954). See also Edwin M. Nakasone, *The Nisei Soldier: Historical Essays of World War II* (White Bear Lake, Minn.: J-Press and E. Nakasone, 1997).

197. Martha Nakagawa, "'De Boys,' an Untold Story," *Pacific Citizen* 129:20 (November 12–18, 1999): 1, 5; and Paul Tsuneishi and Martha Nakagawa, "Remembering the 1800th Engineer Service Battalion," *Pacific Citizen* 129:21 (November 19–25, 1999): 1, 8.

198. Tad Ichinokuchi, ed., *John Aiso and the M.I.S.: Japanese American Soldiers in the Military Intelligence Service, World War II* (Los Angeles: Military Intelligence Club of Southern California, 1988), pp. 60–175.

199. George H. Kerr, *Formosa Betrayed* (Boston: Houghton-Mifflin, 1965), p. 30.

200. Girdner and Loftis, op. cit., pp. 332–35.

201. Tamotsu Shibutani, *The Derelicts of Company K: A Sociological Study of Demoralization* (Berkeley: University of California Press, 1978).

202. Frank Seishi Emi, "Draft Resistance at the Heart Mountain Concentration Camp and the Fair Play Committee," in Gail M. Omura, Russell Endo, Stephen H. Sumida, and Russell C. Leong, eds., *Frontiers of Asian American Studies: Writing, Research, and Commentary* (Pullman: Washington State University Press, 1989), pp. 41–70. See also Daniels, *Asian America,* op. cit., pp. 266–75.

203. S. Frank Miyamoto, "Resentment, Distrust, and Insecurity at Tule Lake," in

Yuji Ichioka, ed., *Views from Within: The Japanese American Evacuation Study* (Los Angeles: Asian American Studies Center, University of California at Los Angeles, 1989), pp. 127–40.

204. Quoted from an essay by Henry Steele Commager published in the September 1947 issue of *Harper's* in Maisie and Richard Conrat, eds., *Executive Order 9066: The Internment of 110,000 Japanese Americans* (San Francisco: California Historical Society, 1972), p. 92.

205. Maki, Kitano, and Berthold, op. cit., p. 184.

206. Irvin Molotsky, "Senate Votes to Compensate Japanese-American Internees," *New York Times*, April 21, 1988, pp. 1, 9. Quoted material from p. 9.

207. "Proposed Marker for Former DOJ Santa Fe Camp Stirs Bitter Memories," *Pacific Citizen* 129:11 (September 10–16, 1999): 1. The stigma of their internment would, as an invisible badge of dishonor, affect the status and opportunities of *Nisei, Sansei,* and *Yonsei* who served in the American military four decades after World War II had ended. See Toshio Whelchel, *From Pearl Harbor to Saigon: Japanese American Soldiers and the Vietnam War* (London: Verso, 1999); and Timothy P. Fong, *The Contemporary Asian American Experience: Beyond the Model Minority* (Upper Saddle River, N.J.: Prentice-Hall, 1998), pp. 16–19, 118–20, 178.

208. See Morton Grodzins, *Americans Betrayed: Politics and the Japanese Evacuation* (Chicago: University of Chicago Press, 1949). See also Dillon S. Myer, *Uprooted Americans: The Japanese Americans and the War Relocation Authority during World War II* (Tucson: University of Arizona Press, 1971), pp. 16–19. Debates over this issue continue to the present day. See, e.g., Peter T. Suzuki, "'For the sake of Inter-University Comity': The Attempted Suppression by the University of California of Morton Grodzins' *Americans Betrayed*," in Ichioka, op. cit., pp. 95–126.

209. Frank J. Taylor, "The People Nobody Wants," *Saturday Evening Post*, May 9, 1942, p. 66. Quoted in Morton Grodzins, *Americans Betrayed: Politics and the Japanese Evacuation*, op. cit., pp. 27–28.

210. Dale McLemore in the *San Francisco Examiner*, January 29, 1942. Quoted in Peter Irons, *Justice at War* (New York: Oxford University Press, 1983), p. 41.

211. Richard White "*It's Your Misfortune and None of My Own*": *A New History of the American West* (Norman: University of Oklahoma Press, 1991), p. 511.

212. Loc. cit.

213. Rev. Yoshiaki Fukuda, op. cit.

214. See Teruko Imai Kumei, "'Skeleton in the Closet': The Japanese American *Hokoku Seinen-dan* and Their 'Disloyal' Activities at the Tule Lake Segregation Center during World War II," *Japanese Journal of American Studies* 7 (1996): 67–102.

215. Maki, Kitano, and Berthold, op. cit., pp. 217–25.

216. Edwin O. Reischauer, *The Japanese* (Cambridge, Mass.: Belknap Press of Harvard University Press, 1977), pp. 357–68. In the years following Japan's economic downturn medical researchers have discovered that as much as one-third of the working-age population is suffering from stress-related chronic fatigue syndrome. Howard W. French, "Saku Journal: A Postmodern Plague Ravages Japan's Workers," *New York Times*, February 21, 2000, p. A4.

217. See Ronald Takaki, *Hiroshima: Why America Dropped the Bomb* (Boston: Little, Brown and Co., 1995). For the after-effects of the atomic bombing of Hiroshima and Nagasaki on United States public policy, domestic life, and popular culture, see Guy Oakes, *The Imaginary War: Civil Defense and American Cold War Culture* (New York: Oxford University Press, 1994).

218. See, e.g., Steven R. Weisman, "Pearl Harbor in the Mind of Japan," *New York Times Magazine,* Sec. 6 (November 3, 1991), pp. 30–33, 42, 47, 68.

219. Callum A. MacDonald, *Korea: The War before Vietnam* (New York: Free Press, 1986), pp. 3–78, 249–64.

220. Robert D. Schulzinger, *A Time for War: The United States and Vietnam, 1941–1975* (New York: Oxford University Press, 1997), pp. 3–181, 305–36.

221. In 1944, sociologist L. L. Bernard (1881–1951) had warned against the effects on domestic life, liberty, and economy should the United States undertake the role of global police officer. L. L. Bernard, *War and Its Causes* (New York: Henry Holt, 1944), pp. 153–54. For a recent analysis of this aspect of the Cold War, see Marc Trachtenberg, *A Constructed Peace: The Making of the European Settlement, 1945–1963* (Princeton, N.J.: Princeton University Press, 1999), pp. 99–100, 384–86, 399–400.

222. David E. Sanger, "50 Years Made China Change, but Not the Fear of It," *New York Times,* October 3, 1999, p. 4; Richard W. Stevenson, "U.S. Reached an Accord to Open China Economy as Worldwide Market," *New York Times,* November 16, 1999, pp. A1, A10; Joseph Kahn, "Executives Make Trade with China a Moral Issue," *New York Times,* February 13, 2000, p. 18; Katharine Q. Seelye, "The Vice President: Cozying Up to Labor, Gore Vows to Shift China Trade Policy," *New York Times,* February 18, 2000, p. A23; David E. Sanger and Katharine Q. Seelye, "Gore Back in Step with White House over China Trade: Caught between Business and Labor over Beijing's Entry in World Trade Group," *New York Times,* February 19, 2000, pp. A1, A4; Steven Greenhouse, "Labor Leaders Stand by Gore Despite His Stance on China Deal," *New York Times,* February 20, 2000, p. 25; David E. Sanger, "Threat Seen to Trade Duel to Let China Joint W.T.O.," *New York Times,* February 24, 2000; Craig S. Smith, "China and Europeans Break Off Talks on W.T.O. Membership," *New York Times,* February 25, 2000, p. A9; Jane Perlez, "U.S. Report Harshly Criticizes China for Deterioration of Human Rights; Russia Also Faulted," *New York Times,* February 26, 2000, p. A7; Erick Eckholm, "China: Rights Criticism," *New York Times,* March 1, 2000, p. A8. On China's military threat to the United States, see Craig S. Smith, "Guided-Missile Ship Acquired by China Heightens Tension," *New York Times,* February 9, 2000, pp. A1, A3; Bruce S. Lemkin, "China's New Missiles Should Raise Alarm," Letter to the editor, *New York Times,* February 11, 2000; p. A30; Tong Yi, "China's Latest Theft," *New York Times,* Op-Ed essay, February 16, 2000, p. A29; and Joseph Kahn and Eric Schmitt, "Clinton to Send China Trade Bill to Congress Soon: Slipping Support Feared—Backers of Normal Commercial Ties See Even Harder Sell Later in Election Year," *New York Times,* March 4, 2000, pp. A1, A15.

223. Pierre Cayrol, *Hong Kong in the Mouth of the Dragon* (Rutland, Vt.: Charles E. Tuttle, 1998).

224. Mark Landler, "Portugal Lowers Its Flag, Handing Macao to China," *New York*

Times, December 20, 1999, p. A14; "Chinese Bring Hope to Macau," *Boca Raton News,* December 21, 1999, p. 8A.

225. Elizabeth Rosenthal, "China's Recovery of Macao Reignites Dreams of Taiwan," *New York Times,* December 18, 1999, p. A7; Charles W. Freeman Jr., "Caught between Two Chinas," *New York Times,* Op-Ed essay, August 2, 1999, p. A19; Walter Goodman, "The Stealth Campaign to Open China," *New York Times,* January 31, 2000, p. B8; Erik Eckholm, "Opposition Candidate in Taiwan Won't Push China on Independence Issue," *New York Times,* January 31, 2000, p. A8; "House Taiwan Boost Unwise and Troubling," editorial, *Boca Raton News,* February 3, 2000, p.8A; Erik Eckholm, "Top Taiwan Party Accuses a Rival of Embezzlement," *New York Times,* February 17, 2000, p. A8; Erik Eckholm, "China Says Taiwan Cannot Continue Delaying Reunion: Use of Force Threatened—Beijing Demands Negotiations as the Island Prepares for a Presidential Election," *New York Times,* February 22, 2000, pp. A1, A10; Erik Eckholm, "Taiwan, Brushing Off Threats Tells Chinese to Be Practical,"*New York Times,* February 23, 2000, p. A10; Timothy Garton Ash, "Taiwan's Election, China's Future," Op-Ed essay, *New York Times,* February 23, 2000, p. A25; "New Tension over Taiwan," editorial, *New York Times,* February 23, 2000, p. A24; Erik Eckholm, "3 Taiwan Contenders All Urge Reform," *New York Times,* February 26, 2000, p. A6; Jane Perlez, "Warning by China to Taiwan Poses Challenge to U.S.—How to Respond Debated: White House, Surprised, Faces Mounting Pressure to Sell Arms to the Taiwanese," *New York Times,* February 27, 2000, pp. 1, 10; Erik Eckholm, "China's Own Witch Hunt," Week in Review section, *New York Times,* February 27, 2000, p. 4; "If Not One China Now, Then When?" Letters to the editor from Robert H. Treadway Jr. and Yu Yuh-chao, *New York Times,* February 27, 2000, p. 16; William Safire, "Great Leap Backward," *New York Times,* February 28, 2000, p. A23; Erik Eckholm and Steven Lee Myers, "Taiwan Asks U.S. to Let It Obtain Top-Flight Arms: Cites Buildup by China—Strong Warnings from Beijing: Political Battlefield for Clinton Administration," *New York Times,* March 1, 2000, pp. A1, A13; "Military Rumblings over Taiwan," Editorial, *New York Times,* March 3, 2000, p. A24.

226. Robert D. Kaplan, "China: A World Power Again," *Atlantic Monthly* 284:2 (August 1999): 16, 18. Quoted material on p. 18. One element of this influence is entailed in the struggle over America's role in deciding who should succeed Tibet's Dalai Lama. See two reports by Barbara Crossette, "Buddhist's Escape from Tibet, by Car, Horse and Plane," *New York Times,* January 31, 2000, p. A4, and "New York Monastery Prepares for a Holy Youth," *New York Times,* February 18, 2000, p. A25. See also Gustav Niebuhr, "Religion Journal: Buddhism Is Reaching Mainstream Status in U.S., Author Says," *New York Times,* January 29, 2000, p. A11.

227. Larry Rohter, "Asia Moves In on the Big Ditch," *New York Times,* December 19, 1999, p. 3.

228. Sterngold, "Two Sides Clash over Bail for Indicted Atom Scientist," op. cit., and "Wen Ho Lee Denied Bail," *Asian Week* 21:17 (December 16–22, 1999): 8; and Vernon Loeb, "Co-Worker Says Leaks Inadvertent," *South Florida Sun Sentinel,* December 29, 1999, p. 3A.

229. Beth McMurtrie, "No Welcome Mat for the Chinese? Visas Seem Harder to Get," *Chronicle of Higher Education* 46:5 (September 24, 1999): A59–A61. For the situation of Chinese students in America in the 1970s and 1980s, see Leo A. Orleans, *Chinese Students in America: Policies, Issues, and Numbers* (Washington, D.C.: National Academy Press, 1988).

230. Barbara Whitaker, "Immigrant Smuggling Draws New Attention," *New York Times*, January 4, 2000, p. A11.

231. See, e.g., Jacques M. Downs, *The Golden Ghetto: The American Commercial Community at Canton and the Shaping of American China Policy, 1784–1844* (Bethlehem, Pa.: Lehigh University Press, 1997), pp. 9–341.

232. See Lian Xi, *The Conversion of Missionaries: Liberalism in American Protestant Missions in China, 1907–1932* (University Park: Pennsylvania State University Press, 1997), pp. 95–130. See also Spence, op. cit., pp. 180–83, 187, 200, 212.

233. Pearl S. Buck, "Missionaries of Empire," in Joseph Barnes, ed., op. cit., pp. 241–66. Quoted material from pp. 261–62.

234. Tyler Dennet, "The Open Door," in Joseph Barnes, ed., op. cit., pp. 269–94. Quoted material from pp. 270, 293–94.

235. John King Fairbank, *Trade and Diplomacy on the China Coast: The Opening of the Treaty Ports, 1842–1854* (Cambridge, Mass.: Harvard University Press, 1964) [1953]), pp. 8–21.

236. Ibid., p. 21.

237. Ibid., p. 5.

238. Ibid., p. 4.

239. Loc. cit.

240. Loc. cit.

241. Ibid., p. 21.

242. Loc. cit.

243. In 1926, Nicholas Spykman (on the first and last pages of "The Social Background of Asiatic Nationalism," *American Journal of Sociology* 33:3 [November 1926]: 396–411) would observe "The revolt of Asia has become a popular topic. Numerous periodicals and a respectable number of books attest to the fact that the Occident is becoming aware of the awakening of the sleeping giant . . . But whatever the political developments of the near future bring, it should be clear that we can reach the meaning and significance of Asiatic nationalism only if we view the movement against the social background of a culture-transformation process."

244. See two works by Harold R. Isaacs, *No Peace for Asia* (Cambridge, Mass.: M.I.T. Press, 1967 [1947]), pp. 17–34; and *Images of Asia: American Views of China and India* (New York: Capricorn Books, 1962), pp. 104 n. 21, 317 n. 65. The ethnophaulism "gook" became an issue in the Republican primary election contest of 2000, after Senator John McCain, a former prisoner of war in Vietnam, and a seeker after his party's nomination for the U.S. presidency, told a South Carolina audience, "I hated the gooks and will continue to hate them as long as I live." See Robert Dreyfuss, "McCain's Vietnam," *Nation* 270:1 (January 3, 2000): 11–16; and Frank Wu, "Racial

Slur Stirs Debate," *Asian Week* 21:27 (March 2–8, 2000): 6; and "McCain Apologizes for Slur," *Pacific Citizen* 130:9 (March 3–9, 2000): 1.

245. Harold Isaacs, *The Tragedy of the Chinese Revolution,* 2d rev. ed. (Stanford, Calif.: Stanford University Press, 1961).

246. Isaacs, *No Peace for Asia,* op. cit., pp. 7–36; *India's Ex-Untouchables* (New York: Harper Torchbooks, 1965).

247. Isaacs, *Images of Asia,* op. cit., pp. 37–408; *The New World of Negro Americans* (New York: John Day Co., 1963); *Idols of the Tribe: Group Identity and Political Change* (New York: Harper and Row, 1975).

248. Isaacs, *No Peace for Asia,* op. cit., p. 33.

249. Isaacs, *Images of Asia,* op. cit., p. 236.

250. "Memorandum by the Central Intelligence Agency," Secret NIE-5, Washington, D.C., December 29, 1950: "National Intelligence Estimate Indochina: Current Situation and Probable Developments—Conclusions," in William Appleman Williams, Thomas McCormick, Lloyd Gardner, and Walter Weber, eds., *America in Vietnam: A Documentary History* (Garden City, N.Y.: Anchor Books, 1985), pp. 119–20.

251. William P. Bundy, "The United States and Communist China," address before the Associated Students of Pomona (California) College, February 12, 1966. In Franz Schurmann and Orville Schell, eds., *Communist China: Revolutionary Reconstruction and International Confrontation, 1949 to the Present* (New York: Random House, 1967), pp. 378–85. Quoted material from pp. 382 and 385.

252. Paul A. Cohen, *History in Three Keys: The Boxers as Event, Experience, and Myth* (New York: Columbia University Press, 1997), p. 235.

253. Thomas A. Bailey, *A Diplomatic History of the American People,* 5th ed. (New York: Appleton-Century-Crofts, 1955), pp. 910–11.

254. Floyd W. Matson, "The Outcry against Chinese Americans," *The Progressive,* September 1955, p. 25. Cited in "Preface to the Third Edition" (1968), tenBroek, Barnhart, and Matson, op. cit., p. vi.

255. Rose Hum Lee, *The Chinese in the United States of America* (Hong Kong: Hong Kong University Press, 1960), p. 115.

256. Ibid., pp. 115–16.

257. Jerome Beatty Jr., "Trade Winds," *Saturday Review,* May 7, 1966. Quoted in Alan R. Bosworth, *America's Concentration Camps* (New York: W. W. Norton, 1967), p. 251.

258. Rose Hum Lee, op. cit., p. 25. See also Yukiko Koshiro, *Trans-Pacific Racisms and the U.S. Occupation of Japan* (New York: Columbia University Press, 1999), pp. 34, 45, 129, 138, 207, 234 n. 43, 278 n. 20.

259. Rose Hum Lee, op. cit., pp. 91–92.

260. Ibid., pp. 103–12, 232–41, 396–404.

261. Ibid., p. 307.

262. Quoted in ibid., p. 308.

263. Ibid., pp. 309–13.

264. The following draws on Jonathan Spence, *To Change China: Western Advisers in China, 1620–1960* (Boston: Little, Brown and Co., 1969), pp. 282–88.

265. Quoted from Morton H. Halperin, *China and the Bomb* (New York: Praeger, 1965), p. 73, in Spence, *To Change China,* op. cit., p. 286.

266. Cohen, op. cit., p. xii.

267. Jonathan G. Utley, "American Views of China, 1900–1915: The Unwelcome but Inevitable Awakening," in Goldstein, Israel, and Conroy, eds., op. cit., p. 115.

268. The following draws on Herbert Blumer, "Race Prejudice as a Sense of Group Position," *Pacific Sociological Review* 1 (spring 1958): 3–7. The quoted material is from the republication of this essay in Stanford M. Lyman and Arthur J. Vidich, *Social Order and the Public Philosophy: An Analysis and Interpretation of the Work of Herbert Blumer* (Fayetteville: University of Arkansas Press, 1988), pp. 196–207.

269. Robert Schmidt, "Crash Landing," November 1999. URL:http://wenholee.org/brillo.htm.

270. Loc. cit.

271. William J. Broad, "Spies vs. Sweat: The Debate over China's Nuclear Advance," *New York Times,* September 7, 1999, pp. A1, A14. Quoted material from p. A1.

272. Paul D. Moore, "China's Subtle Spying," Op-Ed essay, *New York Times,* September 2, 1999, p. A21.

273. Vernon Loeb and Walter Pincus, "New Spy Data Suggests Scientist Is Innocent," *San Jose Mercury News,* November 19, 1999. URL:http://wenholee.org/SJMN111999.htm.

274. James Sterngold, "Coalition Fears an Asian Bias in Nuclear Case," *New York Times,* December 13, 1999, pp. A1, A26. Quoted material from p. A26.

275. For sources on this point, see Stanford M. Lyman, "The 'Chinese Question' and American Labor Historians, *New Politics* 7:4 (winter 2000): 216 n. 278. URL:www.wilpaterson.edu/~newpol. See also Jill Abramson, "A Funds Scandal Shrinks to a Shadow of Itself," Week in Review section, *New York Times,* February 20, 2000, p. 6. On March 2, 2000, Maria Hsia, who had been a principal in the scheme whereby Chinese Buddhist nuns and monks were inveigled to write checks and appear to be donors to the Democratic National Committee, was convicted of five felony counts. Neil A. Lewis, "Longtime Fund-Raiser for Gore Convicted in Donation Scheme: Buddhist Temple Episode Leads to Guilty Verdict," *New York Times,* March 3, 2000, pp. A1, A16.

276. Lisa Lowe, *Immigrant Acts: On Asian American Cultural Politics* (Durham, N.C.: Duke University Press, 1996), pp. 5–6.

277. Editorial, "The Real Danger," *Asian Week* 21:17 (December 16–22, 1999): p. 4.

278. *Report of the Select Committee on U.S. National Security and Military/Commercial Concerns with the People's Republic of China. Submitted by Mr. [Christopher] Cox of California, Chairman,* 105th Congress, 2d Session. Report 105–581. Declassified May 25, 1999, in part pursuant to House Resolution 5, as amended, 106th Congress, 1st Session. Edited by Kenneth deGraffenreid. (Washington, D.C.: Regnery Publishing Co., 1999). Hereafter cited as the *Cox Report.*

279. Richard Hofstadter, *The Paranoid Style in American Politics and Other Essays* (New York: Alfred A. Knopf, 1965).

280. *Cox Report,* op. cit., pp. 31, 33, 35, 36, 68, 69, 70, 71, 72, 73, 74–75, 93, 121, 124.

281. Kenneth E. deGraffenreid, "Editor's Introduction," *Cox Report,* unpaginated first page. Emphasis in original.

282. The following quotes from Caspar W. Weinberger, "Foreword," *Cox Report,* op. cit., 3 pages unpaginated.

283. See, e.g., H. Brett Melendy, *Chinese and Japanese Americans* (New York: Hippocrene Books, 1984), pp. 154–66.

284. Lars-Erik Nelson, "Washington: The Yellow Peril," *New York Review of Books* 46:12 (July 15, 1999): 6–10. Quoted material from p. 6.

285. Earl Derr Biggers, *Charlie Chan: Five Complete Novels* (New York: Avenel Books, 1981). For an excellent discussion, see Sandra M. Hawley, "The Importance of Being Charlie Chan," in Goldstein, Israel, and Conroy, eds., op. cit., pp. 132–47.

286. Quoted in Douglas G. Greene, "Introduction" to Sax Rohmer, *The Insidious Dr. Fu-Manchu: Being a Somewhat Detailed Account of the Amazing Adventures of Nayland Smith in His Trailing of the Sinister Chinaman* (Mineola, N.Y.: Dover Publications, 1997), p. vi.

287. The following draws on Ian Buruma, "What Happened to the Asian Century?" *New York Times,* Op-Ed essay, December 29, 1999, p. A25. Buruma's worries about freedom and human rights in China were soon followed by a statement from Mary Robinson, a high commissioner for human rights in the United Nations: "I am concerned about three areas, expression, freedom of religion, and freedom of association." Erik Eckholm, "High U.N. Official Sees Loss of Rights in China," *New York Times,* March 3, 2000, p. A11.

288. Erik Eckholm, "China's Arrest of Historian Based in U.S. Stirs Protests," *New York Times,* December 31, 1999, p. A5; Elizabeth Rosenthal, "China Frees Scholar Who Worked in U.S.," *New York Times,* January 29, 2000, p. A3; Beth McMurtrie, "Jailed for His Research, a Scholar of China Recalls a 6-Month Ordeal: Dickinson's Yongyi Song Calls His Release a Victory for the Idea of Academic Freedom," *Chronicle of Higher Education* 46:23 (February 11, 2000): A51; "Freed Scholar Gets U.S. Citizenship," *New York Times,* February 21, 2000, p. A11.

289. James Brooke, "Canada Is Leery of Rise in Refugees: Vancouver Astir over Abuse of Immigrant Law by Chinese," *New York Times,* August 29, 1999, p. 6.

290. Whitaker, op. cit.

291. David Shambaugh, "The United States and China: Cooperation or Confrontation?" *Current History,* n.v., 1 (September 1997). Reprinted in Orville Schell and David Shambaugh, eds., *The China Reader: The Reform Era* (New York: Vintage Books, 1999), pp. 470–79. Quoted material from p. 479.

292. David Shambaugh, "China's Military: Real or Paper Tiger," *Washington Quarterly,* n.v.1 (spring 1966). Excerpted in Orville Schell and David Shambaugh, eds., op. cit., pp. 432–47. Quoted material from p. 438.

293. Erik Eckholm, "Cat Burglars Cater to Taste in Beijing," *New York Times,* January 2, 2000, p. 8; Erik Eckholm, "Amid Garbage and Disdain, China Migrants Find a Living," *New York Times,* February 11, 2000, pp. A1, A12. Four days later, Eckholm ("China Reports a Suicide in Tiananmen," *New York Times,* February 16,

2000, p. A8) reported on how Li Xiangshan, a farmer from Hubei province, had exploded a bomb in Beijing's most important public square, killing himself and injuring a bystander. Li had petitioned China's leaders on four previous occasions and was officially regarded as mentally ill. On other recent occasions of such happenings, security officers believed that dissident Uighur separatists from Xinjian province committed these acts.

294. The following draws on Samuel P. Huntington, "The Clash of Civilizations?" *Foreign Affairs* 72:3 (summer 1993): 22–49.

295. See the essays by Fouad Ajami, Kishore Mahbubani, Robert L. Bartley, Liu Binyan, and Jeanne J. Kirkpatrick in "Responses to Samuel P. Huntington's 'The Clash of Civilizations?'" *Foreign Affairs* 72:4 (September–October 1993): 2–27; and two essays by Samuel P. Huntington, "If Not Civilization, What?" *Foreign Affairs* 72:5 (November–December 1993): 186–94; and "The West and the World," *Foreign Affairs* 75:6 (November–December 1996): 28–46.

296. Geramie R. Barmé, *In the Red: On Contemporary Chinese Culture* (New York: Columbia University Press 1999), p. 260.

297. Bao Mi, *Huanghuo,* 3 vols. (Taipei: Fengyun shidai chuban youxian gongsi, 1991). The essay from which Wang quoted is by Li Ming and is entitled "Zongkan Zhongguode weiji" and is printed on pp. 279–313 of volume 3 of *Huanghuo.* See Barmé, op. cit., p. 450 nn. 41–42.

298. Wang Lixiong, "Kewang duoluo-tan zhishifenzide pizihua qingxiang," *Dongfang,* I (1994), p. 18. Translated and quoted in Barmé, op. cit., p. 286.

299. For reasons that can only be guessed at, Wang told an inquiring American reporter that his book was "a philosophical tract against consumerism, not an attack on the Communist regime." Jaime A. FlorCruz, "Secrets of a Hot Novel," *Time* 30 (March 1992). Quoted in Barmé, op. cit., p. 450 n. 42.

300. Qiao Liang, *Mori zhi men* (Beijing: Kunlun chubanshe, 1995).

301. The following draws on Barmé, op. cit., pp. 261, 450 nn. 43, 44, 46.

302. Howard K. Beale, *Theodore Roosevelt and the Rise of America to World Power* (New York: Collier Books, 1956, 1965), p. 142 n. 26.

303. Huntington, "The Clash of Civilizations," op. cit., p. 25.

304. Loc. cit.

305. Robert G. Lee, *Orientals: Asian Americans in Popular Culture* (Philadelphia: Temple University Press, 1999), pp. 206–9.

306. Samuel P. Huntington, "If Not Civilization, What? Paradigms of the Post–Cold War World," op. cit., p. 191.

307. Robert G. Lee, op. cit., p. 217.

308. Rose Hum Lee, op. cit., p. 430.

309. See Grace Yun, ed., *A Look beyond the Model Minority Image: Critical Issues in Asian America* (New York: Minority Rights Group, 1999).

310. Robert G. Lee, op. cit., pp. 145–79.

311. Since the mid-nineties there has been a proliferation of "whiteness" studies. See, e.g., Ruth Frankenberg, *White Women, Race Matters: The Social Construction of*

Whiteness (Minneapolis: University of Minnesota Press, 1993); Theodore Allen, *The Invention of the White Race*, Vol. I: *Racial Oppression and Social Control;* Vol. II: *The Origin of Racial Oppression in Anglo-America* (London: Verso, 1994, 1997); Richard Dyer, *White* (London: Routledge, 1997); Richard Delgado and Jean Stefancic, eds., *Critical White Studies: Looking Behind the Mirror* (Philadelphia: Temple University Press, 1997); Mike Hill, ed., *Whiteness: A Critical Reader* (New York: New York University Press, 1997); Jesse Daniels, *White Lies: Race, Class, Gender, and Sexuality in White Supremacist Discourse* (New York: Routledge, 1997); Ruth Frankenberg, ed., *Displacing Whiteness: Essays in Social and Cultural Criticism* (Durham, N.C.: Duke University Press, 1997); Grace Elizabeth Hale, *Making Whiteness: The Culture of Segregation in the South, 1890–1940* (New York: Pantheon, 1998); Matthew Frye Jacobson, *Whiteness of a Different Color: European Immigrants and the Alchemy of Race* (Cambridge, Mass.: Harvard University Press, 1998); Joe L. Kincheloe et al., eds., *White Reign: Deploying Whiteness in America* (New York: St. Martin's Press, 1998); George Lipsitz, *The Progressive Investment in Whiteness: How White People Profit from Identity Politics* (Philadelphia: Temple University Press, 1998); Valerie Babb, *Whiteness Visible: The Meaning of Whiteness in American Literature and Culture* (New York: New York University Press, 1998. Especially valuable are Alexander Saxton, *The Rise and Fall of the White Republic: Class Politics and Mass Culture in Nineteenth-Century America* (London: Verso, 1990); and David R. Roediger, *The Wages of Whiteness: Race and the Making of the American Working Class,* rev. ed. (London: Verso, 1999).

312. See the debate over "Orientalism" by comparing Edward Said, *Orientalism,* op. cit., with Bernard Lewis, *Islam and the West,* op. cit., pp. 3–42, 99–154. See also Barbara Harlow and Mia Carter, eds., *Imperialism and Orientalism: A Documentary Source Book* (Malden, Mass.: Blackwell, 1999), pp. 49–66.

313. Stanford M. Lyman, "Gunnar Myrdal's *An American Dilemma* after a Half-Century: Critics and Anti-Critics," *International Journal of Politics, Culture and Society* 12:2 (winter 1998): 327–89. See also Charles W. Mills, *The Racial Contract* (Ithaca, N.Y.: Cornell University Press, 1997), pp. 91–133.

314. Robert E. Park, "Race Relations and Certain Frontiers," in E. B. Reuter, ed., *Race and Culture Contacts* (New York: McGraw-Hill, 1934), pp. 57–85. Quoted passage from p. 85.

315. See Stanford M. Lyman, *Color, Culture, Civilization: Race and Minority Issues in American Society* (Urbana: University of Illinois Press, 1994), pp. 1–42, 239–384. See also Leland T. Saito, *Race and Politics: Asian Americans, Latinos, and Whites in a Los Angeles Suburb* (Urbana: University of Illinois Press, 1998), pp. 181–96.

316. Harold Isaacs, *Idols of the Tribe: Group Identity and Political Change,* op. cit., p. 24.

Chapter Three. The "Chinese Question" and America's Labor Historians: A Wrong Turn in a Quest for a Usable Past

1. Andrew Gyory, *Closing the Gate: Race, Politics, and the Chinese Exclusion Act* (Chapel Hill: University of North Carolina Press, 1998).

2. See three works by Peter Kwong, *Chinatown, N.Y.: Labor and Politics, 1930–1950* (New York: Monthly Review Press, 1979); *The New Chinatown* (New York: Hill and Wang, 1987; rev. ed., 1996); *Forbidden Workers: Illegal Chinese Immigrants and American Labor* (New York: New Press, 1997).

3. For John Kuo Wei Tchen, see notes 62, 67–70, 74–77, 135 *infra.* See the following essays by Herbert Hill: "Anti-Oriental Agitation and the Rise of Working-Class Racism," *Transaction: Social Science and Modern Society* 10:2 (January–February 1973): 43–54; "Race, Ethnicity and Organized Labor: The Opposition to Affirmative Action," *New Politics,* n.s., 1:2 (winter 1987): 31–82; "Herbert Hill Replies," *New Politics,* n.s., 1:3 (summer 1987): 61–71; "Myth-Making as Labor History: Herbert Gutman and the United Mine Workers of America," *International Journal of Politics, Culture and Society* 2:2 (winter 1988): 132–200; "Black Labor and Affirmative Action: An Historical Perspective," in Steven Shulman and William Darity Jr., eds., *The Question of Discrimination: Racial Inequality in the U.S. Labor Market* (Middletown, Conn.: Wesleyan University Press, 1989), pp. 190–267; "Black Workers, Organized Labor, and Title VII of the 1964 Civil Rights Act: Legislative History and Litigation Record," in Herbert Hill and James E. Jones Jr., eds., *Race in America: The Struggle for Equality* (Madison: University of Wisconsin Press, 1993), pp. 263–344; "The Problem of Race in American Labor History," *Reviews in American History* 24:2 (June 1996): 189–208; "Black-Jewish Conflict in the Labor Context: Race, Jobs, and Institutional Power," in V. P. Franklin et al., eds., *African Americans and Jews in the Twentieth Century: Studies in Convergence and Conflict* (Columbia: University of Missouri Press, 1998), pp. 264–92: "Lichtenstein's Fictions Revisited: Race and the New Labor History," *New Politics,* n.s., 7:2 (winter 1999): 148–63.

4. Selig Perlman, *A History of Trade Unionism in the United States* (New York: Macmillan, 1922), p. 62.

5. John R. Commons, *Races and Immigrants in America,* 2d ed. (New York: Macmillan, 1920; reprint, New York: Augustus M. Kelley, 1967), pp. 1–106, 198–238; and John R. Commons et al., *History of Labour in the United States,* 4 vols. (New York: Macmillan, 1918–1935), II, pp. 150–51.

6. Philip Taft, *The A.F.L. in the Time of Gompers* (New York: Harper and Brothers, 1957), pp. 302–5.

7. "The original spark for this book," Gyory (op. cit., p. xi) points out, "came from my professor, Herbert Gutman. One day long ago, he remarked, 'This event in North Adams [i.e., the use of Chinese workers as strikebreakers at a Massachusetts shoe factory in 1870] needs to be looked at in a fresh light. Who wants to tackle it?' . . . Herb's spirit and vision infuses every page of this book."

8. In his bibliography, Gyory dissents from three of Herbert Hill's many studies of the relations of racism to the organization of unionism in the United States: "Anti-Oriental Agitation and the Rise of Working-Cass Racism,"op. cit.; "Race and Ethnicity in Organized Labor: The Historical Sources of Resistance to Affirmative Action, *Journal of Intergroup Relations* 12 (winter 1984): 5–49; and "Race, Ethnicity and Organized Labor: The Opposition to Affirmative Action," op. cit.

9. Gyory criticizes three works by Roger Daniels, "American Historians and East Asian Immigrants," *Pacific Historical Review* 43 (August 1974): 449–72; ed., *Anti-Chinese Violence in North America* (New York: Arno Press, 1978); and *Asian America: Chinese and Japanese in the United States since 1850* (Seattle: University of Washington Press, 1988).

10. Gyory critically appraises two works by Ronald Takaki: *Iron Cages: Race and Culture in Nineteenth-Century America* (New York: Knopf, 1979); and *Strangers from a Different Shore: A History of Asian Americans* (New York: Penguin, 1990).

11. Gwendolyn Mink, *Old Labor and New Immigrants in American Political Development: Union, Party, and State, 1875–1920* (Ithaca, N.Y.: Cornell University Press, 1986), p. 73.

12. Gyory, op. cit., p. 12.

13. Mary Roberts Coolidge, *Chinese Immigration* (New York: Henry Holt and Co., 1909).

14. Elmer Clarence Sandmeyer, *The Anti-Chinese Movement in California* (Urbana: University of Illinois Press, 1939).

15. Stuart Creighton Miller, *The Chinese Image in the Eastern United States, 1785–1882,* Ph.D. thesis, Columbia University, 1966; and *The Unwelcome Immigrant: The American Image of the Chinese, 1785–1882* (Berkeley: University of California Press, 1969).

16. Gyory, op. cit., p. 15.

17. Ibid., p.14.

18. Ibid., pp. 14–15.

19. For a spirited exchange between Nick Salvatore and Leon Fink on the value and truth of the Gutman thesis, see Nick Salvatore, "Herbert Gutman's Narrative of the American Working Class: A Reevaluation," *International Journal of Politics, Culture, and Society* 12:1 (fall 1998): 43–80; Leon Fink, "Rules of the Game: Comment on Nick Salvatore's 'Herbert Gutman's Narrative of the American Working Class: A Reevaluation'"; and Nick Salvatore, "A Response to Leon Fink," ibid., 12:4 (summer 1999).

20. Gyory, op. cit., p. 15.

21. See Herbert Hill, "The Problem of Race in American Labor History," op. cit.

22. "The tradition of racial discrimination within trade unions is the great historic failure of organized labor . . . If the failure of organized labor to introduce the spirit of equality and democracy into the workplace has been a heavy burden for Negroes, it is also the tragedy of American labor as a social institution." Herbert Hill, "The Racial Practices of Organized Labor: The Age of Gompers and After," in *Employment, Race, and Poverty: A Critical Study of the Disadvantaged Status of Negro Workers from 1865 to 1965,* ed. Arthur M. Ross and Herbert Hill (New York: Harcourt, Brace and World, 1967), p. 397.

23. Without mentioning the workingmen's or organized labor's attitude toward African Americans, Asians, and other nonwhite and non-Anglos, Karl Marx's son-in-law and daughter, having toured the vistas of the labor movement in the United States,

chose to give thumbnail sketches of eight European and Euro-American "working-class leaders," adding, ". . . the various nationalities of the names we have given in these pages—e.g., Black, Morgan, Mielliez, Macdonald, McGuire, Hruza, Trautwein, Vrooman—show the universality of the Socialist movement in America, and tell of the certainty of its ultimate triumph." Edward and Eleanor Marx-Aveling, *The Working-Class Movement in America,* 2d ed. (London: Swan Sonnenschein and Co., 1891; rpt., New York: Arno and *New York Times,* 1969), p. 212.

24. See Salvatore, op. cit., pp. 65, 67; and Herbert Hill, "Myth-Making as Labor History: Herbert Gutman and the United Mine Workers of America," op. cit., pp. 132–33.

25. Coolidge, op. cit.

26. For Coolidge's role in the development of research on the sex lives of married women, see Rosalind Rosenberg, *Beyond Separate Spheres: Intellectual Roots of Modern Feminism* (New Haven, Conn.: Yale University Press, 1982), pp. 178–206.

27. Mary Roberts Coolidge, *Why Women Are So* (New York: Henry Holt and Co., 1912; rpt., New York: Arno Press, 1972).

28. Mary Roberts Coolidge, *The Rain-Makers: Indians of Arizona and New Mexico* (Boston: Houghton-Mifflin Co., 1929; rpt., New York: AMS Press, 1979; Dane Coolidge and Mary Roberts Coolidge, *The Navajo Indians* (Boston: Houghton-Mifflin Co., 1930; rpt., New York: AMS Press, 1979); and Dane Coolidge and Mary Roberts Coolidge, *The Last of the Seris: The Aboriginal Indians of Kino Bay, Sonora, Mexico* (Glorieta, N.M.: Rio Grande Press, 1971 [1939]).

29. Gyory, op. cit., p. 8.

30. Gyory, op. cit., pp. 62–63, is willing to accept U.S. Consul David H. Bailey's 1871 lurid report on the coolie trade that Coolidge, *Chinese Immigration,* op. cit., p. 49, treated as "a mosaic of falsehood and misrepresentation" and whom she regarded as corrupt and dishonest (pp. 105–6, 308, 419). But even the notorious Sinophobe Frank M. Pixley was led to concede that his own charges of coolieism on the part of the Chinese did not depend on Bailey's report, with which he was unfamiliar, and which, he was told by no less than fellow exclusionist A. A. Sargent, did not refer to the coming of Chinese to America, but rather to "the method of the immigration of these Chinese to the different ports of the world." *Report of the Joint Special Committee to Investigate Chinese Immigration. United States Senate. Forty-fourth Congress* (Washington, D.C.: Government Printing Office, 1877; reprint, New York: Arno Press, 1978), p. 25. And, in the end, Gyory himself, op. cit., p. 63, is forced to admit that "Bailey offered various documents that, though far from conclusive, suggested an underground network in which Americans and Chinese conspired to import laborers to the United States." Yet, in the next sentence, he claims, "These dispatches seemed to offer conclusive evidence of an ongoing 'coolie trade' in which thousands of Chinese immigrants poured into this country as contract laborers . . . [T]hey offered strong support that the 'coolie trade' thrived and prospered." Of course, this is tendentious nonsense. Gyory does not mention the "*Robert Browne* Affair," which occurred in March 1852, and is remarkably similar to the *Amistad* incident. Chinese laborers who

had been inveigled aboard an American merchant ship in the coolie trade revolted, killed the ship's officers, and sailed the ship into Japan. The American consul forced the Chinese back to China where they were hanged. See Earl Swisher, *China's Management of the American Barbarians: A Study of Sino-American Relations, 1841–1861, with Documents* (New Haven, Conn.: Far Eastern Publications, 1953), pp. 199–203. See, in general, Him Mark Lai, Joe Huang, and Don Wong, *The Chinese of America, 1785–1980* (San Francisco: Chinese Cultural Foundation, 1980), pp. 11–19; and Robert J. Schwendinger, *Ocean of Bitter Dreams: Maritime Relations between China and the United States, 1850–1915* (Tucson, Ariz.: Westernlore Press, 1980), pp. 7–198.

31. Gyory, op. cit., p. 8.

32. Herbert Gutman, "Introduction," *Work, Culture and Society in Industrializing America: Essays in American Working Class and Social History* (New York: Alfred A. Knopf, 1976), p. xii.

33. Rose Hum Lee, *The Chinese in the United States of America* (Hong Kong: Hong Kong University Press, 1960), p. 35.

34. B. L. Sung, *Mountain of Gold: The Story of the Chinese in America* (New York: Macmillan, 1967), p. 89.

35. See Herbert Hill, "The Racial Practices of Organized Labor: The Age of Gompers and After," op. cit., pp. 389–97.

36. Peter Kwong, *Forbidden Workers: Illegal Chinese Immigrants and American Labor,* op. cit., p. 16.

37. "An Act to Repeal the Chinese Exclusion Acts, to establish quotas, and for other purposes." H.R.. 3070. Public Law 99. Reprinted in *The Repeal and Its Legacy: Proceedings of the Conference on the 50th Anniversary of the Repeal of the Exclusion Acts,* San Francisco, November 12–14, 1993 (San Francisco: Chinese Historical Society of America, 1994), p. 217.

38. Gyory, op. cit., p. 1.

39. Ibid.

40. L. Ling-chi Wang, "Politics of the Repeal of the Chinese Exclusion Laws," in *The Repeal and Its Legacy,* op. cit., pp. 65–80. Quotation from p. 76.

41. Bill Ong Hing, *Making and Remaking Asian America through Immigration Policy, 1850–1990* (Stanford, Calif.: Stanford University Press, 1993), p. 36.

42. Herbert Gutman, "Work, Culture, and Society in Industrializing America, 1815–1919," in idem, *Work, Culture and Society in Industrializing America: Essays in American Working-Class and Social History,* op. cit., pp. 3–78.

43. See three works by David Montgomery: *Workers' Control in America* (New York: Cambridge University Press, 1979); *Beyond Equality: Labor and the Radical Republicans, 1862–1872* (Urbana: University of Illinois Press, 1981); and *Citizen Worker: The Experience of Workers in the United States with Democracy and the Free Market during the Nineteenth Century* (New York: Cambridge University Press, 1993). However, as I show *infra,* Montgomery offers evidence and argument that stand in sharp contrast to that presented by Gyory.

44. See two works by Leon Fink: *Workingmen's Democracy: The Knights of Labor*

and American Politics (Urbana: University of Illinois Press, 1985); and *In Search of the Working Class: Essays in American Labor History and Political Culture* (Urbana: University of Illinois Press, 1994).

45. Gyory, op. cit., p. 59. Gyory makes no mention of the Chinese immigrants who fought—mostly as part of the Union forces—in the Civil War. In 1996 Ruthanne Lum McCunn ("Chinese in the Civil War: Ten Who Served," *Chinese America: History and Perspectives, 1996,* ed. Marlon K. Hom et al. [San Francisco: Chinese Historical Society of America, 1996], pp. 149–82) showed that, in terms of their proportion to the Chinese population in the United States, their service was substantial. More recently, Thomas P. Lowery and Edward S. Milligan announced discovery of the names of forty-seven Chinese men who served in that war, a higher percentage than from any other ethnic group. Linda Wheeler, "47 Chinese Men Served in U.S. Civil War, New Research Shows," *Washington Post,* May 12, 1999, p. A18.

Despite the fact that Chinese Americans and Japanese Americans fought for the United States in every war in this century, Asian American service personnel continue to experience racist treatment in a variety of forms. See Toshio Whelchel, *From Pearl Harbor to Saigon: Japanese American Soldiers and the Vietnam War* (London: Verso, 1999).

46. Mike Merrill and Herbert Gutman, "Interview with Herbert Gutman," in Herbert Gutman, *Power and Culture: Essays on the American Working Class,* ed. Ira Berlin (New York: New Press, 1987), pp. 336–56.

47. Gyory, op. cit., p. 59.

48. Paul Goodman, *Of One Blood: Abolitionism and the Origins of Racial Equality* (Berkeley: University of California Press, 1998), p. 161.

49. Leon F. Litwack, *North of Slavery: The Negro in the Free States, 1790–1860* (Chicago: University of Chicago Press, 1961), p. 158.

50. Eric L. Hirsch, *Urban Revolt: Ethnic Politics in the Nineteenth-Century Chicago Labor Movement* (Berkeley: University of California Press, 1990), p. 207.

51. Leslie M. Harris, "From Abolitionist Amalgamators to 'Rulers of Five Points': The Discourse of Interracial Sex and Reform in Antebellum New York City," in Martha Hodes, ed., *Sex, Love, Race: Crossing Boundaries in North American History* (New York: New York University Press, 1999), pp. 191–212. See also Sean Wilentz, *Chants Democratic; New York City and the Rise of the American Working Class, 1788–1850* (New York: Oxford University Press, 1986), pp. 255–96; and Graham Hodges, "'Desirable Companions and Lovers': Irish and African Americans in the Sixth Ward, 1830–1870," in Ronald H. Bayor and Timothy J. Meagher, eds., *The New York Irish* (Baltimore: Johns Hopkins University Press, 1996), pp. 107–24.

52. *Dred Scott vs. Sandford,* 19 Howard 393 (1857).

53. *In re Ah Yup,* 5 Sawyer 155 (1878).

54. David R. Roediger, *The Wages of Whiteness: Race and the Making of the American Working Class,* rev. ed. (London: Verso, 1999), pp. 3–18. See also W. E. B. DuBois, *Black Reconstruction in America, 1860–1880: An Essay toward a History of the Part Which Black Folk Played in the Attempt to Reconstruct Democracy in America* (New York: Russell and Russell, 1935), pp. 3–31, 237–324, 711–30.

55. Matthew Frye Jacobson, *Whiteness of a Different Color: European Immigrants and the Alchemy of Race* (Cambridge, Mass.: Harvard University Press, 1998), pp. 13–90; and David R. Roediger, *Towards the Abolition of Whiteness: Essays on Race, Politics, and Working Class History* (London: Verso, 1994), pp. 21–38, 181–98.

56. Noel Ignatiev, *How the Irish Became White* (New York: Routledge, 1995), pp. 10–11.

57. Roediger, *The Wages of Whiteness,* op. cit., p. 136.

58. In a diary entry for July 16, 1863, George Templeton Strong (1820–1875) observed: "Albany, Troy, Yonkers, Hartford, Boston, and other cities have each their Irish anti-conscription Nigger-murdering mob, of the same type with ours. It is a grave business, a *jacquerie* that must be put down by heroic doses of lead and steel." *The Diary of George Templeton Strong,* ed. Alan Nevins and Milton Halsey Thomas, abr. by Thomas J. Pressly (Seattle: University of Washington Press, 1988), p. 243. For the anti-Chinese situation in the New York City draft riots of 1863 and the years thereafter, see Iver Bernstein, *The New York City Draft Riots: Their Significance for American Society and Politics in the Age of the Civil War* (New York: Oxford University Press, 1990), pp. 34, 226–27, 299 n. 132.

59. James Brewer Stewart, *Holy Warriors: The Abolitionists and American Slavery* (New York: Lippincott, 1976; rev. ed., New York: Hill and Wang, 1996), pp. 63–64.

60. John Bernard McGloin, *Eloquent Indian: The Life of James Bouchard, California Jesuit* (Stanford, Calif.: Stanford University Press, 1949), pp. 172–90. For the Protestant reply, see Rev. O. Gibson, *The Chinese in America* (Cincinnati: Hitchcock and Walden, 1877; reprint, New York: Arno Press, 1978), pp. 241–80.

61. Hasia R. Diner, *Erin's Daughters in America: Irish Immigrant Women in the Nineteenth Century* (Baltimore: Johns Hopkins University Press, 1983), pp. 92–93.

62. William Purviance Fenn, *Ah Sin and His Brethren in American Literature* (Peking [Beijing], China: College of Chinese Studies cooperating with California College in China, 1933); L. Perry Curtis, *Apes and Angels: The Irishman in Victorian Caricature,* rev. ed. (Washington, D.C.: Smithsonian Institution Press, 1997), pp. 23–180; Philip P. Choy, Lorraine Dong, and Marlon K. Hom, *The Coming Man: 19th Century American Perceptions of the Chinese* (Seattle: University of Washington Press, 1995), pp. 23–62, 83–160; and John Kuo Wei Tchen, "Quimbo Appo's Fear of Fenians: Chinese-Irish-Anglo Relations in New York City," in Ronald H. Bayor and Timothy J. Meagher, eds., op. cit., pp. 125–52.

63. See two works by Alexander Saxton, *The Indispensable Enemy: Labor and the Anti-Chinese Movement in California* (Berkeley: University of California Press, 1971), pp. 28–30, 37–45; and *The Rise and Fall of the White Republic: Class Politics and Mass Culture in Nineteenth-Century America* (London: Verso, 1990), pp. 269–348.

64. Gyory, ibid., p. 45.

65. Ibid., pp. 44–45.

66. Ibid., p. 45.

67. John Kuo Wei Tchen, *New York before Chinatown: Orientalism, Identity Formation, and Political Culture in the American Metropolis, 1784–1882,* Ph.D. Diss., New York University, 1992. (Ann Arbor: UMI Dissertation Services, 1992), pp. 320–21.

Tchen's monograph has recently been published under the title *New York before Chinatown: Orientalism and the Shaping of American Culture, 1776–1882* (Baltimore: Johns Hopkins University Press, 1999).

68. Ibid., p. 324.

69. Ibid., pp. 324–25.

70. Tchen, "Quimbo Appo . . . ," op. cit.

71. E. P. Thompson, *Customs in Common: Studies in Traditional Popular Culture* (New York: New Press, 1993), pp. 1–15, 97–351, 467–538.

72. Tchen, "Quimbo Appo . . . ," op. cit., p. 140.

73. Ibid., pp. 141–42. See also Forrest G. Wood, *Black Scare: The Racist Response to Emancipation and Reconstruction* (Berkeley: University of California Press, 1968), pp. 53–79; and Eve Allegra Raimon, "Miscegenation, 'Melaleukation' and Public Reception," in *Fear Itself: Enemies Real and Imagined in American Culture,* ed. Nancy Lusignan Schultz (West Lafayette, Ind.: Purdue University Press, 1999), pp. 121–32.

74. Tchen, "Quimbo Appo . . . ," op. cit., p. 147.

75. Ibid., p. 146.

76. Ibid., p. 147.

77. Ibid., p. 147.

78. I have drawn on Howard N. Rabinowitz, *Race Relations in the Urban South, 1865–1890* (New York: Oxford University Press, 1978), pp. 61–96.

79. Eric Foner, *Reconstruction, 1863–1877: America's Unfinished Revolution* (New York: Harper and Row, 1988), p. 479.

80. For these, see three works by Stanford M. Lyman: *Chinese Americans* (New York: Random House, 1974), pp. 29–53; *The Asian in North America* (Santa Barbara, Calif.: American Bibliographic Center, Clio, 1977), pp. 11–150, 277–94; and *Chinatown and Little Tokyo: Power, Conflict, and Community among Chinese and Japanese Immigrants in America* (Millwood, N.Y.: Associated Faculty Press, 1986), pp. 41–56, 69–71, 109–232.

81. For Ng Poon Chew, see Corinne K. Hoexter, *From Canton to California: The Epic of Chinese Immigration* (New York: Four Winds Press, 1976), pp. 133–281; and L. Eve Armentrout Ma, *Revolutionaries, Monarchists, and Chinatowns: Chinese Politics in the Americas and the 1911 Revolution* (Honolulu: University of Hawaii Press, 1990), pp. 33–34, 65, 173 n. 54, 180 n. 60, 181 n. 6.

82. Articles by and about Wong Chin Foo can be found in the *New York Times,* the *Chicago Tribune,* the *North American Review,* the *Chautauquan, Atlantic Monthly,* and *Harper's Weekly Magazine.*

83. See Zhang Qingsong, "The Origins of the Chinese Americanization Movement: Wong Chin Foo and the Chinese Equal Rights League," in K. Scott Wong and Sucheng Chan, eds., *Claiming America: Constructing Chinese American Identities during the Exclusion Era* (Philadelphia: Temple University Press, 1998), pp. 41–63.

84. David Montgomery, *The Fall of the House of Labor: The Workplace, the State, and American Labor Activism, 1865–1925* (Cambridge, U.K.: Cambridge University Press, 1987), pp. 67–68: "No other railroad builders ever accomplished feats of labor as

spectacular as those of the Chinese. After the Central Pacific began hiring them by the thousands in 1865, Chinese workers drove a railbed from San Francisco to Promontory Point in Utah. They carved a path out of the perpendicular cliffs above the American River by lowering one another in wicker baskets to drill holes, set powder, and fire it off. Because the size of the Central Pacific's subsidies from the federal government depended on the track mileage laid before it encountered the westward moving Union Pacific, President Charles Crocker kept his Chinese laborers at work in the dead of winter—even drilling a tunnel through the Donner Summit while their camps were buried in snow. Many of those who were killed in snowslides were not found until the following summer . . . [T]he very existence of the Chinese who had built the railroad was soon obliterated from the American consciousness. When the famous photograph of the joining of the lines from east and west was taken at Promontory Point, all Chinese workers were ushered out of the camera's range."

85. Ibid., p. 94.

86. Ibid., p. 94.

87. Ibid., p. 67.

88. See the articles collected in Roger Daniels, ed., *Anti-Chinese Violence in North America,* op. cit.

89. Montgomery, *The Fall of the House of Labor,* op. cit., p. 85.

90. Ibid., p. 85.

91. Gyory, op. cit., pp. 12, 19–41, 47–70, 96–101, 123–32, 168, 247, 279 nn. 2, 3, 5, 296 n. 37, 314 n. 9.

92. Herbert Hill, "Race and Ethnicity in Organized Labor: The Historical Sources of Resistance to Affirmative Action," *Journal of Intergroup Relations* 12:4 (winter 1984): 14. Quoted in Gyory, op. cit., p. 293 n. 50.

93. Quoted in Gyory, op. cit., p. 293 n. 50, from Mink, op. cit., p. 79.

94. Quoted in Gyory, op. cit., p. 131.

95. Quoted in ibid., p. 132.

96. "An act to execute certain treaty stipulations relating to Chinese," in *The Statutes at Large of the United States of America, from December, 1881, to March, 1883, and Recent Treaties, Postal Conventions, and Executive Proclamations* (Washington, D.C.: Government Printing Office, 1883), 22:58–61. Reprinted in Gyory, op. cit., pp. 261–64. Quotation from p. 264.

97. Coolidge, *Chinese Immigration,* op. cit., pp. 238, 282–84.

98. Gyory, op. cit., Appendix, p. 264.

99. *In re Ah Yup,* 5 Sawyer 155 (1878).

100. Huang Tsen Ming, *The Legal Status of the Chinese Abroad* (Taipei, Taiwan: Chinese Cultural Service, 1954 [1936]), p. 84, citing *Case of the Chinese Wife,* 21 Fed. 785 (1884). For a thorough discussion, see Sucheng Chan, "The Exclusion of Chinese Women, 1870–1943," in idem, ed., *Entry Denied: Exclusion and the Chinese Community in America, 1882–1943* (Philadelphia: Temple University Press, 1991), pp. 94–146.

101. See Don E. Fehrenbacher, *The Dred Scott Case: Its Significance in American Law and Politics* (New York: Oxford University Press, 1978), pp. 335–67.

102. *Restriction of Immigration,* Hearing on H.R.5, H.R. 101, H.R. 561. 68th Congress, 1st session (1924), p. 821. Quoted in Helen Chen, "Chinese Immigration into the United States: An Analysis of Changes in Immigration Policies," in Genny Lim, ed., *The Chinese American Experience: Papers from the Second National Conference on Chinese American Studies* (San Francisco: The Chinese Historical Society of America and the Chinese Culture Foundation of San Francisco, 1980), p. 45.

103. Gyory, op. cit., pp. 33, 273 n. 34.

104. Persia Crawford Campell, *Chinese Coolie Emigration to Countries within the British Empire* (London: P. S. King, 1923; reprint, New York: Negro Universities Press, 1969), pp. 27–36.

105. See Ta Chen, *Chinese Migrations, with Special Reference to Labor Conditions* (Taipei, Taiwan: Ch'eng Wen Publishing Co., 1967 [1923]), pp. 1–19, 111–27, 171–74, 192–97.

106. Watt Stewart, *Chinese Bondage in Peru* (Durham, N.C.: Duke University Press, 1951).

107. The Cuba Commission, *Chinese Emigration: Report of the Commission Sent by China to Ascertain the Condition of Chinese Coolies in Cuba* (Shanghai: Imperial Maritime Customs Press, 1876; reprint, Taipei: Ch'eng-wen Publishing Co., 1970).

108. Walton Look Lai, *Indentured Labor, Caribbean Sugar: Chinese and Indian Migrants to the British West Indies, 1838–1918* (Baltimore: Johns Hopkins University Press, 1993).

109. Ching Chieh Chang, *The Chinese in Latin America: A Preliminary Geographical Survey with Special Reference to Cuba and Jamaica,* Ph.D. Diss., University of Maryland, 1956 (Ann Arbor: University Microfilms, 1970), pp. 12–21; Jan Breman, *Taming the Coolie Beast: Plantation Society and the Colonial Order in Southeast Asia* (New York: Oxford University Press, 1989).

110. For Koopmanschap, see Lucy M. Cohen, *Chinese in the Post–Civil War South: A People without a History* (Baton Rouge: Louisiana State University Press, 1984), pp. 67–70, 80, 89–95, 120–23, 180–81; and Lyman, *Chinatown and Little Tokyo,* op. cit., pp. 240–42, 250–51 nn. 33, 34, 35, 36, 37, 38.

111. Gyory, op. cit., pp. 30–35, 47, 61, 179.

112. Ibid., p. 179.

113. Ibid., p. 33.

114. Ibid., p. 179.

115. The accusations against the Chinese were refuted at the time and in the years that followed passage of the Exclusion law by advocates of the civil rights and liberties of Chinese who regarded them as *persons* protected by the Fourteenth Amendment to the United States Constitution. Among these were attorney Col. F. A. Bee. (See F. A. Bee, compiler, *Memorial: The Other Side of the Chinese Question—Testimony of California's Leading Citizens* [San Francisco: Woodward and Co., Printers, February 1886; Reprint, San Francisco: R. & E. Research Associates, 1971], esp. pp. 50–76); by missionary Esther E. Baldwin (See Mrs. S. L. Baldwin, *Must the Chinese Go? An Examination of the Chinese Question* [New York: H. B. Elkins, 1890. Reprint, San

Francisco: Rand E. Research Associates, 1970]); and, in the year prior to passage of the Exclusion act, former Consul General (1861–1876) in, and former Minister (1876–1880) to, China, George F. Seward; (See George F. Seward, *Chinese Immigration: Its Social and Economical Aspect* [New York: Charles Scribner's Sons, 1881; reprint, New York: Arno Press and the *New York Times*, 1970], pp. 136–421.)

116. This, of course, was the position taken in 1885 by Sigismund Danielewicz, one of the founders of the Sailors' Union of the Pacific, secretary of the International Workingmen's Association (Pacific Coast), and a socialist, when he, alone, opposed a resolution put forward by his fellow union members that denounced the Chinese for "their bad moral habits, their low grades of development, their filth, their vices, their race differences from the Caucasians, and their willing status as slaves" and that called for "their complete removal from all parts of the Pacific Coast, and . . . from San Francisco within sixty days." Asking if the persecution of the Chinese was more justifiable than the oppression visited upon the Jews historically, on the Irish of New York, or on the Germans in other countries, Danielewicz received his answer in the howls and laughter of his comrades. See Saxton, *The Indispensable Enemy* . . . , op. cit., pp. x, 221–23. Danielewicz's name does not appear in the index of Gyory's book.

117. E.g., by the Freedmen's Bureau. See Donald G. Nieman, *To Set the Law in Motion: The Freedmen's Bureau and the Legal Rights of Blacks, 1865–1868*, Millwood, N.Y.: KTO Press, 1979), pp. 35–65, 156–90, 209–21; La Wanda Cox, *Freedom, Racism and Reconstruction: Collected Writings*, ed. Donald G. Nieman (Athens: University of Georgia Press, 1997), pp. 3–62; and Leslie A. Schwalm, *A Hard Fight for We: Women's Transition from Slavery to Freedom in South Carolina* (Urbana: University of Illinois Press, 1997), pp. 199–204, 231–35.

118. Lyman, *Chinatown and Little Tokyo* . . . , op. cit., pp. 247–48 n. 4; and Victor G. and Brett de Bary Nee, *Longtime Californ': A Documentary Study of an American Chinatown* (New York: Pantheon, 1972, 1973), pp. 39–40.

119. See Stanford M. Lyman, "Henry Hughes and the Southern Foundations of American Sociology," in idem, ed., *Selected Writings of Henry Hughes: Antebellum Southerner, Slavocrat, Sociologist* (Jackson: University Press of Mississippi, 1985), pp. 24–25, 43–44.

120. In addition to Cohen, op. cit., a description of Koopmanschap's coolie scheme will be found in John Kuo Wei Tchen, *New York before Chinatown*, op. cit., pp. 288–99.

121. Lyman, "Henry Hughes . . . ," op. cit., pp. 51–53.

122. "About 8,000 Chinese . . . came as indentured laborers to Jamaica and Trinidad before 1893. Most bought out the final years of their indentures, left the plantations, and set up small shops or farms. Like the Indians on Trinidad, many succeeded in retaining their ethnic identity into the 20th century." Jan Rogozinsky, *A Brief History of the Caribbean: From the Arawak and the Carib to the Present* (New York: Penguin-Meridian, 1992), p. 190.

123. See James W. Loewen, *The Mississippi Chinese: Between Black and White*, 2d ed. (Prospect Heights, Ill.: Waveland Press, 1998); Robert Seto Quan, in collaboration with Julian B. Roebuck, *Lotus among the Magnolias: The Mississippi Chinese* (Jackson:

University Press of Mississippi, 1982); and three essays in the special section on "The Chinese: 100 years in the South," in *Southern Exposure* 12:4 (July–August 1984): 17–30: Renee Tajima, "Mississippi Triangle: The Making of a Film"; Adria Bernardi, "Heat in the Delta: Reactions to the Triangle"; and Lucy M. Cohen, "Early Arrivals: Nineteenth-Century Chinese and Their Descendants."

124. Charles J. McClain, *In Search of Equality: The Chinese Struggle against Discrimination in Nineteenth-Century America* (Berkeley: University of California Press, 1994); Hyung Chan Kim, ed., *Asian Americans and the Supreme Court: A Documentary History* (New York: Greenwood Press, 1992).

125. *Rice et al. vs. Gong Lum et al.*, 139 Miss. 760, 104 So. 105 (1925); and *Gong Lum vs. Rice*, 275 U.S. 78 (1927).

126. See, e.g., pp. 16–21 of the minutes of a "Special Session of the Asiatic Exclusion League, convened in San Francisco on Oct. 25, 1908," in *Anti-Movements in America: Proceedings of the Asiatic Exclusion League, 1907–1915*, Advisory ed., Gerald R. Grob (New York: Arno Press, 1977).

127. Him Mark Lai, Joe Huang, and Don Wong, *The Chinese of America, 1785–1980* (San Francisco: Chinese Culture Foundation, 1980), p. 18.

128. For a probing discussion of debt-labor and related forms of contract labor as these forms of migration served to supply agricultural workers and household servants to the colonies in Southeast Asia—and one that distinguishes such contracts from slavery, a matter that Gyory does not take up in any serious way, preferring to let stand the charge that Chinese "coolies" in America were nothing more than slaves—see Bruno Lasker, *Human Bondage in Southeast Asia* (Chapel Hill: University of North Carolina Press, 1950), pp. 113–67.

129. Liping Zhu, *A Chinaman's Chance: The Chinese on the Rocky Mountain Mining Frontier* (Boulder: University Press of Colorado, 1997), p. 22.

130. Ibid., p 23.

131. Gyory, op. cit., pp. 61–63.

132. Zhu, op. cit., p. 23.

133. See, e.g., Wilbur S. Shepperson, *British Emigration to North America: Projects and Opinions in the Early Victorian Period* (Minneapolis: University of Minnesota Press, 1957), pp. 76–114, 192–241; Theodore Saloutos, *The Greeks in the United States* (Cambridge, Mass.: Harvard University Press, 1964), pp. 1–95; Charles Tilly "Transplanted Networks," in Virginia Yans-McLaughlin, ed., *Immigration Reconsidered: History, Sociology, Politics* (New York: Oxford University Press, 1990), pp. 79–95; and, in general, Alan M. Kraut, *The Huddled Masses: The Immigrant in American Society, 1880–1921* (Arlington Heights, Ill.: Harlan Davidson, 1982), pp. 42–109.

134. Lyman, *Chinatown and Little Tokyo* . . . , op. cit., pp. 163–79.

135. Tchen, *New York before Chinatown* . . . , op. cit., pp. 132–48.

136. Oscar Zanetti and Alejandro Garcia, *Sugar and Railroads: A Cuban History, 1837–1959*, trans. Franklin W. Knight and Mary Todd (Chapel Hill: University of North Carolina Press, 1998), pp. 121, 136, 159. Moreover, as Moises Guillermo Leon Azolfeifa, in his Ph.D. dissertation entitled *Chinese Immigrants on the Atlantic Coast of Costa Rica*

([Tulane University, 1987; Ann Arbor: UMI Dissertation Service, 1987], pp. 36–83), points out, the U.S. Exclusion Act of 1882 caused some Chinese to seek such alternative places of work in the Western Hemisphere as Cuba, Mexico, and Costa Rica.

137. Denise Helly, "Introduction," *The Cuba Commission Report: A Hidden History of the Chinese in Cuba* (Baltimore: Johns Hopkins University Press, 1993), p. 20. Emphasis supplied.

138. Two thoroughgoing portraits of the thousands of the immigrant Chinese workmen who virtually single-handedly built the western section of the transcontinental railway will be found in John Hoyt Williams, *A Great and Shining Road: The Epic Story of the Transcontinental Railroad* (Lincoln: University of Nebraska Press, 1988, 1996); and Stephen A. Ambrose, *Nothing Like It in the World: The Men Who Built the Transcontinental Railroad, 1863–1869* (New York: Simon and Schuster, 2000).

139. Robert G. Lee, "The Origins of Chinese Immigration to the United States, 1848–1882," in Thomas W. Chinn and the Chinese Historical Society of America, eds., *The Life, Influence and Role of the Chinese in the United States, 1776–1960.* Proceedings/Papers of the National Conference held at the University of San Francisco, July 10–12, 1975. (San Francisco: Chinese Historical Society of America, 1976), p. 190.

140. Gyory, op. cit., p. 40.

141. Ibid., pp. 41–59.

142. "In the end," Gyory, op. cit., p. 46, concedes, "the NLU's resolution failed to make any distinction between immigration and importation. Delegates resolved only that 'the presence in our country of Chinese laborers in large numbers is an evil entailing want and its consequent train of misery and crime on all other classes of the American people, and should be prevented, by legislation.'" Gyory insists that the "National Labor Union had scant impact on workers' attitudes regarding the Chinese." But that misses the point. The labor union's anti-Chinese stance, in 1869 and later, had its greatest impact on America's policy makers. Gyory seems to be lamenting the absence of plebiscitarian democracy in the labor movement, supposing that if it had been present, organized labor would have opposed the exclusion act. This is chimerical thinking.

143. The following draws on Joel Franks, "Chinese Shoemaker Protest in Nineteenth-Century San Francisco," in Alexander Yamato, Soo-Young Chin, Wendy L. Ng, and Joel Franks, eds., *Asian Americans in the United States* (Dubuque, Iowa: Kendall/Hunt Publishing Co., 1993), I, pp. 137–40, 305–8. Quotations from pp. 305, 306, 307. This essay is based on Joel Franks, *Boot and Shoemakers in Nineteenth-Century San Francisco, 1860–1892: A Study in Class, Culture, Ethnicity and Popular Protest in an Industrializing Community*, Ph.D. diss., University of California, Irvine, 1983 (Ann Arbor: University Microfilms International, 1984).

144. Thus, John R. Commons wrote, citing an article in an encyclopedia as his source, "Chinese coolies came under contract with the Six Companies, who advanced their expenses and looked to their own secret agents and tribunals to enforce repayment with profit." John R. Commons, *Races and Immigrants in America,* op. cit., p. 109. For the background of the Chinese Six Companies, see Him Mark Lai, "Historical

Development of the Chinese Consolidated Benevolent Association/*Huiguan* System," *Chinese America: History and Perspectives, 1987* (San Francisco: Chinese Historical Society of America, 1987), pp. 13–51. See also Lyman, *Chinatown and Little Tokyo,* op. cit., pp. 161–85.

145. Franks, "Chinese Shoemakers . . . ," op. cit., 306, citing E. P. Thompson, "The Moral Economy of the English Crowd," *Past and Present* 50 (1971): 76–136. Thompson's essay is reprinted as "The Moral Economy of the English Crowd in the Eighteenth Century," in E. P. Thompson, *Customs in Common: Studies in Traditional Popular Culture,* op. cit., pp. 185–258.

146. Indeed, Gyory, op. cit., pp. 57–58, is so interested in granting credence to the workingmen's denunciation of the Chinese shoemakers as servile contract laborers that he denigrates abolitionist leader William Lloyd Garrison's charge that the Knights of St. Crispin were "dictatorial," that organized labor's leaders were "political demagogues," and that Sampson's contract with Kwong, Chong, Wing, and Co. had been made "in the usual manner, under lawful conditions." Garrison's statement that he saw no reason "why Chinamen should not be as freely induced to add their skill and labor to our capital stock," is quoted by Gyory, but without mentioning the great abolitionist's later denunciation of the impending exclusion act as a law inspired by a "caste spirit—vulgar, conceited, and contemptible" and a violation of "those fundamental principles which as a nation we profess to be guided by." (Henry Mayer, *All on Fire: William Lloyd Garrison and the Abolition of Slavery* [New York: St. Martin's Press, 1998], p. 624). In effect, Gyory, by using the term *importation,* misrepresents and impugns Garrison's motives: "Of the wide range of attitudes abolitionists expressed, Garrison's pro-importation stance garnered the most support." Lest anyone suppose that Garrisons' ideals and those of such other abolitionists as Julia Ward Howe might have had any weight with the white workingmen, Gyory concludes, "Abolitionists had recently split over women's rights and their split over the Chinese issue further rent this aging band of reformers. They no longer spoke with a single voice on human rights or, even more specifically, on racial matters. Once the crusading vanguard for freedom and racial justice, abolitionists no longer served as the conscience of the nation." Gyory would have us believe that the white working class—except for its Pacific Coast members and its organizational leaders—had stepped into the breach.

147. Herbert G. Gutman, "Labor History and the 'Sartre Question,'" in *Power and Culture,* op. cit., pp. 326–28.

148. Paul C. P. Siu, *The Chinese Laundryman: A Study in Social Isolation,* ed. John Kuo Wei Tchen (New York: New York University Press, 1987).

149. Roediger, "Afterword to the Revised Edition," *The Wages of Whiteness,* op. cit., p. 188.

150. The following draws on two essays by Herbert Hill: "Myth-Making as Labor History: Herbert Gutman and the United Mine Workers of America," op. cit., quotation from p. 142; and "Lichtenstein's Fictions Revisited: Race and the New Labor History," op. cit. The essay by Gutman to which Hill refers is entitled "The Negro and the United Mine Workers of America." It first appeared in Julius Jacobson, ed., *The*

Negro and the American Labor Movement (Garden City, N.Y.: Doubleday, Anchor, 1968), pp. 49–127 and is reprinted in Gutman, *Work, Culture and Society,* op. cit., pp. 121–208. The biography to which Hill refers is Nelson Lichtenstein, *The Most Dangerous Man in Detroit: Walter Reuther and the Fate of American Labor* (New York: Basic Books, 1995).

151. See Stanford M. Lyman, "The Race Question and Liberalism: Casuistries in American Constitutional Law," *International Journal of Politics, Culture, and Society* 5:2 (winter 1991): 183–248.

152. Lyman, *Chinese Americans,* op. cit., pp. 105–18.

153. Montgomery, *The Fall of the House of Labor,* op. cit., p. 85.

154. Ibid., p. 86.

155. Ibid., p. 86. Montgomery cites with apparent approval, Saxton, *The Indispensable Enemy,* op. cit., pp. 214–18.

156. Calvin Winslow, "Introduction," in idem, ed., *Waterfront Workers: New Perspectives on Race and Class* (Urbana: University of Illinois Press, 1998), p. 9.

157. Montgomery, *The Fall of the House of Labor,* op. cit., p. 335.

158. Gyory, op. cit., p. 94.

159. Shih-shan Henry Tsai, *The Chinese Experience in America* (Bloomington: Indiana University Press, 1986), pp. 67–76. Nor does Gyory deal with the protests over these riots lodged by the Chinese government against the United States and the demand for an indemnity for these violations of the Burlingame Treaty. See Coolidge, *Chinese Immigration,* op. cit., pp. 190–91; Shih-shan Henry Tsai, *China and the Overseas Chinese in the United States, 1868–1911* (Fayetteville: University of Arkansas Press, 1983), pp. 60–123.

160. Gyory, op. cit., p. 287 n. 4.

161. Ibid., pp. 94–95.

162. For accounts of the Rock Springs massacre, see anon., *The Chinese Massacre at Rock Springs, Wyoming Territory, September 2, 1885* (Boston: Franklin Press, Rand Avery and Co., 1886); Paul Crane and Alfred Larson, "The Chinese Massacre," *Annals of Wyoming* 12:1 (January 1940): 47–55. Reprinted without new pagination in Roger Daniels, ed., *Anti-Chinese Violence in North America,* op. cit., and Craig Storti, *Incident at Bitter Creek: The Story of the Rock Springs Chinese Massacre* (Ames: Iowa State University Press, 1991). A comprehensive account of anti-Chinese actions in this area will be found in William Wei, "The Anti-Chinese Movement in Colorado: Interethnic Competition and Conflict on the Eve of Exclusion," *Chinese America: History and Perspectives, 1995,* Marlon K. Hom, et al., eds. (San Francisco: Chinese Historical Society of America, 1995), pp. 179–97.

163. Storti, op. cit., pp. 170–74.

164. *Immigrants in Industries, Part 25: Japanese and Other Immigrant Races in the Pacific Coast and Rocky Mountain States—Diversified Industries* (Washington, D.C.: Government Printing Office, 1911. Reprint, New York: Arno Press, 1970), III, p. 280.

165. Storti, op. cit., p. 170.

166. *Immigrants in Industries,* op. cit., III, p. 280.

167. Ibid., p. 291. Emphasis supplied.

168. Ibid., pp. 292, 282.

169. Hill, "Myth-Making as Labor History: Herbert Gutman and the United Mine Workers of America," op. cit., pp. 182 and 182n.

170. Yuji Ichioka, *The* Issei: *The World of the First Generation of Japanese Immigrants, 1885–1924* (New York: Free Press, 1988), p. 125.

171. Frederick Rudolph, "Chinamen in Yankeedom: Anti-Unionism in Massachusetts in 1870," *American Historical Review* 53:1 (October 1947): 1–29. Quotation from p. 29.

172. David Montgomery, *Citizen Worker,* op. cit., p. 142. Emphasis supplied.

173. Perlman, op. cit., p. 62 n. 1.

174. Commons et al., op. cit., II, p. 149.

175. This and what follows in this paragraph, quote Gyory, op. cit., pp. 246–47.

176. Ibid., p. 247.

177. Gyory, op. cit., p. 314 n. 9.

178. Lucy E. Salyer, "*Laws Harsh as Tigers": Chinese Immigrants and the Shaping of Modern Immigration Law* (Chapel Hill: University of North Carolina Press, 1995).

179. See John R. Wunder, *Inferior Courts, Superior Justice: A History of the Justices of the Peace on the Northwest Frontier, 1853–1889* (Westport, Conn.: Greenwood Press, 1979), pp. 153–63; Christian G. Fritz, *Federal Justice in California: The Court of Ogden Hoffman, 1851–1891* (Lincoln: University of Nebraska Press, 1991), pp. 210–49; and Charles J. McClain and Laurene Wu McClain, "The Chinese Contribution to the Development of American Law," in Chan, ed., op. cit., pp. 3–24.

180. Corinne K. Hoexter, *From Canton to California: The Epic of Chinese Immigration,* op. cit., pp. 188–99; Ng Poon Chew and Patrick J. Healy, "Fighting Exclusion," in Yamato et al., eds., *Asian Americans in the United States,* op. cit., II, pp. 75–76; L. Eve Armentrout Ma, op. cit., pp. 32–37, 100–114; C. F. Remer, *A Study of Chinese Boycotts with Special Reference to Their Economic Effectiveness* (Taipei, Taiwan: Cheng-Wen Publishing Co., 1966 [1933]), pp. 29–39; and Kuang-sheng Liao, *Antiforeignism and Modernization in China, 1860–1980* (Hong Kong: Chinese University Press, 1984), pp. 58–59, 73–77, 94–97.

181. Salyer, op. cit., pp. 102, 301 n. 13.

182. Gyory, op. cit., pp. 97–99.

183. Ibid., p. 107.

184. Ibid., pp. 219–21, 310 n. 22.

185. Samuel Gompers, *Seventy Years of Life and Labor: An Autobiography* (New York: E. P. Dutton and Co., 1925), I, pp. 216–17.

186. Stuart B. Kaufman, ed., *The Samuel Gompers Papers,* Vol. 1: *The Making of a Union Leader, 1850–86* (Urbana: University of Illinois Press, 1986), p. 114.

187. Ibid., pp. 218, 242. Emphasis supplied.

188. Ibid., p. 454.

189. Stuart B. Kaufman and Peter J. Albert, eds., *The Samuel Gompers Papers,* Vol. 3: *Unrest and Depression, 1891–94* (Urbana: University of Illinois Press, 1989), pp. 370–72 n. 4.

190. Ibid., p. 292.

191. Letter to Adlai Stevenson, in Kaufman and Albert, eds., op. cit., pp. 488–89.

192. Letter to Thomas Reed, in Stuart B. Kaufman, Peter Albert, and Grace Palladino, eds., *The Samuel Gompers Papers,* Vol. 4: *A National Labor Union Takes Shape* (Urbana: University of Illinois Press, 1991), pp. 487–88.

193. See Thomas J. McCormick, *China Market: America's Quest for Informal Empire, 1893-1901* (Chicago: Quadrangle Books, 1967), pp. 21–52; and Delber L. McKee, *Chinese Exclusion versus the Open Door, 1900–1906: Clashes over China Policy in the Roosevelt Era* (Detroit, Mich.: Wayne State University Press, 1977).

194. Letter to Sofus Jensen, in Kaufman, Albert, and Palladino, eds., op. cit., 4: pp. 342, 342 nn. 1–3. For a comprehensive analysis of the Chinese in this industry, see Robert A. Nash, "The 'China Gangs' in the Alaska Packers Association Canneries, 1892–1935," in *The Life, Influence and the Role of the Chinese in the United States, 1776–1960,* op. cit., pp. 257–83.

195. See *Reports of the Immigration Commission. Immigrants in Industries . . . ,* op. cit., Vol. 23, 24, 25.

196. Excerpts from Samuel Gompers's Testimony before the Committee on Immigration of the U.S. Senate, in Kaufman, Albert, and Palladino, eds., *The Samuel Gompers Papers,* Vol. 5: *An Expanding Movement at the Turn of the Century, 1898–1902* (Urbana: University of Illinois Press, 1996), pp. 466–67.

197. Ibid., p. 471.

198. Ibid.

199. *Some Reasons for Chinese Exclusion. Meat vs. Rice. American Manhood against Asiatic Coolieism. Which Shall Survive?* Published by the AFL in 1901, reprinted as U.S. Senate Document 102 in 1902. Reissued in 1908 by the Asiatic Exclusion League which identifies Samuel Gompers and Hermann Gudstadt as its authors. There is disagreement as to the proper spelling of the name of Gompers's coauthor. In his autobiography, *Seventy Years of Life and Labor* (vol 1, pp. 231, 251, 304, 337; vol. 2, pp. 161, 316, 588), Gompers spells it as "Hermann Gudstadt." In Kaufman, Albert, and Palladino, eds., *The Samuel Gompers Papers* (vol. 5, pp. 538–39; 6, p. 562) there is provided a brief biography of "Herman Gutstadt (1853–1918?)." I have adopted Gompers's spelling.

200. Gompers and Gudstadt, op. cit., p. 22.

201. Quoted in Philip Taft, *The A. F. of L. in the Time of Gompers* (New York: Harper and Brothers, 1957), pp. 304–5.

202. California Bureau of Labor Statistics, *Biennial Report,* 1885–1886, p. 46. Quoted and cited in *Freedom, Racism, and Reconstruction: Collected Writings of La Wanda Cox,* ed. Donald G. Nieman (Athens: University of Georgia Press, 1997), p. 325 n. 40.

203. Carey McWilliams, *Factories in the Fields: The Story of Migratory Farm Labor in California* (Boston: Little, Brown and Co, 1939), pp. 74–80. See also LaWanda Cox, "The American Agricultural Wage Earner, 1865–1900: The Emergence of a Modern Labor Problem," in *Freedom, Racism, and Reconstruction,* op. cit., pp. 24–26.

204. I have drawn on the Reports of the Immigration Commission, *Immigrants in Industry,* Part 25, vol. 24, op. cit., pp. 3–82. See also Gilbert G. Gonzalez, *Labor and*

Community: Mexican Citrus Worker Villages in a Southern California County, 1900–1950 (Urbana: University of Illinois Press, 1994), pp. 26–29.

205. See Dudley O. McGovney, "The Anti-Japanese Land Laws of California and Ten Other States," *California Law Review* 35 (1947): 7–60. These laws applied to Chinese aliens residing in those States also. It took two separate higher court judicial proceedings to invalidate these laws. See *Oyama vs. California* 332 U.S. 81 (1943) and *Sei Fujii vs. State* 217 Pac. (2d) 481 (1950).

206. The following draws on the endnotes attached to "Fred Wheeler to Frank Morrison, Los Angeles, Cal., June 2, 1903," in Stuart B. Kaufman, Peter J. Albert, Grace Palladino, eds., *The Samuel Gompers Papers,* Vol. 6: *The American Federation of Labor and the Rise of Progressivism* (Urbana: University of Illinois Press, 1997), pp. 149–51. For detailed accounts of the Oxnard incident, see Ichioka, op. cit., pp. 96–102; and Tomas Almaguer, *Class, Race, and Capitalist Development: The Social Transformation of a Southern California County, 1848–1903,* Ph.D. diss., University of California, Berkeley, 1979 (Ann Arbor, Mich.: University Microfilms International, 1999), pp. 262–309.

207. Quoted in Ichioka, op. cit., p. 102.

208. Gompers, *Seventy Years of Life and Labor,* op. cit., I, pp. 304–5.

209. Ibid., II, pp. 160–65.

210. Ibid., II, p. 163.

211. Ibid., II, pp. 163–64.

212. Mink, op. cit., pp. 236, 239.

213. Richard Hofstadter, *The Paranoid Style in American Politics and Other Essays* (New York: Alfred A. Knopf, 1965), p. 3.

214. Gompers, *Seventy Years of Life and Labor,* op. cit., II, p. 173.

215. Ibid., II, pp. 173–74.

216. *Report of the Proceedings of the Fourteenth Annual Convention of the American Federation of Labor,* 1894, p. 70. Quoted in Taft, *The A. F. of L. in the Time of Gompers,* op. cit., p. 303.

217. Jacob A. Riis, *How the Other Half Lives: Studies among the Tenements of New York* (New York: Sagamore Press, 1957), p. 76.

218. Gyory, op. cit., pp. 97–99, 131–34, 163, 186, 222, 293 n. 50.

219. A thumbnail biography of Strasser will be found in Kaufman, Albert, and Palladino, eds., op. cit., 6: pp. 586–87.

220. See Seymour Martin Lipset, *American Exceptionalism: A Double-Edged Sword* (New York: W. W. Norton, 1996), pp. 77–175; and Deborah L. Madsen, *American Exceptionalism* (Jackson: University Press of Mississippi, 1998), pp. 1–121.

221. Roediger, *The Wages of Whiteness,* op. cit.; Ignatiev, *How the Irish Became White,* op. cit.

222. Timothy Messer-Kruse, *The Yankee International: Marxism and the American Reform Tradition, 1848–1876* (Chapel Hill: University of North Carolina Press, 1998), p. 229.

223. Ibid.

224. Before 1874, as Ira Cross pointed out long ago (*A History of the Labor Movement*

in California, University of California Publications in Economics, vol. 14 [Berkeley: University of California Press, 1935], pp. 136–37), "The consumer had no way of knowing whether the goods which he bought were made by white labor or by Chinese labor. In 1874 the cigarmakers, who had suffered most seriously from the effects of Chinese competition, originated the idea of attaching a label to their products by means of which it would be possible to distinguish white-labor cigars from Chinese-labor cigars. The label was white and was pasted across the box. Shortly thereafter the shoemakers also adopted a white-labor label . . . At a meeting of . . . the Workingmen's Party of California on October 2, 1878, William Wallaz, an ardent trade unionist and later one of the leaders of the local union movement, said that the adoption of the cigarmakers' label had thrown more than 1,000 Chinese out of work and had made room for 200 or 300 additional white cigarmakers in San Francisco."

225. Messer-Kruse, op. cit., p. 231.

226. Gyory, op. cit., pp. 131–32 and 293 n. 50.

227. Mink, op. cit., p. 79.

228. "An Article in the *New York Tribune* [November 5, 1878]," in Kaufman, ed., op. cit., 1:, pp. 124–25. Quotation from p. 125.

229. "An Article in the *New York World* [November 9, 1877]," in ibid., pp. 112–16.

230. Ibid., pp. 115–16 n. 17. Emphasis supplied.

231. August Sartorius von Waltershausen, *The Worker's Movement in the United States, 1879–1885,* trans. Harry Drost et al., ed. David Montgomery and Marcel van der Linden (New York: Cambridge University Press, 1998).

232. August Sartorius von Waltershausen, "Die Chinesen in den Vereinigten Staaten von Amerika," *Zeitschrift für die gesammte Staatswissenschaft* (Tubingen) 39:2 (1883): 320–431.

233. David Montgomery, "Introduction," in Sartorius, *The Worker's Movement* . . . , op. cit., p. 23.

234. Ibid., pp. 44–46, 61–62 . For an English translation of Ratzel's memoir of his trip across the United States (1873–1874), including a paragraph describing the Chinese workers in San Francisco as a "dull, stolid group" whom "you cannot escape . . . [E]verywhere they are busy in the same somewhat slow, careful, cautious yet diligent manner and always seem to be the same limited passive beings with the same yellow, slant-eyed, expressionless, beardless dozen or so faces," see Friedrich Ratzel, *Sketches of Urban and Cultural Life in North America,* trans. and ed. Stewart A. Stehlin (New Brunswick, N.J.: Rutgers University Press, 1988), p. 283.

235. Marcel van der Linden and Gregory Zieren, "August Sartorius von Waltershausen (1852–1938), German Political Economy, and American Labor," in Sartorius, op. cit., pp. 51–52.

236. August Sartorius von Waltershausen, "Boycotten, ein neues Kampfmittel der amerikanische Gewerkvereine," *Jahrbucher für Nationalökonomie und Statistik,* Neue Folge, Band II (1885), pp. 1–18. Translated as "Boycotts; A New Trade Union Weapon in the United States," in Sartorius, op. cit., pp. 153–70.

237. Ibid., p. 163.

238. For Woodhull, see Johanna Johnston, *Mrs. Satan: The Incredible Saga of Victoria C. Woodhull* (New York: G. P. Putnam's Sons, 1967); Barbara Goldsmith, *Other Powers: The Age of Suffrage, Spiritualism, and the Scandalous Victoria Woodhull* (New York: Alfred A. Knopf, 1998; and Lois Beachy, *The Woman Who Ran for President: The Many Lives of Victoria Woodhull,* trans. Gloria Steinem (New York: Penguin, 1996); Victoria Woodhull, *Victoria Woodhull Reader* (Weston, Mass.: M and S Press, 1975). For Andrews, see Madeline B. Stern, *The Pantarch: A Biography of Stephen Pearl Andrews* (Austin: University of Texas Press, 1968); Stephen Pearl Andrews, *The Science of Society* (Weston, Mass.: M and S Press, 1970 [1851]); and Charles Shively, ed., *Love, Marriage and Divorce, and the Sovereignty of the Individual: A Discussion between Henry James, Horace Greeley, and Stephen Pearl Andrews, and a Hitherto Unpublished Manuscript, Love, Marriage and the Condition of Woman by Stephen Pearl Andrews* (Weston, Mass.: M and S Press, 1975).

239. Messer-Kruse, op. cit., pp. 226–31.

240. Goldsmith, op. cit., pp. 29, 77, 101–2, 178–82, 325; Stern, op. cit., pp. 120–21.

241. Saul K. Padover, ed. and trans., *Karl Marx on the First International* (New York: McGraw-Hill, 1973), pp. 225–31; Hans Gerth, ed. and trans., *The First International: Minutes of the Hague Congress in 1872 with Related Documents* (Madison: University of Wisconsin Press, 1958), pp. 177–78, 194–95, 248, 264–67; and Arthur J. Vidich and Stanford M. Lyman, *American Sociology: Worldly Rejections of Religion and Their Directions* (New Haven, Conn.: Yale University Press, 1985), pp. 165–66 n. 8.

242. Goldsmith, op. cit., pp. 331–33. See also Amanda Frisken, "'Shameless Prostitute and a Negro': Miscegenation Fears in the Election of 1872," in Nancy Lusignan Schultz, ed., op. cit., pp. 133–48.

243. Messer-Kruse, op. cit., pp. 244–45.

244. John R. Commons et al., *History of Labour in the United States,* op. cit., II, pp. 217–18, 270–74, 302–9, 400–404.

245. Messer-Kruse, op. cit., pp. 207–16, 231–33, 244–60.

246. Taft, *The A. F. of L. in the Time of Gompers,* op. cit., pp. 10, 22–28, 34–35, 63–66, 86–90. A brief biography of Powderly can be found in Kaufman, Albert, and Padillo, eds., op. cit. vol. 6, p. 582.

247. Gyory, op. cit., pp. 107, 119, 123.

248. On this crucial point, which Gyory misses altogether in his overly class-oriented approach, see Richard T. Ely, *The Labor Movement in America* (New York: Thomas Y. Crowell and Co., 1886; reprint, New York: Arno Press, 1969), pp. 310–24; and Ken Fones-Wolf, *Trade Union Gospel: Christianity and Labor in Industrial Philadelphia, 1865–1915* (Philadelphia: Temple University Press, 1989); and Herbert G. Gutman, "Protestantism and the American Labor Movement: The Christian Spirit in the Gilded Age," *Work, Culture and Society in Industrializing America,* op. cit., pp. 79–117.

249. McGloin, op. cit., pp. 172–87.

250. Robert Seagar II, "Some Denominational Reactions to Chinese Immigration to California," *Pacific Historical Review* 23 (February 1959): 49–66. For the life and work of Donaldina Mackenzie Cameron (1868–1969), a Presbyterian missionary who took as

her calling the rescue of Chinese women impressed into prostitution in Chinatown, see Carol Green Wilson, *Chinatown Quest: The Life Adventures of Donaldina Cameron,* rev. ed. (Stanford, Calif.: Stanford University Press, 1950); and Mildred Crowl Martin, *Chinatown's Angry Angel: The Story of Donaldina Cameron* (Palo Alto, Calif.: Pacific Books Publishers, 1986 [1977]) .

251. William Speer, *The Oldest and the Newest Empire: China and the United States* (Hartford, Conn.: S. S. Scranton and Co., 1870), pp. 3–6, 462–530, 554–662; Rev. O. Gibson, op. cit., pp. 158–332, 345–73; Ira M. Condit, op. cit., pp. 90–224.

252. Fones-Wolf, op. cit., pp. 64–121.

253. Robert G. Lee, *Orientals: Asian Americans in Popular Culture* (Philadelphia: Temple University Press, 1999), p. 66.

254. Quoted from "The Chinese Evil, Master Workman Powderly Speaks Out, Urges Reenactment of the Exclusion Law by Congress," *San Francisco Chronicle,* January 8, 1892, in Jules Becker, *The Course of Exclusion, 1882–1924: San Francisco Newspaper Coverage of the Chinese and Japanese in the United States* (San Francisco: Mellen Research University Press, 1992), p. 13.

255. Quoted from "The Chinese Evil . . . ," in Robert McClellan, *The Heathen Chinee: A Study of American Attitudes toward China, 1890–1905* (Columbus: Ohio State University Press, 1971), p. 13.

256. Salyer, op. cit., p. 102.

257. Terence V. Powderly, "Exclude Anarchist and Chinaman," *Collier's Weekly* 28 (December 14, 1901): p. 7. Quoted in McClellan, op. cit., p. 20.

258. Powderly, "Exclude Anarchist and Chinaman," quoted in Becker, op. cit., pp. 99–100.

259. Ibid., p. 100.

260. Salyer, op. cit., p. 301 n. 13.

261. Gompers, *Seventy Years of Life and Labor,* op. cit., II, pp. 151–73.

262. Hoexter, op. cit., pp. 133–281.

263. Armentrout Ma, op. cit., pp. 32–34, 178 n. 13, 193 n. 11.

264. *New York Times,* December 9, 1905, p. 2. Quoted in Hoexter, op. cit., pp. 197–98.

265. Hoexter, op. cit., pp. 196–99.

266. Tien-lu Li, *Congressional Policy of Chinese Immigration, or Legislation Relating to Chinese Immigration to the United States* (South Nashville, Tenn.: Publishing House of the Methodist Episcopal Church, 1916), p. 118.

267. Gyory's statement can be accessed on the internet at Amazon.com.UK.

268. Philip P. Choy, Lorraine Dong, and Marlon K. Hom, *The Coming Man: 19th-Century American Perceptions of the Chinese,* op. cit.

269. Floyd W. Matson, "The Outcry against Chinese-Americans," *The Progressive* (September 1955): 25. Cited in Jacobus tenBroek, Edward N. Barnhart, and Floyd Matson, "Preface to the Third Printing," *Prejudice, War and the Constitution* (Berkeley: University of California Press, 1968), p. vi.

270. Jerome Beatty Jr., "Trade Winds," *Saturday Review,* May 7, 1966. Quoted in Alan R. Bosworth, *America's Concentration Camps* (New York: W. W. Norton, 1967), p. 251.

271. Choy, Dong, and Hom, op. cit., p. 172.

272. Loren W. Fessler, ed., *Chinese in America: Stereotyped Past, Changing Present,* compiled by China Institute in America, Inc. (New York: Vantage Press, 1983), p. 267.

273. Ronald Takaki, "Who Killed Vincent Chin?" in *A Look beyond the Model Minority Image: Critical Issues in Asian America,* ed. Grace Yun (New York: Minority Rights Group, 1989), pp. 23–29.

274. Choy, Dong, and Hom, op. cit., p. 162. For a comprehensive report on this issue, see Sam Chu Lin et al., "The Bloody Legacy of Hate Crimes: From Vincent Chin to Joseph Ileto, the Killing Continues," *Asian Week* 20:51 (August 19–25, 1999): 13–15.

275. Richard Austin Thompson, *The Yellow Peril, 1890–1924* (New York: Arno Press, 1978), pp. 1–62.

276. Morrison G. Wong, "Chinese Americans," in Pyong Gap Min, ed., *Asian Americans: Contemporary Trends and Issues* (Thousand Oaks, Calif.: Sage Publications, 1995), pp. 58–94.

277. Wong, op. cit., pp. 76–79.

278. Perla Ni And Ap, "Los Alamos Case Perplexes APAs," *Asian Week* 20:29 (March 18, 1999): 8; Jeff Gerth and James Resin, "1998 Report Told of Lab Breaches and China Threat: A Bomb Data Vulnerable," *New York Times,* May 2, 1999, pp. 1, 8; David Johnson, "Committee Told of Beijing Cash for Democrats," *New York Times,* May 12, 1999, pp. A1, A20; Tim Golden and Jeff Gerth, "China Sent Cash to U.S. Bank, With Suspicions Slow to Rise," *New York Times,* May 12, 1999, pp. A1, A20; David Johnston, "Friend of President Admits to Violating Fund-Raising Laws, *New York Times,* May 22, 1999, pp. A1, A9; Jeff Gerth, "Note Hints Fund-Raiser Knew of Bribery Issue, *New York Times,* May 22, 1999, p. A9; Jeff Gerth and James Risen, "Spying Charges against Beijing Are Spelled Out by House Panel," *New York Tiimes,* May 26, 1999, pp. A1, A15; John M. Broder, "President's Sober Response Assures Public of Counterespionage Measures," *New York Times,* May 26, 1999, p. A15; Tim Weiner, "How Right Is Report? Caveats by Experts," *New York Times,* May 26, 1999, p. A16; James Risen, "Fund-Raising Figure Had Spy Case Role," *New York Times,* May 26, 1999, p. A16; David Johnston, "Guilty Plea Set by Fund-Raiser for Democrats," *New York Times,* May 26, 1999, pp. A1, A24; Hoyt Zia, "Well, Is He a Spy—Or Not?" *New York Times,* May 26, 1999, Op-Ed, p. A31. Finally, Dr. Lee was released, the government's case against him having fallen apart. After fifty-eight counts were dropped, he pleaded guilty to one minor charge. See Matthew Purdy, "The Making of a Suspect: The Case of Wen Ho Lee," *New York Times,* February 4, 2001, pp. 1, 18–19; and Matthew Purdy with James Sterngold, "The Persecution Unravels: The Case of Wen Ho Lee," *New York Times,* February 5, 2001, pp. A1, A15.

279. Fox Butterfield and Joseph Kahn, "Chinese Intellectuals in U.S. Say Spying Case Unfairly Casts Doubt on Their Loyalties," *New York Times,* May 16, 1999, p. 26. See also Bill Mesler, "The Spy Who Wasn't," *Nation* 269: 5 (August 9–16, 1999): 13–17. Ling-Chi Wang, "China Spy Scandal Taps Reservoir of Racism," on the internet. URL: w.w.w.minorities-jb.com/asian/news/spying3c.html.

280. Caspar W. Weinberger, "Foreword," *Report of the Select Committee on U.S. National Security and Military Commercial Concerns with the People's Republic of China.* 105th Congress, Report 105–851. May 25, 1999 (Lanham, Md.: Regnery Publishing, 1999), p. vi. Moreover, Lars-Erik Nelson points out that "most irresponsibly, the Cox report suggests that every Chinese visitor to this country, every Chinese scholar, every Chinese student, every Chinese permanent resident, and even every Chinese-American citizen is a spy, potential spy, or 'sleeper agent,' merely waiting for the signal to rise up and perform some unimaginable act of treachery." Lars-Erik Nelson, "Washington: The Yellow Peril," *New York Review of Books* 46:12 (July 15, 1999): 6–10. Quotation from p. 6.

281. Charles C. Mann, "The Mole in the Machine," *New York Times Magazine,* Sec. 7 (July 25, 1999), pp. 32–35. Quoted material from p. 33.

282. Mia Tuan, *Forever Foreigners or Honorary Whites? The Asian Ethnic Experience Today* (New Brunswick, N.J.: Rutgers University Press, 1998).

283. Lisa Lowe, *Immigrant Acts: On Asian American Cultural Politics* (Durham, N.C.: Duke University Press, 1996), pp. 5–6.

284. Op. cit., p. xi.

285. Herbert G. Gutman, "Protestantism and the American Labor Movement: The Christian Spirit in the Gilded Age," *American Historical Review* 72 (October 1966): 74–101. Reprinted in Gutman, *Work, Culture and Society,* op. cit., pp. 79–117.

286. Kimberly L. Phillips, "Making a Church Home: African-American Migrants, Religion, and Working-Class Activism," in Eric Arnesen, Julie Greene, and Bruce Laurie, eds., *Labor Histories: Class, Politics, and the Working-Class Experience* (Urbana: University of Illinois Press, 1998), pp. 230–56.

287. Julie Greene, Bruce Laurie, and Eric Arnesen, "Introduction," in Arnesen, Greene, and Laurie, op. cit., pp. 8–10.

288. "Class was perhaps overworked in the 1960s and 1970s, and it has become merely boring. It is a concept long past its sell-by date." Quoted from E. P. Thompson, "The Making of a Ruling Class," *Dissent* (summer 1993): 380, in Nick Salvatore, "Herbert Gutman's Narrative of the American Working Class: A Reevaluation," *International Journal of Politics, Culture and Society* 12:1 (fall 1998): 75.

289. Gutman, "Protestantism and the American Labor Movement," op. cit. See also Herbert G. Gutman, "Enslaved Afro-Americans and the 'Protestant' Work Ethic," in Berlin, ed., *Power and Culture,* op. cit., pp. 298–325.

290. David R. Roediger, "The Greatness of Herbert Gutman," in idem, *Towards the Abolition of Whiteness: Essays on Race, Politics, and Working-Class History* (London: Verso, 1994), pp. 39–46. Quoted material from p. 41.

291. Hill, "Myth-Making . . . ," op. cit.; Salvatore, "Herbert Gutman's Narrative . . . ," op. cit., pp. 66–68.

292. Salvatore, "Herbert Gutman's Narrative . . . ," op. cit.

293. Gutman, "Protestantism and the American Labor Movement," in *Work, Culture and Society,* op. cit., p. 88.

294. Salvatore, "Herbert Gutman's Narrative . . . ," op. cit., p. 66.

295. Gyory, op. cit., p. xi.

296. Herbert Gutman, "Labor History and the 'Sartre Question,'" *Power and Culture,* op. cit., pp. 326–28. See also Laurence J. McCaffrey, *The Irish Catholic Diaspora in America* (Washington, D.C.: Catholic University of America Press, 1997); and L. A. O'Donnell, *Irish Voice and Organized Labor in America: A Biographical Study* (Westport, Conn.: Greenwood Press, 1997).

297. A fictional account of the Chinese danger to America will be found in P. W. Dooner, *Last Days of the Republic* (San Francisco: Alta California Publishing House, 1880).

298. Franklin Ng, "The Sojourner, Return Migration, and Immigration History," in idem, ed., *The History and Immigration of Asian Americans* (New York: Garland Publishing Co., 1998), pp. 87–105. Quoted material from p. 100.

Chapter Four. The Lost Tribes of Israel as a Problem in History and Sociology

1. Stanford M. Lyman, *Postmodernism and a Sociology of the Absurd and Other Essays on the 'Nouvelle Vague' in American Social Science* (Fayetteville: University of Arkansas Press, 1997).

2. See, e.g., "Is the Bible Right After All? BAR Interviews William Dever, Part 2," *Biblical Archaeology Review* 22:5 (September–October 1996): 30–37, 74–77; and "Face to Face: Biblical Minimalists Meet Their Challengers," *Biblical Archaeology Review* 23:4 (July–August 1997): 26–42, 66–67.

3. J. Maxwell Miller, "Israel, History of" in *The Oxford Companion to the Bible,* ed. Bruce M. Metzger and Michael D. Coogan (New York: Oxford University Press, 1993), pp. 329–32. Quotation from p. 331.

4. William Foxwell Albright, "The Biblical Period," in Louis Finkelstein, ed., *The Jews: Their History, Culture, and Religion,* 3d ed. (New York: Harper and Row, 1960), I, pp. 3–69. Quotation from pp. 40–41.

5. David Norman Smith, "The Social Construction of Enemies: Jews and the Representation of Evil," *Sociological Theory* 14:3 (November 1996): 203–40. Quotation from p. 234.

6. Smith provides a representative list of the protagonists in this debate in ibid., pp. 235–40.

7. Ibid., p. 225.

8. Loc. cit.

9. Lyman, op. cit., pp. 9–65.

10. Mark Peter Jones, "Posthuman Agency: Between Theoretical Traditions," *Sociological Theory* 14:3 (November 1996): 290–309.

11. See David A. Hollinger, *Science, Jews and Secular Culture: Studies in Mid-Twentieth-Century American Intellectual History* (Princeton, N.J.: Princeton University Press, 1996).

12. Ian Buruma, "Poland's New Jewish Question," *New York Times Magazine,* Sec. 6 (August 3, 1997): 34–41, 55–57.

13. Deborah Ramirez, "Judaism Reborn in Cuba," *South Florida Sun Sentinel,* August 3, 1997, pp. 1A, 14A–15A.

14. Tamar Garb, "Introduction: Modernity, Identity, Textuality," in Linda Nochlin and Tamar Garb, eds., *The Jew in the Text: Modernity and the Construction of Identity* (London: Thames and Hudson, 1995), pp. 20–30. Quotation from p. 23.

15. See James Clifford, "Diasporas," *Cultural Anthropology* 9:3 (1994): 302–38, esp. pp. 321–28.

16. Garb, op. cit., p 29.

17. "II Kings 17: 21–23," in *Tanakh: The Holy Scriptures. The New JPS Translation according to the Traditional Hebrew Text* (Philadelphia: Jewish Publication Society, 1985), pp. 595–96.

18. Mattis Kantor, *The Jewish Time Line Encyclopedia,* updated ed. (Northvale, N.J.: Jason Aronson, 1992), pp. 50–53.

19. Samuel Kurinsky, *The Eighth Day: The Hidden History of the Jewish Contribution to Civilization* (Northvale, N.J.: Jason Aronson, 1994), p. 235.

20. James D. Purvis, "Samaria, District of," in Paul J. Achtemeier, ed., *Harper's Bible Dictionary* (San Francisco: Harper and Row, 1985), p. 897.

21. Gabriel Sivan, "Sambatyon," in R. J. Zwi Werblowsky and Geoffrey Wigoder, eds., *The Oxford Dictionary of the Jewish Religion* (New York: Oxford University Press, 1997), pp. 604–5.

22. "XI Isaiah 11–12" in *Tanakh,* op. cit., p. 641.

23. "III Amos 14" in *Tanakh,* op. cit., p. 1020.

24. "IX Amos 9" in *Tanakh,* op. cit., p. 1030.

25. "IX Amos 14–15" in *Tanakh,* op. cit., p. 1031.

26. "XI Ezekiel 16–18," "XLVII Ezekiel 13–14," in *Tanakh,* op. cit., pp. 905–77.

27. "XLII Ezekiel 21–23" in *Tanakh,* op. cit., pp. 977–78.

28. On the life of Aqiva ben Josef, see "Akiba, Rabbi," in Louis Jacobs, *The Jewish Religion: A Companion* (New York: Oxford University Press, 1995), pp. 19–20; and Isaac B. Gottlieb, Aqiva Ben Josef," in Werblosky and Wigoder, eds., op. cit., p. 59. For the myths surrounding the life and teachings of Aqiva, see Nathan Ausubel, ed., *A Treasury of Jewish Folklore: Stories, Traditions, Legends, Humor, Wisdom and Folk Songs of the Jewish People* (New York: Crown Publishers, 1948, 1975), pp. 33–36, 42.

29. "Safra, Behukotai 8," quoted in Rabbi Eliyahu Avichail, *The Tribes of Israel: The Lost and the Dispersed,* trans. M. Gross (Jerusalem, Israel: Amishav, 5750 [1990]), p. 11.

30. Loc. cit.

31. "Moses Ben Nachman," in *The Standard Jewish Encyclopedia,* editor-in-chief Dr. Geoffrey Wigoder, 7th ed. (New York: Facts on File, 1992), p. 678; Michael A. Singer, "Nahmanides, Moses," in Werblowsky and Wigoder, eds., op. cit., pp. 490–91; "Nahmanides," in Jacobs, op. cit., p. 361.

32. Quoted in Avichail, op. cit., pp. 22–23.

33. "Pseudo-Jonathan Targum," in Werblowsky and Wigoder, eds., op. cit., p. 55. On the meaning and usages of Targums, see "Targum," in ibid., pp. 675–76; and "Targum" in Wigoder, ed., op. cit., p. 905. Robert P. Gordon observes (in "Translations:

Targums," in Metzger and Coogan, op. cit., pp. 754–55): "All translations of the Bible are necessarily interpretive to a degree, but the Targums differ in that they are interpretive as a matter of policy, and often to an extent that far exceeds the bounds of 'translation' or even 'paraphrase.'"

34. Quoted in Avichail, op. cit., p. 11.

35. Indeed, R. Aqiva used the rhythmic flow of the Sambatyon as one of his proofs that the Jewish day of the Sabbath was the correct one, telling the tyrant Rufus who had inquired about the matter: "It is proved by the fact that the river Sambatyon, which [flows so swiftly] on weekdays [that] it pulls up the stones [from] its bed, does not pull them up on the Sabbath, when it rests." Hayim Nahman Bialik and Yehoshua Hans Ravnitzky, eds., *The Book of Legends: Sefer Ha-Aggadah—Legends from the Talmud and Midrash,* trans. William G. Braude (New York: Schocken Books, 1992), p. 492.

36. Sivan, op. cit., p. 604. See also Nathan Ausubel, "The Ten Lost Tribes: Introduction," in Ausubel, ed., op. cit., pp. 515–17. See also ibid., pp. 526–29, wherein there is presented an English translation of a popular Yiddish folktale, based on *Gelilot Erez Yisroel,* a fanciful travel book published in Lublin in 1634, that purports to tell of the author's (Gershom ben Eliezer Halevi Judels's) travels from Salonika to Abyssinia via Palestine and Arabia, during which he encountered "The Little Red Jews on the Other Side of the Sambatyon."

37. Bialik and Ravnitsky, eds., op. cit., p. 135.

38. Ibid., pp. 134, 384.

39. "Case as to Eldad the Danite," in Elkan Nathan Adler, eds., *Jewish Travellers in the Middle Ages: 19 Firsthand Accounts* (New York: Dover Publications, 1987), pp. 15–21. Quotation from p. 19.

40. "And this is my name, Eldad ben Mahali ben Ezekiel ben Hezekiah ben Aluk ben Abner ben Shemiah ben Hater ben Hur ben Elkanah ben Hillel ben Tobias ben Pedath ben Ainon ben Naaman ben Taam ben Taami ben Onam ben Gaul ben Shalom ben Caleb ben Omram ben Dumain ben Obadiah ben Abraham ben Joseph ben Moses ben Jacob ben Kappur ben Ariel ben Asher ben Job ben Shallum ben Elihu ben Ahaliab ben Ahisamch ben Hushim ben Dan ben Jacob our father, on whom be peace and on all Israel." "The Letter of Eldad the Danite," in Elkan Nathan Adler, ed., op. cit., pp. 14–15.

41. Elkan Nathan Adler, "Introduction to the Letter of Eldad the Danite," in Adler, ed., op. cit., pp. 5, 15.

42. "The Letter of Eldad the Danite, in Adler, ed., op. cit., pp. 5–15.

43. Ibid., p. 14. See also "Eldad Ha-Dani Visits the Ten Lost Tribes," in B. Halper, ed., *Post-Biblical Hebrew Literature* (Philadelphia: Jewish Publication Society of America, 1921). Partially reprinted in Ausubel, ed., op. cit., pp. 517–20. A portion of Eldad's letter can also be found in Robert Silverberg, *The Realm of Prester John* (Garden City, N.Y.: Doubleday, 1972), p. 51.

44. Robert R. Wilson, "Prophetess," in Achtemeier, op. cit., p. 889.

45. "II Kings 22:14" in *Tanakh,* op. cit., p. 606.

46. Adrien Janis Bledstein, "Is Judges a Woman's Satire of Men Who Play God?" in

A Feminist Companion to Judges, ed. Athalya Brenner (Sheffield, England: Sheffield Academic Press, 1993), p. 53. Cited in Jonathan Kirsch, *The Harlot by the Side of the Road: Forbidden Tales of the Bible* (New York: Ballantine Books, 1997), pp. 254, 324.

47. Richard Elliott Friedman, *Who Wrote the Bible?* (Englewood Cliffs, N.J.: Prentice-Hall, 1987), pp. 103, 117. Cited in Kirsch, op. cit., p. 254.

48. Daniel Sperber, "Yohanan Bar Nappaha," in Werblosky and Wigoder, eds., op. cit., p. 748.

49. The following draws on Avichail, op. cit., pp. 25–28.

50. Erich Kahler, "Forms and Features of Anti-Judaism," originally published in the November 1939 issue of *Social Research* and reprinted in his *The Jews among the Nations* (New Brunswick, N.J.: Transaction Publishers, 1989), pp. xv–li. Quotation from p. xvi.

51. "Tribes, Lost Ten," in Wigoder, ed., op. cit., p. 928.

52. Shmuel Ahituv and Shalom Paul, "Tribes of Israel," in Werblowsky and Wigoder, eds., op. cit., p. 704.

53. The following draws on Richard J. Coggins, "The Origins of the Jewish Diaspora," in R. E. Clements, ed., *The World of Ancient Israel: Sociological, Anthropological and Political Perspectives* (Cambridge, U.K.: Cambridge University Press, 1991) [1989]), pp. 163–81. Quotations from p. 164.

54. Kahler, op. cit., pp. xvi–xvii.

55. Michael Grant, *The History of Ancient Israel* (New York: Charles Scribner's Sons, 1984), p. 164. However, if any historical credence is to be given to the claim by the unknown author of the book of *Tobit,* one of the fifteen books that form the *Apocrypha,* none of which is accepted as part of the Hebrew canon of scriptures, and which "is best understood as a romance of Diaspora Judaism," the eponymous autobiographer, a member of the tribe of Naphtali "carried away captive to Nineveh . . . [obtained] favor and good standing with Shalmaneser . . . [for whom he used] to go into Media, and by for him there." (I *Tobit:* 10–15). Tobit ran afoul of Shalmaneser's successor, Sennacherib, only to be restored to an honorable place in the kingdom after Sennacherib had been assassinated and his more friendly son, Esar-haddon, enthroned in his place. The latter appointed Tobit's nephew, Ahikar, to be his cup-bearer and accountant. The story suggests the possibility that some Israelites did well in Assyrian captivity without giving up their faith. Moreover, XIV *Tobit* 3–9 predicts: "All of our kindred, inhabitants of the land of Israel, will be scattered and taken as captives from the good land; and the whole land of Israel will be desolate, even Samaria and Jerusalem . . . But God . . . will bring them back into the land of Israel; and they will rebuild the temple of God, but not like the first one until the period when the times of fulfillment shall come. After this they all will return from their exile and will rebuild Jerusalem in splendor; and in it the temple of God will be rebuilt, just as the prophets of Israel have said . . . Then the nations in the whole world will all be converted and worship God in truth . . . All the Israelites who are saved in those days and are truly mindful of god will be gathered together, they will go to Jerusalem and live in safety forever in the land of Abraham . . . but those who commit sin and injustice will vanish from all the earth." "Tobit," *The Apocryphal/Deuterocanonical Books of the Old*

Testament, rev. std. version, in Bruce M. Metzger and Roland E. Murphy, eds., *The New Oxford Annotated Bible with Apocryphal Deuterocanonical Books* (New York: Oxford University Press, 1994), pp. iii–xiii AP, 1–19 AP. Quotations from pp. 1AP, 3 AP, 18 AP.

56. "II Kings 25: 27–30."

57. Grant, op. cit., p. 164.

58. Loc. cit.

59. "I–X Ezra," "I–XIII Nehemiah," in *Tanakh,* op. cit., pp. 1493–1530.

60. Philip Stern, "Dispersion, Diaspora," in Metzger and Coogan, op. cit., p. 169.

61. "I Maccabees 15: 1–24," in Metzger and Murphy, eds., op. cit., pp. 224–25 AP.

62. "I–II Maccabees," in Metzger and Murphy, eds., op. cit., pp. 217–58. For a discussion of this matter, see Irving M. Zeitlin, *Ancient Judaism: Biblical Criticism from Max Weber to the Present* (Cambridge, U.K.: Polity Press, 1984), pp. 273–74.

63. Werner Keller, *Diaspora: The Post-Biblical History of the Jews* (New York: Harcourt, Brace and World, 1966), p. 7.

64. Zeitlin, op. cit., p. 258.

65. Loc. cit.

66. Hayim Tadmor, "The Period of the First Temple, the Babylonian Exile and the Restoration," in H. H. Ben-Sasson, ed., *A History of the Jewish People* (Cambridge, Mass.: Harvard University Press, 1976), pp. 89–182. Quotation from pp. 137–38.

67. "Samaritans," in Jacobs, op. cit., pp. 441–42; "Samaritans," in Achtemeier, op. cit., pp. 963–66; "Samaritans," in Werblowsky and Wigoder, op. cit., pp. 603–4; "Samaritans," in Wigoder, op. cit., p. 826.

68. Tadmor, op. cit., p. 170.

69. "II Kings 17:24" in *Tanakh,* op cit., p. 596.

70. "II Kings 17:25" in *Tanakh,* op. cit., pp. 596–97.

71. "II Kings 17:29–33" in *Tanakh,* op. cit., p. 596.

72. "I–X Ezra" in *Tanakh,* op. cit., pp. 1493–1507; "I–XIII Nehemiah" in *Tanakh,* op. cit., pp. 1509–30.

73. "I Ezra 5–11," "II Ezra 64," "I Nehemiah 2–20" in *Tanakh,* op. cit., pp. 1493–95, 1509–11. See also Paul Johnson, *A History of the Jews* (New York: Harper and Row, 1987), p. 86.

74. For a biography of Josephus, see Mireille Hadas-Lebel, *Flavius Josephus: Eyewitness to Rome's First-Century Conquest of Judea,* trans. Richard Miller (New York: Macmillan, 1993).

75. Flavius Josephus, "The Antiquities of the Jews," pp. 22–426, in *Josephus: Complete Works,* trans. William Whiston (Grand Rapids, Mich.: Kregel Publications, 1960). Quotation from Book IV, Ch. XIV: 1–3, pp. 211–12.

76. Book X, Ch. IX:7, in ibid., p. 222.

77. Book XI, Ch. II:1, in ibid., p. 229.

78. Loc. cit.

79. Book XI, Ch. II:1–2, in ibid., p. 229.

80. Book XI, Chs. II, III, IV, in ibid., pp. 229–34. See also Zeitlin, op. cit., pp. 269–74.

81. Thus, the minor tractate *Kutim,* usually found in standard editions of the Talmud Bavli, is wholly devoted to a critique of the Samaritans, opening with "The usages of the Samaritans are at times like those of the heathens, at times like those of the Israelites" (Avraham Walfish, "Kutim," in Werblowsky and Wigoder, eds., op. cit., p. 407), and closing with "When will we accept them? When they deny belief in Mount Gerizim and confess Jerusalem and the resurrection of the dead." ("Samaritans," in Wigoder, ed., op. cit., p. 826.)

82. Book XI, Ch. V:4 in Josephus, op. cit., p. 235. See also "Book of Ezra," in *Tanakh,* op. cit., pp. 1493–1507; "Book of Nehemiah," in *Tanakh,* op. cit., pp. 1509–30; and "2 Esdras," in Metzger and Murphy, op. cit., pp. 300–340.

83. Zeitlin (op. cit., p. 276) is of the opinion that these wives were not "pagans." It "should be noted that though the wives are described as foreign, they are nowhere accused of paganism, i.e., worshipping their original gods after marriage. Therefore, the mixed marriages, far from being a symptom of assimilation or decline, might have been quite the opposite—a result of the growing Jewish influence in that generation upon the surrounding peoples. The number of Judaizing families that wished to become a part of Israel [sic] was on the rise. The foreign wives were not pagans but Judaized women. *In these terms Ezra's expulsion of these wives is a parallel to Zerubabel's rejection of the Samaritans* . . . What, then, is the best explanation for Ezra's decision? Most probably it was his fear that the mixed marriages were an abomination in Yahweh's eyes. (Emphasis supplied.) However, my reading of Nehemiah 13:23 (in *Tanakh,* op. cit., p. 1530) wherein this governor of Jerusalem censured, cursed, flogged, tore out the hair and abjured those who married "foreign" women does not lead me to share in Zeitlin's judgment on this matter.

84. Book XI, Ch. IV:9, in Josephus, op. cit., p. 234.

85. Loc. cit. According to Menahem Mansoor, *Jewish History and Thought: An Introduction* (Hoboken, N.J.: KTAV Publishing House, 1991), p. 19b: "In 538 [B.C.E.] the first group [of Jewish returnees] (approximately fifty thousand persons) traveled under the leadership of a Jewish noble named Sheshbazzar. A person named Zerubbabel is also mentioned"; p. 19c: "Some scholars believe that Zerubbabel is just another name for Sheshbazzar; others believe that Zerubbabel is Sheshbazzar's successor. According to one account, Zerubbabel, a grandson of Jehoiachin and, therefore, of Davidic descent, tried to revive the ceremonial religious practices in Jerusalem by setting up an altar and by reinstating observance of the festivals. He also made efforts to being the rebuilding of the Temple. After his reign the high priests assumed more religious and political power in Jerusalem."

86. "XIII Nehemiah 28," in *Tanakh,* op. cit., p. 1530. See also *Tadmor,* op. cit., pp. 177–78.

87. "IV Nehemiah 4–16," in *Tanakh,* op. cit., pp. 1513–14.

88. Book XI, Ch. V:8, in Josephus, op cit., pp. 236–37.

89. Max Weber, *Ancient Judaism,* trans. and ed. Hans H. Gerth and Don Martindale (Glencoe, Ill.: Free Press, 1952), pp. 361–62.

90. Book XI, Ch. VIII:6, in ibid., p. 244.

91. Book XI, Ch. VIII:7, in ibid., p. 245.

92. Book XII, Ch. I:1, in ibid., p. 245.

93. See, e.g., Gudrun Krämer, *The Jews in Modern Egypt, 1914–1952* (Seattle: University of Washington Press, 1989), pp. 12–18.

94. Book XII, Ch. V:5, in ibid., p. 257.

95. Book XVIII, Ch. IV:1–2, in ibid., pp. 380–81.

96. Flavius Josephus, "The Wars of the Jews; or The History of the Destruction of Jerusalem," in Josephus, *Complete Works,* op. cit., Book I, Ch. II:5–7, p. 431.

97. Mansoor, op. cit., pp. 11n and 19. According to the unsigned entry on "Samaritans" in Wigoder, op. cit., p. 826, Samaritan religious practices differ significantly from those of the Judean faith: "Samaritan religion is a form of primitive Judaism, except that the whole Bible of the S[amaritans] is the Pentateuch, which is the same as the Jewish version but represents a pre-Masoretic text with Samaritan variants; claiming, for instance, in the Ten Commandments that the place chosen by God for His sanctuary is Mt. Gerizim . . . [and] maintain[ing] that their text is the original and that the Jewish one was altered by Ezra . . . *Pesah* (Passover) can only be celebrated on Mt. Gerizim where the lambs are sacrificed, roasted and hastily eaten. On the seventh day of *Matzot* (i.e., unleavened bread) they make a *Hag* (pilgrimage) to the mountain, reciting sections of the Pentateuch. *Hag Shavuot* (Pentecost) always falls on a Sunday (the morrow of the seventh Sabbath after *Pesah*). *Yom Teruah* ("The Day of Trumpet-Call") is not called *Rosh Ha-Shanah.* At *Hag Sukkot* (Tabernacles), the *lulav* and *etrog* are unknown. Twice a year at the semi-festivals of Tsimmut *Pesah* (Shevat 15) and *Tsimmut Sukkot* (Av 15) the Samaritan priests supply calendars for the ensuing six months. The priests and levites never allowed a class of lay religious scholars to develop as in Judaism. There is practically no halakhic development of the 613 precepts, which are kept literally, but a rigid *Haggadah* compensated for lack of Halakhic activity. Moses is the one prophet in Samaritan eyes."

98. Louis H. Feldman, *Jew and Gentile in the Ancient World: Attitudes and Interactions from Alexander to Justinian* (Princeton, N.J.: Princeton University Press, 1993), p. 45.

99. "Two nations my soul detests, and the third is not even a people; those who live in Seir, and the Philistines, and the foolish people that live in Shechem." *L Sirach* 25–26 in Metzger and Murphy, eds., op. cit., p. 158AP.

100. Alfred Edersheim, *Sketches of Jewish Social Life,* updated ed. (Peabody, Mass.: Hendrickson Publishers, 1994), p. 14. The Judaeo-Samaritan rivalry over temple centers for diasporic Jewry is illustrated by what might be called the Elephantine Temple affair. As Cyrus H. Gordon and Gary A. Rendsburg (*The Bible and the Ancient Near East,* 4th ed. [New York: W. W. Norton, 1997], pp. 309–10) analyze a dispute that arose in 410 B.C.E., when Jedoniah, the leader of the Egyptian Jewish community in Elephantine, appealed to Jerusalem for permission and aid in rebuilding the local temple that had been destroyed by Egyptian and Persian marauders, no reply came from the Judean capital: "What was . . . the undeniable fact [was] that Jerusalem depended on the exiles of Babylonia for support so that the High Priest could scarcely afford to deny the right

of Jews outside Israel to have a place of worship. Disapproving of the Elephantine Temple, but not daring to maintain the principle of Jerusalem exclusivism, perhaps the best way out was to leave Jedoniah's letter unanswered." But then Jedoniah wrote a plea for recognition and authorization to the sons of Sanballat, the Samaritan builder of the temple on Mount Gerizim, which, Gordon and Rendsburg point out, "shows that, as seen from Egypt, the Samaritans no less than the Judeans were recognized as coreligionists of the Elephantine Jews, who had left Israel before the irreparable break on Judeo-Samaritan relations had developed." The Jerusalem authorities gave in after three years, permitting Jedoniah and his followers to rebuild their temple. See also Grant, op. cit., pp. 270–72.

101. Menahem Stern, "The Period of the Second Temple," in Ben-Sassoon, ed., op. cit., p. 260.

102. Dr. David A. Law, *From Samaria to Samarkand: The Ten Lost Tribes of Israel* (Lanham, Md.: University Press of America, 1992).

103. Ibid., pp. 24–25.

104. Ibid., p. 46.

105. Chaim Raphael, *The Road from Babylon: The Story of Sephardi and Oriental Jews* (New York: Harper and Row, 1985), p. 23.

106. Ibid., p. 222. For a brief but cautious history and analysis of the Jews in Bukhara, a city in Central Asia that might have been Assyria's "Hador," i.e., a city of lost-ten-tribe exile, see Donna Carr, *The Jews of Bukhara* (1997), available on the internet: URL: http://www.grtnet.com/~byblos/bukhara.html

107. Rabbi Adin Steinsaltz, "Heritage and Inheritance," address at the annual dinner of the Institute for Jewish Studies in the C.I.S., Jerusalem, Israel (September 25, 1996). Available on the internet: URL: http://www.judaica.ru/english/articles/morashen.html

108. Max Weber, *Ancient Judaism,* trans. and ed. Hans H. Gerth and Don Martindale (Glencoe, Ill.: Free Press, 1952).

109. The other three are "*The Protestant Ethic and the Spirit of Capitalism,* trans. Talcott Parsons (New York: Charles Scribner's Sons, 1930); *The Religion of China: Confucianism and Taoism,* trans. and ed. Hans H. Gerth (Glencoe, Ill.: Free Press, 1951); and *The Religion of India: The Sociology of Hinduism and Buddhism,* trans. and ed. Hans H. Gerth and Don Martindale (Glencoe, Ill.: Free Press, 1958).

110. Weber, *Ancient Judaism,* op. cit., p. 361.

111. Ibid., pp. 361–62.

112. Ibid., p. 362.

113. For a fuller treatment, see Gary A. Abraham, *Max Weber and the Jewish Question: A Study of the Social Outlook of His Sociology* (Urbana: University of Illinois Press, 1992).

114. Weber, *Ancient Judaism,* op. cit., p. 362.

115. James D. Purvis, "Exile and Return: From the Babylonian Destruction to the Reconstruction of the Jewish State," in Hershel Shanks, ed., *Ancient Israel: A Short History from Abraham to the Roman Destruction of the Temple* (Englewood Cliffs, N.J.: Prentice-Hall, 1988), p. 174.

116. See David Kessler, *The Falashas: A Short History of the Ethiopian Jews,* 3d ed. (London: Frank Cass, 1996), pp. xvii, 17, 45–47, 72, 108, 177; and Teshome G. Wagaw, *For Our Soul: Ethiopian Jews in Israel* (Detroit, Mich.: Wayne State University Press, 1993), p. 254n.6.

117. Max Weber, *The Religion of China,* op. cit., p. 23.

118. See Chaim Herzog and Mordechai Gichon, *Battles of the Bible* (London: Greenhill Books, 1997), pp. 125–262.

119. Weber, *The Religion of China,* op. cit., p. 23.

120. Loc. cit.

121. "Genesis XXXII: 25–33," in *Tanakh,* op. cit., p. 52.

122. "Genesis XLVIII: 3–7," in *Tanakh,,* op. cit., p. 78.

123. "Genesis XXVII: 1–46," in *Tanakh,* op. cit., pp. 40–42.

124. "Genesis XLVIII: 12–20," in *Tanakh,* op. cit., p. 79.

125. "Genesis XLIX: 8–10, in *Tanakh,* op. cit., p. 80. However, the English translators of *Tanakh* substitute "So that tribute shall come to him / And the homage of peoples be his," for the phrase "Until he comes to Shiloh." The Hebrew phrase "shai loh" may, following Isaiah 18:7, be translated "tribute to him."

126. "Genesis XXIX:3–4," and "XXX:1–8" in *Tanakh,* op. cit., pp. 80 and 46.

127. Daniel J. Elazar, *Covenant and Polity in Biblical Israel: Biblical Foundations and Jewish Expressions of the Covenant Tradition in Politics* (New Brunswick, N.J.: Transaction Publishers, 1995), I, pp. 123–226.

128. "Judges I–XXI" in *Tanakh,* op. cit., pp. 377–416; and Elazar, op. cit., p. 157.

129. See James L. Kugel, *The Bible As It Was* (Cambridge, Mass.: Belknap Press of Harvard University Press, 1997), pp. 274–82, for an interpretation of Jacob's blessing as prophecy.

130. Cyrus Gordon and Gary A. Rendsburg, op. cit., p. 265.

131. "Judges I–XIX," and "First Samuel I–XIII" in *Tanakh,* op. cit., pp. 377–437.

132. Larry G. Herr, "The Iron Age II Period: Emerging Nations," *Biblical Archaeologist* 40:3 (September 1997): 114–83. Quotation from p. 120.

133. "First Samuel XVI–XXXIII:II" and "Second Samuel I–V" in *Tanakh,* op. cit., pp. 442–78.

134. Herr, op. cit., pp. 120–21.

135. Tomoo Ishida, "Solomon's Succession to the Throne of David—A Political Analysis," in *Studies in the Period of David and Solomon and Other Essays,* ed. Tomoo Ishida (Tokyo, Japan: Yamakawa-Shuppansha, 1982), pp. 175–88.

136. Hayim Tadmor, "Traditional Institutions and the Monarchy: Social and Political Tensions in the Time of David and Solomon," in Ishida, ed., op. cit., pp. 239–58.

137. Kiyoshi K. Sacon, "A Study of the Literary Structure of 'The Succession Narrative,'" in Ishida, op. cit., pp. 27–54. Quotation from p. 54.

138. Herr, op. cit., p. 132.

139. "First Kings XII:16," in *Tanakh,* op. cit., p. 542.

140. Herr, op. cit., p. 132.

141. Ibid., p. 134.

142. "Haggai I:1; II:2, 20–23," in *Tanakh,* op. cit., pp. 1079, 1080–81.

143. "Zechariah VIII:13," in *Tanakh,* op. cit., p. 1090.

144. Flavius Josephus, "The Wars of the Jews," in Josephus, op. cit., pp. 427–606; Heinrich Graetz, "The Diaspora Suffering and Spirit," in *Ideas of Jewish History,* ed. Michael A. Meyer (Detroit, Mich.: Wayne State University Press, 1987), pp. 229–44.

145. Gordon and Rendsburg, op. cit., p. 297.

146. Elazar, op. cit., p. 334.

147. "Ezekiel XXXVII:20–28," in *Tanakh,* op. cit., p. 958.

148. "The Letter of Eldad the Danite—Being his letter to the Jews of Spain according to the text printed in Italy about 1480," in Elkan Nathan Adler, ed., op. cit., pp. 4–21.

149. "The Epistle of R. Chisadi, Son of Isaac (of Blessed Memory) To the King of the Khozars (ca. 960)," in Adler, ed., op. cit., pp. 22–36.

150. "The book of travels, which was compiled by Rabbi Benjamin, the son of Jonah, of the land of Navarre," excerpt in Adler, ed., op. cit., pp. 38–63. Quotation from p. 53. See also Sandra Benjamin, *The World of Benjamin of Tudela: A Medieval Mediterranean Travelogue* (Madison, Wisc.: Fairleigh Dickinson University Press, 1995).

151. Rabbi Judah the Pious bar Samuel, "narrative put together from . . . notes [of Rabbi Petachia of Ratisbon (1170–1187)]" in Adler, ed., op. cit., pp. 64–91. Quotation from p. 71.

152. See Wolf Leslau, trans. and ed., *Falasha Anthology: The Black Jews of Ethiopia* (New York: Schocken Books, 1969 [1951]), pp. xxxviii–xliii; Louis Rapoport, *The Lost Jews: Last of the Ethiopian Falashas* (New York: Stein and Day, 1980), pp. 57–184; James Quirin, *The Evolution of the Ethiopian Jews: A History of the Beta Israel Falasha to 1920* (Philadelphia: University of Pennsylvania Press, 1992), pp. 7–39; Steven Kaplan, *The Beta Israel (Falasha) in Ethiopia—From Earliest Times to the Twentieth Century* (New York: New York University Press, 1992); Teshome G. Wagaw, *For Our Soul: Ethiopian Jews in Israel* (Detroit, Mich.: Wayne State University Press, 1993), pp. 1–29; and David Kessler, *The Falashas: A Short History of the Ethiopian Jews,* 3d rev. ed. (London: Frank Cass, 1996), pp. ix–xxxi, 1–57.

153. "Letter of Elijah of Ferrara (1434)," in Adler, op. cit., pp. 151–55. Quotation from pp. 153–54.

154. *Cathay and the Way Thither—Being a Collection of Medieval Notices of China,* trans. and ed. Colonel Sir Henry Yule, new ed. rev. by Henri Cordier, 2 vols. (Taipei, Republic of China: Ch'eng-Wen Publishing Co., 1966); and Eileen Power, "The Opening of the Land Routes to Cathay," in *Travel and Travellers of the Middle Ages,* ed. Arthur Percival Newton (New York: Barnes and Noble, 1968), pp. 124–58.

155. Sir E. Denison Ross, "Prester John and the Empire of Ethiopia," in Newton, ed., op. cit., pp. 174–94; and Robert Silverberg, *The Realm of Prester John* (Garden City, N.Y.: Doubleday, 1972).

156. Albert Einstein and Erich Kahler, "The Jews and Arabs in Palestine: A Disputation with Philip Hitti." Appendix, in Kahler, op. cit., pp. 121–49. Quotation from p. 145.

157. Chaim Raphael, *The Sephardi Story: A Celebration of Jewish History* (London: Vallentine Mitchell & Co., 1993), p. 222.

158. Paul Johnson, *A History of the Jews* (New York: Harper and Row, 1987), p. 250.

159. Louis H. Feldman, *Jew and Gentile in the Ancient World: Attitudes and Interactions from Alexander to Justinian* (Princeton, N.J.: Princeton University Press, 1993), p. 47.

160. The following draws on "The Red Book of the Peoples of the Russian Empire," a document on the internet: URL: *http://www.eki.ee/books/redbook/introduction.html-ssi*

161. URL: http://www.getnet.com/~byblos/bukhara.html

162. URL: http://www.eki/books/redbook/georgian_jews.html-ssi

163. URL: http://www.eki.ee/books/redbook/mountain_jews.html-ssi

164. The Jewish Agency for Israel, "Rescue from Chechnya," URL: http://www.macom.co.il/Jafi/communications/Archive/chechnya.html

165. URL: http://www.virtual.co.il/communities/wjcbook/russia/index.html

166. URL: http://www.virtual.co.il/communities/wjcbook/ukraine/index.html

167. URL: http://www.cyberroad.com/poland/jews.html

168. URL: http://www.virtual.co.il/communities/wjcbook/lithuan/index.html

169. Yukiko, Sugihara, *Visas for Life,* trans. Hiroki Sugihara with Anne Hoshiko Akabori, ed. Loni Silver and Eric Saul (San Francisco: Edwards Brothers, 1993).

170. Marvin Tokayer and Mary Swartz, *The Fugu Plan: The Untold Story of the Japanese and the Jews during World War II* (New York: Paddington Press, 1979), p. 180.

171. Loc. cit.

172. Stanford M. Lyman, "Postmodernism and the Construction of Ethnocultural Identity: The Jewish-Indian Theory and the Lost Tribes of Israel," *Sociological Spectrum* 17:3 (July–September 1997): 259–82.

Chapter Five. Postmodernism and the Construction of Ethnocultural Identity: The Jewish-Indian Theory and the Lost Tribes of Israel

1. Sanford Budick, "Crises of Alterity: Cultural Untranslatability and the Experience of Secondary Others," in Sanford Budick and Wolfgang Iser, eds., *The Translatability of Cultures: Figurations of the Space Between* (Stanford, Calif.: Stanford University Press, 1996), pp. 1–24. Quotation from p. 6.

2. See, e.g., Michael Grant, *The History of Ancient Israel* (New York: Charles Scribner's Sons, 1984), pp. 121, 164, 272.

3. Erich Kahler, "Forms and Features of Anti-Judaism," originally published in the November 1939 issue of *Social Research* and reprinted in the rev. ed. of his *The Jews among the Nations* (New Brunswick, N.J.: Transaction Publishers, 1989), pp. xv–li. Quotation from p. xvi.

4. Loc. cit.

5. Ibid., p. xvii.

6. Daniel J. Elazar, *Covenant and Polity in Biblical Israel: Biblical Foundations and Jewish Expressions* (New Brunswick, N.J.: Transaction Publishers, 1995, pp. 155–60. See also Michael Walzer, *Exodus and Revolution* (New York: Basic Books, 1985).

7. Anatoly M. Khazanov, *Nomads and the Outside World,* 2d ed., trans. Julia Crookenden (Madison: University of Wisconsin Press, 1994), p. 98.

8. Cf. Kahler, op. cit., pp. 1–30.

9. Avi Erlich, *Ancient Zionism: The Biblical Origins of the National Idea* (New York: Free Press, 1995), p. 199.

10. Tamar Garb, "Introduction: Modernity, Identity, Textuality," in Linda Nochlin and Tamar Garb, eds., *The Jew in the Text: Modernity and the Construction of Identity* (London: Thames and Hudson, 1995), pp. 20–30. Quotation from p. 29.

11. Rabbi Eliyahu Avichail, *The Tribes of Israel: The Lost and the Dispersed,* trans. M. Gross (Jerusalem, Israel: Amishav, 1990).

12. See, e.g., Werner Keller, *Diaspora: The Post-Biblical History of the Jews* (New York: Harcourt, Brace and World, 1969); Howard M. Sachar, *Diaspora: An Inquiry into the Contemporary Jewish World* (New York: Harper and Row, 1985); Etan Levine, ed., *Diaspora: Exile and the Contemporary Jewish Condition* (New York: Steimatzky-Shapolsky, 1986).

13. Fredric Jameson, *Postmodernism or the Cultural Logic of Late Capitalism* (Durham, N.C.: Duke University Press, 1991), pp. 297–418.

14. Homi K. Bhabha, *The Location of Culture* (London: Routledge, 1984), p. 217.

15. Cf. Angelika Bammer, ed., *Displacements: Cultural Identities in Question* (Bloomington: Indiana University Press, 1994).

16. See R. Clayton Brough, *The Lost Tribes: History, Doctrine, Prophecies, and Theories about Israel's Lost Ten Tribes* (Bountiful, Utah: Horizon Publishers, 1979, 1994).

17. Marc Augé, *Non-Places: Introduction to an Anthropology of Supermodernity,* trans. John Howe (London: Verso, 1995).

18. Peter Jackson, *Maps of Meaning: An Introduction to Cultural Geography* (London: Routledge, 1989, 1994).

19. See Don Handelman and Elihu Katz, "State Ceremonies of Israel: Remembrance Day and Independence Day," in Shlomo Deshen, Charles S. Liebman, and Moshe Shokeid, eds., *Israeli Judaism: The Sociology of Religion in Israel,* Studies of Israeli Society, vol. 7 (New Brunswick, N.J.: Transaction Publishers, 1995), pp. 75–85.

20. Maurice Natanson, "History as a Finite Province of Meaning," in idem, *Literature, Philosophy, and the Social Sciences: Essays in Existentialism and Phenomenology* (The Hague: Martinus Nijhoff, 1968), pp. 172–77. See also Stanford M. Lyman, "History and Sociology: Some Unresolved Epistemological Problems," *International Journal of Politics, Culture and Society* 9:1 (fall 1995): 29–56.

21. Carl Becker, "What Are Historical Facts?" in Phil L. Snyder, ed., *Detachment and the Writing of History: Essays and Letters of Carl L. Becker* (Ithaca, N.Y.: Cornell University Press, 1958), p. 61. Quoted in Yael Zerubavel, *Recovered Roots: Collective Memory and the Making of Israeli National Tradition* (Chicago: University of Chicago Press, 1995), p. 3.

22. Stanford M. Lyman and Marvin B. Scott, *A Sociology of the Absurd,* 2d. ed. (Dix Hills, N.Y.: General Hall, 1989), pp. 35–50.

23. Ibid., pp. 22–34, 51–59, 182–90.

24. See Wolf Leslau, trans. and ed., *Falasha Anthology: The Black Jews of Ethiopia* (New York: Schocken Books, 1969); Michael Ashkenazi and Alex Weingrod, eds.,

Ethiopian Jews and Israel (New Brunswick, N.J.: Transaction Books, 1987); Steven Kaplan, *The Beta Israel (Falasha) in Ethiopia: From Earliest Times to the Twentieth Century* (New York: New York University Press, 1992).

25. Ronald H. Isaacs and Kerry M. Olitzky, eds., *Critical Documents of Jewish History: A Sourcebook* (Northvale: Jason Aronson, 1995), pp. 212–26.

26. Avichail, op. cit., pp. 56–62.

27. Cf. Cynthia Hay, "What Is Sociological History?" in Stephen Kendrick, Pat Straw, and David McCrone, eds., *Interpreting the Past, Understanding the Present* (New York: St. Martin's Press, 1990), pp. 20–37.

28. Mikhail N. Epstein, *After the Future: The Paradoxes of Postmodernism and Contemporary Russian Culture,* trans. Anesa Miller-Pogacar (Amherst: University of Massachusetts Press, 1995), pp. 330–31.

29. Frederick J. Teggart, *Theory of History* (New Haven, Conn.: Yale University Press, 1925), pp. 82–86, 107–49, 180–94.

30. See Alfred Schutz, "Type and Eidos in Husserl's Late Philosophy," *Collected Papers III: Studies in Phenomenological Philosophy* (The Hague: Martinus Nijhoff, 1966), pp. 93–98.

31. Harold Garfinkel, *Studies in Ethnomethodology* (Englewood Cliffs, N.J.: Prentice-Hall, 1967).

32. See Alfred Schutz, "Some Structures of the Life-World," *Collected Papers III,* op. cit., pp. 116–32.

33. See Irving Rouse, *The Tainos: Rise and Decline of the People Who Greeted Columbus* (New Haven, Conn.: Yale University Press, 1992); and William F. Keegan, *The People Who Discovered Columbus: The Prehistory of the Bahamas* (Gainesville: University Press of Florida, 1992).

34. Lee Eldridge Huddleston, *Origin of the American Indians: European Concepts, 1492–1729* (Austin: University of Texas Press, 1967).

35. Stanford M. Lyman, *Civilization: Contents, Discontents, Malcontents, and Other Essays in Social Theory* (Fayetteville: University of Arkansas Press, 1990), pp. 22–75.

36. Cecil Roth, *A Life of Menasseh ben Israel: Rabbi, Printer, and Diplomat* (Philadelphia: Jewish Publication Society of America, 1934), pp. 176–273.

37. Ibid., pp. 176–81.

38. Ibid., p. 184.

39. See Henry L. Feingold, *Zion in America: The Jewish Experience from Colonial Times to the Present* (New York: Hippocrene Books, 1974), pp. 3–5, 25–27, 65–67.

40. See, e.g., Charles Even, *The Lost Tribes of Israel, or The First of the Red Men* (Philadelphia: Lippincott and Co., 1861; reprint, New York: Arno Press, 1977).

41. James Adair, *The History of the American Indians* (London: Edward and Charles Dilly, 1775; republished as *Adair's History of the American Indians,* ed. Samuel Cole Williams (New York: Promontory Press, 1930); and Lewis Spence, *North American Indians* (London: Studio Editions, 1994 [1914]), pp. 3–4.

42. Roth, op. cit., pp. 225–73.

43. Menasseh Ben Israel, *The Hope of Israel,* trans. Moses Wall (London: Hannah

Allen, 1651). Excerpts will be found in *A Treasury of Jewish Folklore,* ed. Nathan Ausubel (New York: Crown Publishers, 1975), pp. 520–26. Quotations from pp. 520–21.

44. Ibid., p. 521.

45. Roth, op. cit., p. 65.

46. Ibid., pp. 191–202.

47. Daniel 12:7, in ibid., p. 206, and in the King James version.

48. In *Tanakh: The Holy Scriptures: The New JPS Translation According to the Traditional Hebrew Text* (Philadelphia: Jewish Publication Society, 1985), p. 1492, the passage from Daniel 12:7 is translated as "and when the breaking of the power of the holy people comes to an end, then shall all these things be fulfilled."

49. Roth, op. cit., p. 207.

50. Ibid., pp. 274–84.

51. Ibid., pp. 231–32.

52. Ibid., p. 232.

53. Loc. cit.

54. Ibid., p. 283.

55. Ibid., pp. 225–73.

56. See Lloyd P. Gartner, *The Jewish Immigrant in England, 1870–1914* (London: George Allen and Unwin, 1960); Stephen Aris, *But There Are No Jews in England* (New York: Stein and Day, 1970); David Feldman, *Englishmen and Jews: Social Relations and Political Culture, 1840–1914* (New Haven, Conn.: Yale University Press, 1994); and two works by Chaim Bermant, *Troubled Eden: An Anatomy of British Jewry* (New York: Basic Books, 1970); and *London's East End: Point of Arrival* (New York: Macmillan, 1975).

57. See Bernard Wasserstein, *Britain and the Jews of Europe, 1939–1945* (London: Institute of Jewish Affairs and the Clarendon Press of Oxford, 1979); and Monty Noam Penkower, *The Jews Were Expendable: Free World Diplomacy and the Holocaust* (Urbana: University of Illinois Press, 1983). For Canada's response, see Irving Abella, *None Is Too Many: Canada and the Jews of Europe, 1933–1948* (New York: Random House, 1982). For the United States, see two works by David Wyman, *Paper Walls: America and the Refugee Crisis, 1938–1941* (New York: Pantheon, 1968, 1985); and *The Abandonment of the Jews: America and the Holocaust, 1941–1945* (New York: Pantheon, 1984); Arthur D. Morse, *While Six Million Died: A Chronicle of American Apathy* (Woodstock, N.Y.: Overlook Press, 1983); Henry L. Feingold, *The Politics of Rescue: The Roosevelt Administration and the Holocaust, 1938–1945* (New York: Holocaust Library, 1970); Leonard Dinnerstein, *America and the Survivors of the Holocaust* (New York: Columbia University Press, 1982).

58. See Nicola Caracciolo, *Uncertain Refuge: Italy and the Jews during the Holocaust,* trans. and ed. Florette Rechnitz Koffler and Richard Koffler (Urbana: University of Illinois Press, 1995).

59. See Yukiko Sugihara, *Visas For Life,* trans. Hiroki Sugihara with the assistance of Anne Hoshiko Akabori, ed. Lani Silver and Eric Saul (San Francisco: Pre-Publication edition, Edu-Comm. Plus, 1995); and Marvin Tokayer and Mary Swartz, *The Fugu Plan: The Untold Story of the Japanese and the Jews during World War II* (New York: Paddington Press, 1979).

60. Huddleston, op. cit., pp. 33–40, 128–38.

61. Ibid., p. 131.

62. Simon Schama, *Landscape and Memory* (New York: Alfred A. Knopf, 1995), p. 24.

63. Adair, op. cit., pp. 16–230, 481–97.

64. Bernard W. Sheehan, *Seeds of Extinction: Jeffersonian Philanthropy and the American Indian* (New York: W. W. Norton, 1974), p. 59.

65. See Ronald Numbers, *The Creationists: The Evolution of Scientific Creationism* (New York: Alfred A. Knopf, 1992).

66. On the vicissitudes and variations in the curse of Ham in English thought, see Winthrop D. Jordan, *White over Black: American Attitudes toward the Negro, 1550–1812* (Chapel Hill: University of North Carolina Press, 1968), pp. 17–20, 35–62, 84, 111, 158, 243–46, 525.

67. Theodore Dwight Bozeman, *To Live Ancient Lives: The Primitivist Dimension in Puritanism* (Chapel Hill: University of North Carolina Press, 1988), pp. 202–59, 271–80.

68. For a summary, see John Canup, *Out of the Wilderness: The Emergence of an American Identity in Colonial New England* (Middletown, Conn.: Wesleyan University Press, 1990), pp. 55–87.

69. See Maria Eugenia Aubet, *The Phoenicians and the West: Politics, Colonies, and Trade,* trans. Mary Turton (Cambridge, U.K.: Cambridge University Press, 1996), pp. 8–20, 121–29, 290–93.

70. Ibid., pp. 79–85.

71. Ibid., p. 73.

72. Loc. cit.

73. Sacvan Bercovitch, *The American Jeremiad* (Madison: University of Wisconsin Press, 1978), p. 75n.

74. Sheehan, op. cit., pp. 59–60.

75. Ibid., p. 111.

76. See William G. McLoughlin, *Cherokee Renascence in the New Republic* (Princeton, N.J.: Princeton University Press, 1986, 1992), pp. 277–78, 367–403, 416–17, 450–51; Francis Paul Prucha, *American Indian Treaties: The History of a Political Anomaly* (Berkeley: University of California Press, 1994), pp. 178–81.

77. David Williams, *The Georgia Gold Rush: Twenty-Niners, Cherokees, and Gold Fever* (Columbia: University of South Carolina Press, 1993), p. 150 n. 32.

78. See William G. McLoughlin, *After the Trail of Tears: The Cherokees' Struggle for Sovereignty, 1839–1880* (Chapel Hill: University of North Carolina Press, 1993), pp. 13–20, 42–55, 145–59, 175–87, 210–48, 265, 274, 307.

79. Henry L. Feingold, *Zion in America,* op. cit., p. 55.

80. Peter Grose, *Israel in the Mind of America* (New York: Alfred A. Knopf, 1983), p. 8.

81. Ibid., p. 9.

82. Howard M. Sachar, *A History of the Jews in America* (New York: Alfred A. Knopf, 1992), pp. 45–48.

83. Hasia R. Diner, *A Time for Gathering: The Second Migration, 1820–1880* (Baltimore: Johns Hopkins University Press, 1992), pp. 40–42, 153.

84. For modernist sociological views of these prophecies, see two essays in *The*

World of Ancient Israel: Sociological, Anthropological and Political Perspectives, ed. R. E. Clements (Cambridge, U.K.: Cambridge University Press, 1989): R. J. Coggins, "The Origins of the Jewish Diaspora," pp. 163–84; and R. P. Carroll, "Prophecy and Society," pp. 203–26.

85. Feingold, op. cit., p. 66; Seymour Martin Lipset and Earl Raab, *Jews and the New American Scene* (Cambridge, Mass.: Harvard University Press, 1995), pp. 112–13.

86. Natanson, op. cit., pp. 172–77.

87. Pierre Vidal-Naquet, *The Jews: History, Memory, and the Present,* trans. and ed. David Ames Curtis (New York: Columbia University Press, 1996), p. 250.

88. Bernard Lewis, *Cultures in Conflict: Christians, Muslims, and Jews in the Age of Discovery* (New York: Oxford University Press, 1995), p. 70.

89. See, e.g., Charles Taylor et al., *Multiculturalism: Examining the Politics of Recognition,* ed. Amy Gutman (Princeton, N.J.: Princeton University Press, 1994).

90. See Ellen Schiff, *From Stereotype to Metaphor: The Jew in Contemporary Drama* (Albany: State University of New York Press, 1982); and Patricia Erens, *The Jew in American Cinema* (Bloomington: Indiana University Press, 1984).

91. See Neal Gabler, *An Empire of Their Own: How the Jews Invented Hollywood* (New York: Crown Publishers, 1988); and Andrew R. Heinze, *Adapting to Abundance: Jewish Immigration, Mass Consumption, and the Search for American Identity* (New York: Columbia University Press, 1990), pp. 203–18.

92. Arthur Kroker and David Cook, *The Postmodern Scene: Excremental Culture and Hyper-Aesthetics,* 2d ed. (Montreal: New World Perspectives, 1991), p. 272.

93. Homi K. Bhabha, op. cit., p. 152.

94 . See Lester D. Friedman, ed., *Unspeakable Images: Ethnicity and the American Cinema* (Urbana: University of Illinois Press, 1991).

95. Lester D. Friedman, *Hollywood's Image of the Jew* (New York: Frederick Ungar, 1982), p. 227.

96. Herbert Marcuse, *An Essay on Liberation* (Boston: Beacon Press, 1969), pp. 25–26.

97. Sanford Pinsker, "Mel Brooks and the Cinema of Exhaustion," in *From Hester Street to Hollywood: The Jewish-American State and Screen,* ed. Sarah Blacher Cohen (Bloomington: Indiana University Press, 1983), pp. 245–56. Quotation from p. 250.

98. Avichail, op. cit., pp. 63–176.

99. Harold Garfinkel, "Remarks on Ethnomethodology," in *Directions in Sociolinguistics: The Ethnography of Communication,* ed. John J. Gumperz and Dell Hymes (New York: Holt, Rinehart, and Winston, 1972), pp. 301–24, esp. p. 312 n. 3. See also Stanford M. Lyman, "Marginalizing the Self: A Study of Citizenship, Color, and Ethnoracial Identity in American Society," *Symbolic Interaction* 16:4 (winter 1993): 379–93.

100. Georg Simmel, "The Stranger," in *The Sociology of Georg Simmel,* trans. and ed. Kurt H. Wolff (Glencoe, Ill.: Free Press, 1950), pp. 402–8.

101. Rudolf Glanz, "The Wandering Jew in America," in *The Wandering Jew: Essays in the Interpretation of a Christian Legend,* ed. Galit Hasan-Rokem and Alan Dundes (Bloomington: Indiana University Press, 1986), pp. 105–18. Quotation from p. 116.

102. Friedman, *Hollywood's Image . . .*, op. cit., p. 228.

103. Jean-Francois Lyotard, *The Differend: Phrases in Dispute,* trans. Georges Van Den Abbeele (Minneapolis: University of Minnesota Press, 1988), p. xi.

104. David J. Hess, *Science in the New Age: The Paranormal, Its Defenders, and American Culture* (Madison: University of Wisconsin Press, 1993), p. 37.

105. Loc. cit.

106. Karl Marx, "The Eighteenth Brumaire of Louis Bonaparte," in *The Portable Karl Marx,* ed. Eugene Kamenka (New York: Penguin Books, 1983), pp. 287–323.

Chapter Six. Social Reality as Theater: Dramas, Narratives, and the Postmodern Challenge

1. Lester Embree, ed., *A Construction of Alfred Schutz's "Sociological Aspects of Literature"* (1955), unpublished draft, 1994.

2. Stanford M. Lyman and Marvin B. Scott, *The Drama of Social Reality* (New York: Oxford University Press, 1975).

3. See Stanford M. Lyman, *Postmodernism and a Sociology of the Absurd and Other Essays on the "Nouvelle Vague" in American Social Science* (Fayetteville: University of Arkansas Press, 1997).

4. Madan Sarup, *An Introductory Guide to Post-Structuralism and Postmodernism* (Athens: University of Georgia Press, 1989), p. 41.

5. Jacques Derrida, *Positions,* trans. Alan Bass (Chicago: University of Chicago Press, 1981), esp. pp. 37–96.

6. William Graham Sumner, *Folkways: A Study of the Sociological Importance of Usages, Manners, Customs, Mores, and Morals* (Boston: Ginn and Co., 1940 [1906]), pp. 13–15.

7. Stanford M. Lyman and Marvin B. Scott, *A Sociology of the Absurd,* rev. ed. (Dix Hills, N.Y.: General Hall, 1989), pp. 22–50, 182–90.

8. Jacques Derrida, *Aporias,* trans. Thomas Dutoit (Stanford, Calif.: Stanford University Press, 1993), p. 1.

9. Derrida, *Positions,* op. cit., p. 82.

10. Ibid., p. 43.

11. Jacques Derrida, *Dissemination,* trans. Barbara Johnson (Chicago: University of Chicago Press, 1981), pp. 95–117.

12. Jacques Derrida, "Difference" an address given before the Société francaise de philosophie, January 27, 1968, translated into English by Alan Bass and published in Jacques Derrida, *Margins of Philosophy* (Chicago: University of Chicago Press, 1982), pp. 1–28. Quotation from p. 13.

13. Ibid., p. 17.

14. Loc. cit.

15. Frederic Jameson, "Postmodernism, or the Cultural Logic of Late Capitalism," *New Left Review* 146 (July–August 1984): 53–92. Quotation from p. 83. Quoted in Pauline Marie Rosenau, *Postmodernism and the Social Sciences: Insights, Inroads, and Intrusions* (Princeton, N.J.: Princeton University Press, 1992), p. 69.

16. Embree, ed., op. cit., pp. 9–13.

17. Fredric Jameson, *Postmodernism, or, the Cultural Logic of Late Capitalism* (Durham, N.C.: Duke University Press, 1991), p. 31.

18. Henry Louis Gates Jr., *Figures in Black: Words, Signs, and the "Racial" Self* (New York: Oxford University Press, 1987), pp. 196–224.

19. Toni Morrison, *Playing in the Dark: Whiteness and the Literary Imagination,* The William E. Massey Sr. Lectures in the History of American Civilization, 1990 (Cambridge, Mass.: Harvard University Press, 1992). For further discussion of Gates's and Morrison's postmodern analyses, see Stanford M. Lyman, *Color, Culture, Civilization: Race and Minority Issues in American Society* (Urbana: University of Illinois Press,1994), pp. 25–27, 349–84.

20. See Maurice Natanson, *Anonymity: A Study in the Philosophy of Alfred Schutz* (Bloomington: Indiana University Press, 1986).

21. Roland Barthes, *Image-Music-Text: Essays,* trans. Stephen Heath (New York: Hill and Wang, 1977), pp. 143–48.

22. Alfred Schutz, "Mozart and the Philosophers," in idem, *Collected Papers II: Studies in Social Theory,* ed. Arvid Brodersen (The Hague: Martinus Nijhoff, 1964), pp. 179–200. Quotation from p. 195.

23. Ibid., p. 196.

24. Alfred Schutz, "Meaning Structures of Drama and Opera," in idem, *Life Forms and Meaning Structure,* trans. and annotated by Helmut Wagner (London: Routledge, 1982), pp. 180–207. Quotation from p. 181.

25. Richard Grathoff, ed., *Philosophers in Exile: The Correspondence of Alfred Schutz and Aron Gurwitsch,* trans. J. Claude Evans (Bloomington: Indiana University Press, 1989).

26. Alfred Schutz, "The Stranger: An Essay in Social Psychology," *American Journal of Sociology* 49:6 (May 1944): 499–507. Reprinted in Schutz, *Collected Papers II,* op. cit., pp. 91–105.

27. Aron Gurwitsch to Alfred Schutz, July 16, 1944. In Grathoff, ed., op. cit., pp. 69–72.

28. Schutz, "The Stranger" in *Collected Papers II,* op. cit., p. 105.

29. Grathoff, ed., op. cit., pp. 70, 71, 72.

30. See Aron Gurwitsch, "On Contemporary Nihilism," *Review of Politics* 7 (1945): 170–98. Reprinted in *Essays in Memory of Aron Gurwitsch,* ed. Lester Embree (Washington, D.C.: Center for Research in Phenomenology and University Press of America, 1983), pp. 523–50.

31. Ibid., p. 524.

32. Loc. cit.

33. Ibid., p. 526.

34. Ibid., p. 539.

35. Ibid., p. 529.

36. Lester Embree, "Notes on the Specification of 'Meaning' in Schutz," *Human Studies: A Journal for Philosophy and the Social Sciences* 14:2–3 (July 1991): 207–18.

37. Ibid., p. 216.

38. Richard Grathoff, ed., *The Theory of Social Action: The Correspondence of Alfred Schutz and Talcott Parsons* (Bloomington: Indiana University Press, 1978, p. 36.

39. Cf. Fredric Jameson, *The Prison-House of Language: A Critical Account of Structuralism and Russian Formalism* (Princeton, N.J.: Princeton University Press, 1972).

40. Stanford M. Lyman, "Animal Faith, Puritanism, and the Schutz-Gurwitsch Debate: A Commentary." Paper presented at the Alfred Schutz Memorial Symposium, New School for Social Research, New York City, November 30–December 1, 1989. In *Human Studies* 14:2–3 (July 1991): 199–206. Quotation from p. 200.

41. Loc. cit.

42. Loc. cit.

43. See Martin Esslin, *The Theatre of the Absurd*, rev. ed. (Garden City, N.Y.: Doubleday, Anchor, 1969).

44. Richard Schechner, *Public Domain: Essays on the Theatre* (New York: Avon Books, 1969), pp. 144–54 et passim.

45. Karl Marx, "Theses on Feuerbach," in *Marx and Engels: Basic Writings on Politics and Philosophy*, ed. Lewis S. Feuer (Garden City, N.Y.: Doubleday, Anchor, 1959), pp. 243–45. Quotation from p. 245.

46. Alfred Schutz, *The Phenomenology of the Social World*, trans. George Walsh and Frederick Lehnert (Evanston, Ill.: Northeastern University Press, 1967), pp. 139–214.

47. See Don H. Zimmerman and Melvin Pollner, "The Everyday World as Phenomenon," in Jack D. Douglas, ed., *Understanding Everyday Life: Toward the Reconstruction of Sociological Knowledge* (Chicago: Aldine Publishing Co., 1970), pp. 80–103.

48. Talcott Parsons, *The Social System* (Glencoe, Ill.: Free Press, 1951), pp. 249–325, 480–535.

49. Seymour Martin Lipset, *The First New Nation: The United States in Historical and Comparative Perspective*, rev. ed. (New York: W. W. Norton, 1979), pp. 99–204.

50. Cf. Georg Simmel, "How Is Society Possible?" in *Georg Simmel, 1858–1918: A Collection of Essays, with Translations and a Bibliography*, ed. Kurt H. Wolff (Columbus: Ohio State University Press, 1959), pp. 337–56.

51. Peter McHugh, "On the Failure of Positivism," in Douglas, op. cit., pp. 320–35. Quotation from p. 335.

52. Cf. Herbert Blumer, *Symbolic Interaction: Perspective and Method* (Englewood Cliffs, N.J.: Prentice-Hall, 1969), pp. 1–89.

53. Pauline Marie Rosenau, op. cit., pp. 21, 42–61.

54. Barthes, op. cit., pp. 142–48.

55. Rosenau, op. cit., pp. 43–44.

56. Ibid., p. 57.

57. Lyman and Scott, *The Drama of Social Reality*, op. cit., pp. 1–3, 101–14, 159–62, 163–70.

58. Kenneth Burke, "Interaction: Dramatism," *International Encyclopedia of the Social Sciences* 7(1968): 446. See also Bernard L. Brock, ed., *Kenneth Burke and*

Contemporary European Thought: Rhetoric in Transition (Tuscaloosa: University of Alabama Press, 1995).

59. Cf. two studies by Jean-Francois Lyotard, *The Postmodern Condition: A Report on Knowledge,* trans. Geoff Bennington and Brian Massumi (Minneapolis: University of Minnesota Press, 1984, 1991); and *The Postmodern Explained: Correspondence, 1982–1985,* trans. and ed. Julian Pefanis and Morgan Thomas (Minneapolis: University of Minnesota Press, 1993).

60. Jean Baudrillard, *In the Shadow of the Silent Majorities, or, The End of the Social and Other Essays,* trans. Paul Foss, John Johnston, and Paul Patton (New York: Semiotext(e), 1983), pp. 1–94.

61. Keith Tester, *The Life and Times of Post-Modernity* (London: Routledge, 1993), p. 152.

62. Georg Simmel, "The Stranger," in *The Sociology of Georg Simmel,* trans. and ed. Kurt H, Wolff (Glencoe, Ill.: Free Press, 1950), pp. 402–8. See also Margaret Mary Wood, *The Stranger: A Study in Social Relationships* (New York: AMS Press, 1969 [1934]).

63. Alfred Schutz, "The Stranger," op. cit.

64. Robert E. Park, "Human Migration and the Marginal Man," in Ernest W. Burgess, ed., *Personality and the Social Group* (Chicago: University of Chicago Press, 1929; reprint, Freeport, N.Y.: Books for Libraries Press, 1969), pp. 64–77.

65. Everett V. Stonequist, *The Marginal Man: A Study in Personality and Culture Conflict* (New York: Charles Scribner's Sons, 1937; reprint, New York: Russell and Russell, 1961).

66. H. F. Dickie-Clarke, *The Marginal Situation: A Sociological Study of a Coloured Group* (London: Routledge, 1966); Sister Frances Jerome Woods, *Marginality and Identity: A Colored Creole Family through Ten Generations* (Baton Rouge: Louisiana State University Press, 1972); Noel P. Gist and Anthony Gary Dworkin, eds., *The Blending of Races: Marginality and Identity in World Perspective* (New York: Wiley-Interscience, 1972); Noel P. Gist and Roy Dean Wright, *Marginality and Identity: Anglo-Indians as a Racially Mixed Minority in India* (Leiden, The Netherlands: E. J. Brill, 1973); Janice E. Perlman, *The Myth of Marginality: Urban Poverty and Politics in Rio de Janeiro* (Berkeley: University of California Press 1976, 1979); Abdolmaboud Ansari, *Iranian Immigrants in the United States: A Case Study of Dual Marginality* (Millwood, N.J.: Associated Faculty Press, 1988); John P. Meier, *A Marginal Jew: Rethinking the Historical Jesus* (New York: Doubleday, Vol. I, 1991; Vol. II, 1994; Vol. III, forthcoming). Sociological studies of Chinese in America have often focused on their marginality. See, e.g., Stanford M. Lyman, *The Asian in North America* (Santa Barbara, Calif.: American Bibliographic Center, Clio Press, 1977), pp. 11–66, 103–18, 151–200; Paul C. P. Siu, *The Chinese Laundryman: A Study of Social Isolation,* ed. John Kuo Wei Tchen (New York: New York University Press, 1987); Robert Seto Quan in collaboration with Julian B. Roebuck, *Lotus among the Magnolias: The Mississippi Chinese* (Jackson: University Press of Mississippi, 1982); James W. Loewen, *The Mississippi Chinese: Between Black and White,* 2d ed. (Prospect Heights, Ill.: Waveland Press, 1988).

67. See two works by Aron Gurwitsch, *The Field of Consciousness* (Pittsburgh: Duquesne University Press, 1964), p. 4; *Marginal Consciousness,* ed. Lester Embree (Athens: Ohio University Press, 1985).

68. Blumer, op. cit., p. 10.

69. Ibid., p. 15.

70. Kenneth Bock, *Human Nature Mythology* (Urbana: University of Illinois Press, 1994).

71. Ibid., p. 80.

72. Ibid., p. 113.

73. Ibid., pp. 101–16.

74. Pico della Mirandola, *On the Dignity of Man,* trans. Charles Glenn Wallis (Indianapolis, Ind.: Bobbs-Merrill, 1965), pp. 3–17.

75. Bock, op. cit., p. 114.

76. Ibid., p. 116.

77. Cf. Stephen Park Turner and Jonathan H. Turner, *The Impossible Science: An Institutional Analysis of American Sociology* (Newbury Park, Calif.: Sage Publications, 1990).

78. Richard Rorty, *Philosophy and the Mirror of Nature* (Princeton, N.J.: Princeton University Press, 1979).

79. McHugh, op. cit., pp. 322–24.

80. Rosenau, op. cit., pp. 77–108.

81. Rorty, op. cit., pp. 357–94.

82. Burke, op. cit.

83. See Tom Burns, *Erving Goffman* (London: Routledge, 1992), pp. 106–40.

84. Peter Berger, *Invitation to Sociology: A Humanistic Perspective* (Garden City, N.Y.: Doubleday, Anchor, 1963), pp. 122–50, 164–76.

85. Rom Harré, *Social Being: A Theory for Social Psychology* (Totowa, N.J.: Rowman and Littlefield, 1979), pp. 45–62, 189–232; R. Harré and P. F. Secord, *The Explanation of Social Behaviour* (Totowa, N.J.: Rowman and Littlefield, 1972), pp. 147–226; Peter Marsh, Elizabeth Rosser, and Rom Harré, *The Rules of Disorder* (London: Routledge, 1978); Rom Harré and Grant Gillett, *The Discursive Mind* (Thousand Oaks, Calif.: Sage Publications, 1994), pp. 97–180.

86. In addition to Richard Schechner's *The Public Domain,* op. cit., see five studies by the same author: "Drama, Script, Theatre, and Performance," *Drama Review* 17:3 (September 1973): 5–36; *Environmental Theater* (New York: Hawthorn Books, 1973); *Essays on Performance Theory, 1970–1976* (New York: Drama Book Specialists, 1977); idem and Mady Schuman, eds., *Ritual, Play, and Performance: Readings in the Social Sciences/Theatre* (New York: Seabury Press, 1976); *Between Theater and Anthropology* (Philadelphia: University of Pennsylvania Press, 1985).

87. See, among many others by the same author, Victor W. Turner, "Dewey, Dilthey, and Drama: An Essay in the Anthropology of Experience," in idem and Edward M. Bruner, eds., *The Anthropology of Experience* (Urbana: University of Illinois Press, 1986), pp. 33–44.

88. Nicolas Evreinoff, *The Theatre in Life,* ed. and trans. A. I. Nazaroff (New York: Benjamin Blom, 1970 [1920]). See also Stanford M. Lyman, "Evreinoff, Our Contemporary," in Japanese, the foreword to H. Shimizu's Japanese translation of Evreinoff's *Theatre in Life* (Tokyo: Shinyo-sha, 1983), pp. 1–17.

89. Lyman and Scott, *A Sociology of the Absurd,* op. cit., pp. 21–190; *The Drama of Social Reality,* op. cit., pp. 1–3, 101–62. See also T. R. Young, *The Drama of Social Life: Essays in Post-Modern Social Psychology* (New Brunswick, N.J.: Transaction Publishers, 1990), pp. 169–356.

90. For a brief but useful summary, see Christopher Lloyd, *Explanation in Social History* (Oxford, U.K.: Basil Blackwell, 1986), pp. 263–78.

91. See Paul Ricoeur, "The Model of the Text: Meaningful Action Considered as a Text," *Social Research* 38:3 (autumn 1971): 529–62.

92. Schechner, *The Public Domain,* op. cit., pp. 189–91, 222–25; Lyman and Scott, *A Sociology of the Absurd,* op. cit., pp. 61–68, 215–16.

93. Schechner, *The Public Domain,* op. cit., pp. 63–67.

94. Schutz, *Life Forms and Meaning Structure,* op. cit., p. 181.

95. See Lyman and Scott, *The Drama of Social Reality,* op. cit., pp. 101–15. See also two studies by Alan F. Blum, "Theorizing," in Douglas, ed., op. cit., pp. 305–23; and *Theorizing* (London: Heinemann, 1974).

96. Schutz, *Life Forms and Meaning Structures,* op. cit., pp. 52–76.

97. Ibid., p. 62.

98. Ibid., p. 109.

99. Alfred Schutz, "Lecture XVI: The Social Stratification of Language" (January 12, 1953), *Problems of a Sociology of Language: A Lecture Course,* ed. Lester Embree. Unpublished MS, pp. 50–52.

100. Ibid., p. 52.

101. Lyman and Scott, *A Sociology of the Absurd,* op. cit., pp. 2–20.

102. Schutz, "The Social Stratification of Language," op. cit., pp. 50–52.

103. See Homi K. Bhabha, "DissemiNation: Time, Narrative, and the Margins of the Modern Nation," in idem, ed., *Nation and Narration* (London: Routledge, 1990), pp. 291–322; Patricia M. Lengermann and Jill Niebrugge-Brantley, "Feminist Sociological Theory: The Near-Future Prospects," in *Frontiers of Social Theory: The New Syntheses,* ed. George Ritzer (New York: Columbia University Press, 1990), pp. 316–44; and four works by Steven Seidman, "The End of Sociological Theory: The Postmodern Hope," and "Postmodern Anxiety: The Politics of Epistemology," pp. 131–46 and 180–90 in *Sociological Theory* 9:2 (fall 1991); *Embattled Eros: Sexual Politics and Ethics in Contemporary America* (New York: Routledge, 1992), pp. 1–16, 97–144, 187–215; "Symposium: Queer Theory/Sociology: A Dialogue," *Sociological Theory* 12:2 (July 1994): 166–77.

104. Schutz, "The Social Stratification of Language," op. cit., p. 52.

105. Harré and Secord, op. cit., pp. 209–15.

106. See, of course, the classical statement of the twentieth-century crisis: Edmund Husserl, *The Crisis of European Sciences and Transcendental Phenomenology,* trans. David Carr (Evanston, Ill.: Northwestern University Press, 1970).

107. Maurice Natanson, "History as a Finite Province of Meaning," in idem, *Literature, Philosophy and the Social Sciences: Essays in Existentialism and Phenomenology* (The Hague, Netherlands: Martinus Nijhoff, 1968), pp. 172–77.

108. Ibid.

109. For a fascinating investigation that questions the postmodern critique insofar as it applies to law and jurisprudence in the West, see Gillian Rose, *Dialectic of Nihilism: Post-Structuralism and Law* (Oxford, U.K.: Basil Blackwell, 1984).

110. For three studies of how the law and the courts are engaged in the construction and legitimation of Otherhood, see Stanford M. Lyman, "The Race Question and Liberalism: Casuistries in American Constitutional Law," *International Journal of Politics, Culture, and Society* 5:2 (winter 1991): 183–247; "The Chinese before the Courts: Ethnoracial Construction and Marginalization," *International Journal of Politics, Culture, and Society* 6:3 (spring 1993): 443–62; "Marginalizing the Self: A Study of Citizenship, Color, and Ethnoracial Identity in American Society," *Symbolic Interaction* 16:4 (winter 1993): 379–94.

111. Michael D. Barber, *Social Typifications and the Elusive Other: The Place of Sociology of Knowledge in Alfred Schutz's Phenomenology* (Lewisburg, Pa.: Bucknell University Press, 1988), p. 100.

Chapter Seven. Cinematic Ideologies and Societal Dystopias: Filmmaking in the United States, Japan, Germany, and the Soviet Union, 1900–1996

1. Hugo Münsterberg, *The Photoplay: A Psychological Study* (New York: D. Appleton and Co., 1916. Republished as *The Film: A Psychological Study—The Silent Photoplay in 1916* (New York: Dover Publications, 1970). For a discussion of Münsterberg's contributions to sociology and social psychology, see Arthur J. Vidich and Stanford M. Lyman, *American Sociology: Worldly Rejections of Religion and Their Directions* (New Haven, Conn.: Yale University Press, 1985), pp. 87–101.

2. See Steven Starker, *Evil Influences: Crusades against the Mass Media* (New Brunswick, N.J.: Transaction Publishers, 1989), pp. 89–106; Leonard J. Leff and Jerold L. Simmons, *The Dame in the Kimono: Hollywood Censorship and the Production Code from the 1920s to the 1960s* (New York: Grove Weidenfeld, 1990), and Frank Wald, *Sin and Censorship: The Catholic Church and the Motion Picture Industry* (New Haven, Conn.: Yale University Press, 1996).

3. Herbert Blumer, *Movies and Conduct* (New York: Macmillan, 1933).

4. Herbert Blumer and Philip M. Hauser, *Movies, Delinquency and Crime* (New York: Macmillan, 1933).

5. Herbert Blumer, "Moulding of Mass Behavior through the Motion Picture," *Publications of the American Sociological Society* 29 (August 1935): 115–27. Quotation from p. 119. For a discussion, see Stanford M. Lyman and Arthur J. Vidich, *Social Order and the Public Philosophy: An Analysis and Interpretation of the Work of Herbert Blumer* (Fayetteville: University of Arkansas Press, 1988), pp. 36–42.

6. J. P. Mayer, *Sociology of Film: Studies and Documents* (London: Faber and Faber,

1946), p. 9. Mayer regarded this book as the sequel to his *Max Weber and German Politics: A Study in Political Sociology,* 2d ed. (London: Faber and Faber, 1946).

7. I. C. Jarvie, *Movies and Society* (New York: Basic Books, 1970).

8. I. C. Jarvie, *Movies as Social Criticism: Aspects of Their Social Psychology* (Metuchen, N.J.: Scarecrow Press, 1978).

9. I. C. Jarvie, *Philosophy of the Film: Epistemology, Ontology, Aesthetics* (New York: Routledge, 1987).

10. See Leo Lowenthal, *Literature and Mass Culture,* Communication in Society, vol. 1 (New Brunswick, N.J.: Transaction Publishers, 1984), pp. 1–240; and Paul R. Gorman, *Left Intellectuals and Popular Culture in Twentieth-Century America* (Chapel Hill: University of North Carolina Press, 1996).

11. See, e.g., Douglas Kellner, *Media Culture: Cultural Studies, Identity and Politics between the Modern and the Postmodern* (London: Routledge, 1995); and Stuart Hall, "What Is This 'Black' in Black Popular Culture?" in *Stuart Hall: Critical Dialogues in Cultural Studies,* ed. David Morley and Kuan-Hsing Chen (New York: Routledge, 1996), pp. 465–75. In general, see Stephan Fuchs and Steven Ward, "Deconstruction: Making Facts in Science, Building Cases in Law," *American Sociological Review* 59:4 (August 1994): 481–500.

12. See Fred Inglis, *Media Theory: An Introduction* (Cambridge, Mass.: Basil Blackwell, 1990), pp. 74–91; and Norman K. Denzin, *Symbolic Interaction and Cultural Studies: The Politics of Interpretation* (Oxford, U.K.: Blackwell, 1992).

13. Kevin Brownlow, *Behind the Mask of Innocence—Sex, Violence, Prejudice, Crime: Films of Social Conscience in the Silent Era* (New York: Alfred A. Knopf, 1990).

14. Tom Conley, *Film Hieroglyphs: Ruptures in Classical Cinema* (Minneapolis: University of Minnesota Press, 1991).

15. Lee Lourdeaux, *Italian and Irish Filmmakers in America* (Philadelphia: Temple University Press, 1990).

16. J. Hoberman, *Bridge of Light: Yiddish Film between Two Worlds* (New York: Museum of Modern Art and Schocken Books, 1991).

17. See Neal Gabler, *An Empire of Their Own: How the Jews Invented Hollywood* (New York: Crown Publishers, 1988); and Andrew R. Heinze, *Adapting to Abundance: Jewish Immigrants, Mass Consumption, and the Search for American Identity* (New York: Columbia University Press, 1990), pp. 203–18.

18. See Ellen Schiff, *From Stereotype to Metaphor: The Jew in Contemporary Drama* (Albany: State University of New York Press, 1982); Lester D. Friedman, *Hollywood's Image of the Jew* (New York: Frederick Ungar Publishing Co., 1982); Sarah Blacher Cohen, ed., *From Hester Street to Hollywood: The Jewish-American Stage and Screen* (Bloomington: Indiana University Press, 1983); Patricia Erens, *The Jew in American Cinema* (Bloomington: Indiana University Press, 1984); and David Desser, "The Cinematic Melting Pot: Ethnicity, Jews, and Psychoanalysis," in *Unspeakable Images: Ethnicity and the American Cinema,* ed. Lester D. Friedman (Urbana: University of Illinois Press, 1991), pp. 379–403.

19. See the text as well as the bibliography in Stanford M. Lyman, "Race, Sex, and

Servitude: Images of Blacks in American Cinema," *International Journal of Politics, Culture and Society* 4:1 (fall 1990): 49–77.

20. See Kobena Mercer, *Welcome to the Jungle: New Positions in Black Cultural Studies* (New York: Routledge, 1994), pp. 53–68; and Michael Banton, "Type-casting," *Times Literary Supplement*, January 9, 1976, p. 29.

21. Parker Tyler, *Screening the Sexes: Homosexuality in the Movies* (New York: DaCapo Press, 1993. Original publication, 1972).

22. Vito Russo, *The Celluloid Closet: Homosexuality in the Movies*, rev. ed. (New York: Harper and Row, 1987). See three works by Richard Dyer: ed., *Gays and Film* (London: British Film Institute, 1977); *Heavenly Bodies: Film Stars and Society* (New York: St. Martin's Press, 1986), pp. 141–94; and *The Matter of Images: Essays on Representation* (London: Routledge, 1993).

23. See three essays by Stanford M. Lyman, "From Matrimony to Malaise: Men and Women in the American Film, 1930–1980," *International Journal of Politics, Culture, and Society* 1:2 (winter 1987): 73–100; "Anhedonia: Gender and the Decline in Emotions in American Film, 1930–1988," *Sociological Inquiry* 60:1 (February 1990): 1–19; "The Road to Anhedonia: Patterns of Emotional Control in American Films, 1930–1988," *Social Perspectives on Emotion*, vol. 1, ed. David D. Franks and Viktor Gekas (Greenwich, Conn.: JAI Press, 1992), pp. 161–87, and the bibliographies contained therein.

24. See Noël Carroll, *The Philosophy of Horror or Paradoxes of the Heart* (New York: Routledge, 1990); Cecil Helman, *The Body of Frankenstein's Monster: Essays in Myth and Medicine* (New York: W. W. Norton, 1991); Manuela Dunn Mascetti, *Vampire: The Complete Guide to the World of the Undead* (New York: Viking Studio Books, 1992); Michael Sevastakis, *Songs of Love and Death: The Classical American Horror Film of the 1930s* (Westport, Conn.: Greenwood Press, 1993); Ken Gelder, *Reading the Vampire* (London: Routledge, 1994); and Nina Auerbach, *Our Vampires, Ourselves* (Chicago: University of Chicago Press, 1995).

25. J. P. Telotte, *Voices in the Dark: The Narrative Pattern of Film Noir* (Urbana: University of Illinois Press, 1989).

26. J. P. Telotte, *Dreams of Darkness: Fantasy and the Films of Val Lewton* (Urbana: University of Illinois Press, 1985).

27. J. P. Telotte, *Replications: A Robotic History of the Science Fiction Film* (Urbana: University of Illinois Press, 1995). See also Annette Kuhn, ed., *Alien Zone: Cultural Theory and Contemporary Science Fiction* (London: Verso, 1990).

28. Lary May, *Screening Out the Past: The Birth of Mass Culture and the Motion Picture Industry* (New York: Oxford University Press, 1980).

29. Alvah Bessie, *Inquisition in Eden* (New York: Macmillan, 1965); quoted in Eric Bentley, ed., *Thirty Years of Treason: Excerpts from Hearings before the House Committee on Un-American Activities, 1938–1968* (New York: Viking Press, 1971), p. xix. For a thoroughgoing history and analysis, see Larry Ceplair and Steven Englund, *The Inquisition in Hollywood: Politics in the Film Community* (Berkeley: University of California Press, 1983). See also Victor S. Navasky, *Naming Names* (New York: Viking Press, 1980).

30. Andrew Sarris, *Politics and Cinema* (New York: Columbia University Press, 1978), p. 15.

31. Jerry Christensen, *Reel Politics: American Political Movies from Birth of a Nation to Platoon* (New York: Basil Blackwell, 1987), p. 66.

32. Ibid., p. 68.

33. Ibid., p. 211.

34. Norman K. Denzin, *The Cinematic Society: The Voyeur's Gaze* (London: Sage Publications, 1995), pp. 165–67.

35. Weber observed [in "Science as a Vocation," in *From Max Weber: Essays in Sociology,* trans. and ed., by Hans H. Gerth and C. Wright Mills (New York: Oxford University Pres, 1946), pp. 145, 147]: "[P]olitics is out of place in the lecture-room . . . When speaking in a political meeting about democracy, one does not hide one's personal standpoint; indeed, to come out clearly and take a stand is one's damned duty. The words one uses in such a meeting are not means of scientific analysis but means of canvassing votes and winning over others. They are not plowshares to loosen the soil of contemplative thought; they are swords against the enemies; such words are weapons. It would be an outrage, however, to use words in this fashion in a lecture or in the lecture-room . . . The primary task of a useful teacher is to teach his students to recognize 'inconvenient' facts." In "Politics as a Vocation" (Ibid. p. 121), Weber pointed out: "No ethics in the world can dodge the fact that in numerous instances [for] the attainment of 'good' ends . . . one must be willing to pay the price of using morally dubious means or at least dangerous ones—and facing the possibility or even the probability of evil ramifications . . . The decisive means for politics is violence."

36. C. Wright Mills, *The Sociological Imagination* (New York: Oxford University Press, 1959), p. 226.

37. Cf. Robert Jewett and John Shelton Lawrence, *The American Monomyth* (Garden City, N.Y.: Doubleday, Anchor, 1977).

38. Denzin, *The Cinematic Society,* op. cit., p. 166.

39. Loc. cit.

40. Loc. cit.

41. Loc. cit.

42. Ibid., p. 167.

43. Ibid., p. 188.

44. See Jack Shadoian, *Dreams and Dead Ends: The American Gangster/Crime Film* (Cambridge, Mass.: MIT Press, 1977), pp. 174–90.

45. Ralph Willetts, "The Nation in Crisis: Hollywood's Response to the 1940's," in *Cinema, Politics and Society in America,* ed. Philip Davies and Brian Neve (New York: St. Martin's Press, 1981), pp. 59–75. Quotation from p. 74.

46. Inez Hedges, *Breaking the Frame: Film Language and the Experience of Limits* (Bloomington: Indiana University Press, 1991), pp. 142–43.

47. See Stephen Prince, *The Warrior's Camera: The Cinema of Akira Kurosawa* (Princeton, N.J.: Princeton University Press, 1991), pp. 127–42 et passim.

48. See, however, Geoffrey O'Brien, *The Phantom Empire* (New York: W. W.

Norton, 1993); and Robert Sklar, *Film: An International History of the Medium* (New York: Harry N. Abrams, Publishers, 1993).

49. See Barry Keith Grant, ed., *Film Genre Reader* (Austin: University of Texas Press, 1986).

50. See Albert Bermel, *Farce: A History from Aristophanes to Woody Allen* (Carbondale: Southern Illinois University Press, 1990), pp. 137–235, 362–417; and Elizabeth Kendall, *The Runaway Bride: Hollywood Romantic Comedies of the 1930s* (New York: Alfred A. Knopf, 1990).

51. See Gerald Mast, *Can't Help Singing: The American Musical on Stage and Screen* (Woodstock, N.Y.: Overlook Press, 1987).

52. See Jenny Calder, *There Must Be a Lone Ranger: The American West in Film and in Reality* (New York: Taplinger, 1975); John G. Cawelti, *The Six-Gun Mystique* (Bowling Green, Ohio: Bowling Green University Popular Press, n.d.); Christopher Frayling, *Spaghetti Westerns: Cowboys and Europeans from Karl May to Sergio Leone* (London: Routledge, 1981); George N. Fenin and William K. Everson, *The Western: From Silents to the Seventies* (New York: Penguin, 1977); Jack Nachbar, ed., *Focus on the Western* (Englewood Cliffs, N.J.: Prentice-Hall, 1974); and Rita Parks, *The Western Hero in Film and Television: Mass Media Mythology* (Ann Arbor: UMI Research Press, 1982).

53. See John Gabree, *Gangsters: From Little Caesar to the Godfather* (New York: Pyramid Publications, 1973); Carlos Clarens, *Crime Movies: An Illustrated History* (New York: W. W. Norton, 1980); and Rupert Wilkinson, *American Tough: The Tough Guy Tradition and American Character* (New York: Harper and Row, 1986). Studies of actors who became identified with the gangsters, detectives, rebels, misfits, or outcasts include: Robert Sklar, *City Boys: Cagney, Bogart, Garfield* (Princeton, N.J.: Princeton University Press, 1992); and Graham McCann, *Rebel Males: Clift, Brando, Dean* (New Brunswick, N.J.: Rutgers University Press, 1993). By far the most incisive of such analyses is Jack Shadoian, *Dreams and Dead Ends: the American Gangster/Crime Film* (Cambridge, Mass.: MIT Press, 1977). See also John McCarty, *Hollywood Gangland: The Movies' Love Affair with the Mob* (New York: St. Martin's Press, 1993).

54. See Alain Silver and Elizabeth Ward, eds., *Film Noir: An Encyclopedic Reference to the American Style* (Woodstock, N.Y.: Overlook Press, 1979); and Bruce Crowther, *Film Noir: Reflections in a Dark Mirror* (New York: Continuum, 1989).

55. See G. William Jones, *Black Cinema Treasures: Lost and Found* (Denton: University of North Texas Press, 1991); four works by Thomas Cripps, *Slow Fade to Black: The Negro in American Film, 1900–1942* (New York: Oxford University Press, 1977); *Black Film as Genre* (Bloomington: Indiana University Press, 1978); "The Dark Spot in the Kaleidoscope: Black Images in American Film," in *The Kaleidoscopic Lens: How Hollywood Views Ethnic Groups,* ed. Randall M. Miller (Englewood, N.J.: Jerome S. Ozer, Publisher, 1980), pp. 15–35; and *Making Movies Black: The Hollywood Message Movie from World War II to the Civil Rights Era* (New York: Oxford University Press, 1993); Norman K. Denzin, *Images of Postmodern Society: Social Theory and Contemporary Cinema* (London: Sage, 1991), pp. 125–36; two works by Donald Bogle,

Toms, Coons, Mulattoes, Mammies, and Bucks: An Interpretive History of Blacks in American Films (New York: Viking Press, 1973; expanded ed., New York: Continuum, 1989); and *Blacks in American Films and Television: An Illustrated Encyclopedia* (London: Simon and Schuster, Fireside, 1988). See also Peter Noble, *The Negro in Films* (London: Skelton Robinson, 1948; reissued Port Washington, N.Y.: Kennikat Press, 1969); Edward Mapp, *Blacks in American Films: Today and Yesterday* (Metuchen, N.J.: Scarecrow Press, 1972); Gary Null, *Black Hollywood: The Negro in Motion Pictures* (Secaucus, N.J.: Citadel Press, 1975, 1980); Lindsay Patterson, ed., *Black Films and Film-Makers: A Comprehensive Anthology from Stereotype to Superhero* (New York: Dodd, Mead and Co., 1975); Daniel J. Leab, *From Sambo to Superspade: The Black Experience in Motion Pictures* (Boston: Houghton Mifflin Co., 1975); James Murray, *To Find an Image: Black Films from Uncle Tom to Superfly* (Indianapolis, Ind.: Bobbs-Merrill, 1973); James R. Nesteby, *Black Images in American Films, 1896–1954* (Washington, D.C.: University Press of America, 1982); Allen L. Woll and Randall M. Miller, "Afro-Americans," *Ethnic and Racial Images in American Film and Television: Historical Essays and Bibliography* (New York: Garland Publishing Co., 1987), pp. 39–178; Mbye B. Cham and Claire Andrade-Watkins, eds., *Blackframes: Critical Perspectives on Black Independent Cinema* (Cambridge, Mass.: MIT Press, 1988); Ed Guerrero, *Framing Blackness: The African American Image in Film* (Philadelphia: Temple University Press, 1993); and Manthia Diawara, ed., *Black American Cinema* (New York: Routledge, 1993). For a controversial study of the impact that the Jewish immigrants had on "blackface" imagery, see Michael Rogin, *Blackface, White Noise: Jewish Immigrants in the Hollywood Melting Pot* (Berkeley: University of California Press, 1996). See also Teshome H. Gabriel, "Thoughts on Nomadic Aesthetics and Black Independent Cinema: Traces of a Journey," in *Out There: Marginalization and Contemporary Cultures,* ed. Russell Ferguson, Martha Gever, Trinh T. Minh-ha, and Cornel West (Cambridge, Mass.: MIT Press, 1990), pp. 395–410.

56. See Dorothy Jones, *The Portrayal of China and India on the American Screen, 1896–1955* (Cambridge, Mass.: Center for International Studies, October 1955); Harold R. Isaacs, *Images of Asia: American Views of China and India* (New York: Capricorn Books, 1962), passim; William K. Everson, *The Detective in Film* (Secaucus, N.J.: Citadel Press, 1972), pp. 72–85; Jon Tuska, *The Detective in Hollywood* (Garden City, N.Y.: Doubleday, 1978), pp. 105–58; Eugene Franklin Wong, *On Visual Media Racism: Asians in the American Motion Pictures* (New York: Arno Press, 1978); Richard Oehling, "The Yellow Menace: Asian Images in American Film," in Randall M. Miller, ed., op. cit., pp. 182–206; Woll and Miller, op. cit., pp. 189–201; Gina Marchetti, *Romance and the Yellow Peril: Race, Sex, and Discursive Strategies in Hollywood Fiction* (Berkeley : University of California Press, 1993); James S. Moy, *Marginal Sights: Staging the Chinese in America* (Iowa City: University of Iowa Press, 1993); and two works by Darrell Y. Hamamoto, *Nervous Laughter: Television Situation Comedy and Liberal Democratic Ideology* (New York: Praeger, 1989), pp. 95–97, 146–47; and *Monitored Peril: Asian Americans and the Politics of TV Representation* (Minneapolis: University of Minnesota Press, 1994); Norman K. Denzin, "Chan Is Missing: The Asian Eye Examines Cultural

Studies," *Symbolic Interaction* 17:1 (spring 1994): 63–89. See also Robert C. Schmitt, *Hawaii in the Movies, 1898–1959* (Honolulu: Hawaiian Historical Society, 1988). For biographical information on one of Hollywood's most famous film stars, see Sessue Hayakawa, *Zen Showed Me the Way,* ed. Croswell Bowen (Indianapolis, Ind.: Bobbs-Merrill, 1960), and Paul L. Montgomery, "Sessue Hayakawa Is Dead at 83: Silents Star Was in 'River Kwai': Japanese Aristocrat Acted in More Than 120 Movies—Nominated for '57 Oscar," *New York Times,* November 25, 1973, p. 83b. For a haunting biographical sketch of Anna May Wong (Wong Liu Tsong, 1907–1961), a tragic victim of Hollywood stereotypy, see Lisa See, *On Gold Mountain* (New York: St. Martin's Press, 1995), pp. 225–30.

57. See Allen Woll, "Bandits and Lovers: Hispanic Images in American Films," in Randall M. Miller, ed., op. cit., pp. 54–72; Woll and Miller, op. cit., pp. 243–59; and George Hadley-Garcia, *Hispanic Hollywood: The Latins in Motion Pictures* (Secaucus, N.J.: Citadel-Carol Publishing Co., 1990); and Martha Gil-Montero, *Brazilian Bombshell: The Biography of Carmen Miranda* (New York: Donald I. Fine, 1989). See also Carl J. Mora, *Mexican Cinema: Reflections of a Society, 1896–1980* (Berkeley: University of California Press, 1982), pp. 22–24, 33–34, 80–88, 135–37.

58. See Gretchen Bataille and Charles Silet, "The Entertaining Anachronism: Indians in American Film," in Randall M. Miller, ed., op. cit., pp. 36–53; Woll and Miller, op. cit., pp. 327–41; Ralph and Natasha Friar, *The Only Good Indian: The Hollywood Gospel* (New York: Drama Book Specialists/Publishers, 1972); Robert F. Berkhofer Jr., *The White Man's Indian: Images of the American Indian from Columbus to the Present* (New York: Alfred A. Knopf, 1978), pp. 71–112; Raymond William Stedman, *Shadows of the Indian: Stereotypes in American Culture* (Norman: University of Oklahoma Press, 1982); Edward Countryman, "John Ford's "Drums along the Mohawk: The Making of an American Myth," in *Presenting the Past: Essays on History and the Public,* ed. Susan Porter Benson, Stephen Brier, and Roy Rosenzweig (Philadelphia: Temple University Press, 1986), pp. 87–102; and the several essays on the cinematic and televised imagery of Native Americans in S. Elizabeth Bird, ed., *Dressing in Feathers: The Construction of the Indian in American Popular Culture* (Boulder, Colo.: Westview Press, 1996), pp. 79–95, 195–279.

59. See Barbara Deming, *Running Away from Myself: A Dream Portrait of America Drawn from the Films of the Forties* (New York: Grossman, 1969); Joan Mellen, *Women and Their Sexuality in the New Film* (New York: Dell-Laurel, 1973); Marjorie Rosen, *Popcorn Venus* (New York: Avon, 1973); Norman Zierold, *Sex Goddesses of the Silent Screen* (Chicago: Henry Regnery, 1973); Kathryn Kay and Gerald Peary, eds., *Women and the Cinema: A Critical Anthology* (New York: E. P. Dutton, 1977); Brandon French, *On the Verge of Revolt: Women in American Films of the Fifties* (New York: Frederick Ungar, 1978); Sumiko Higashi, *Virgins, Vamps and Flappers: The American Silent Movie Heroine* (Montreal: Eden Press Women's Publications, 1978); two works by E. Ann Kaplan, ed., *Women in Film Noir* (London: British Film Institute, 1978, 1980); and *Women and Film: Both Sides of the Camera* (New York: Methuen, 1983); Annette Kuhn, *Women's Pictures: Feminism and Cinema* (London: Routledge and Kegan Paul, 1982);

Rosalind Coward, *Female Desires: How They Are Sought, Bought and Packaged* (New York: Grove Press, 1985); two works by Mary Ann Doane, *The Desire to Desire, The Woman's Film of the 1940s* (Bloomington: Indiana University Press, 1987); and *Femmes Fatales: Feminism, Film Theory and Psychoanalysis* (New York: Routledge, 1991); Molly Haskell, *From Reverence to Rape: The Treatment of Women in the Movies* (Baltimore: Penguin Books, 1974; 2d ed., Chicago: University of Chicago Press, 1987); Christine Gledhil, ed., *Home Is Where the Heart Is: Studies in Melodrama and the Woman's Film* (London: British Film Institute, 1987); four works by Norman K. Denzin, *Hollywood Shot by Shot: Alcoholism in American Cinema* (New York: Aldine de Gruyter, 1991); *Images of Postmodern Society,* op. cit., pp. 107–24; *The Cine-Matic Society,* op. cit., pp. 139–89; "Women at the Keyhole: Fatal Female Visions," *Symbolic Interaction* 18:2 (summer 1995): 165–90; S. Paige Baty, *American Monroe: The Making of a Body Politic* (Berkeley: University of California Press, 1995). See also Andrea Fontana and Stanford M. Lyman, "Norma Jeane and Jimmy Deane: Nostalgic Signifiers of the Postmodern Era," in *Studies in Symbolic Interaction,* vol. 18., ed. Norman K. Denzin (Greenwich, Conn.: JAI Press, 1995), pp. 157–70.

60. Yvonne Tasker, *Spectacular Bodies: Gender, Genre and the Action Cinema* (London: Routledge, 1993); Pat Kirkham and Janet Thumim, eds., *You Tarzan: Masculinity, Movies and Men* (New York: St. Martin's Press, 1993); and Joan Mellen, *Big Bad Wolves: Masculinity in the American Film* (New York: Pantheon, 1977).

61. See, for example, three studies devoted to the imagery of American adolescents in the 1950s: David M. Considine, *The Cinema of Adolescence* (Jefferson, N.C.: McFarland, 1985); James Gilbert, *A Cycle of Outrage: America's Reaction to the Juvenile Delinquent in the 1950s* (New York: Oxford University Press, 1986); and Thomas Doherty, *Teenagers and Teenpics: The Juvenilization of American Movies in the 1950s* (Boston: Unwin Hyman, 1988).

62. See, e.g., Leonard Quart and Albert Auster, *American Film and Society since 1945* (New York: Praeger, 1984); Paul Monaco, *Ribbons in Time: Movies and Society since 1945* (Bloomington: Indiana University Press, 1987); Andrew Dowdy, *The Films of the Fifties: The American State of Mind* (New York: William Morrow, 1973, 1975); Peter Biskind, *Seeing Is Believing: How Hollywood Taught Us to Stop Worrying and Love the Fifties* (New York: Pantheon, 1983); David E. James, *Allegories of Cinema: American Film in the Sixties* (Princeton, N.J.: Princeton University Press, 1989); and Seth Cagin and Philip Dray, *Hollywood Films of the Seventies: Sex, Drugs, Violence, Rock 'n' Roll and Politics* (New York: Harper and Row, 1984); Douglas Brode, *The Films of the Eighties* (New York: Citadel Press, 1990).

63. Carlos Clarens, *An Illustrated History of the Horror Film* (New York: G. P. Putnam's Sons, 1967); Peter Haining, ed., *The Ghouls* (London: W. H. Allen, 1971); Edward Edelson, *Great Monsters of the Movies* (Garden City, N.Y.: Doubleday, 1973); David Pirie, *A Heritage of Horror: The English Gothic Cinema, 1946–1972* (New York: Avon, 1973); Leslie Halliwell, *The Dead That Walk: Dracula, Frankenstein, The Mummy, and Other Favorite Movie Monsters* (New York: Continuum, 1988); Vera Dika, *Games of Terror: Halloween, Friday the 13th, and the Films of the Stalker Cycle* (Cranbury, N.J.:

Associated University Presses, 1990); Walter Kendrick, *The Thrill of Fear: 250 Years of Scary Entertainment* (New York: Grove Weidenfeld, 1991), pp. xviii–xxii, 74, 153, 163, 199, 206–60; four works by James B. Twitchell: *Dreadful Pleasures: An Anatomy of Modern Horror* (New York: Oxford University Press, 1985); *Preposterous Violence: Fables of Aggression in Modern Culture* (New York: Oxford University Press, 1989); *The Living Dead: A Study of the Vampire in Romantic Literature* (Durham, N.C.: Duke University Press, 1981); and *Carnival Culture: The Trashing of Taste in America* (New York: Columbia University Press, 1992); and three volumes by David J. Skal: *Hollywood Gothic: The Tangled Web of Dracula from Novel to Stage to Screen* (New York: W. W. Norton, 1990); *The Monster Show: A Cultural History of Horror* (New York: W. W. Norton, 1993); and, with Elias Savada, *Dark Carnival: The Secret World of Tod Browning, Hollywood's Master of the Macabre* (New York: Anchor Books, 1995). See also Peter Underwood, *Karloff: The Life of Boris Karloff—with an Appendix of the films in which he appeared* (New York: Drake Publishers, 1972); and R. H. W. Dillard, "Even a Man Who Is Pure at Heart: Poetry and Danger in the Horror Film," in *Man and the Movies,* ed. W. R. Robinson with assistance of George Garrett (Baton Rouge: Louisiana State University Press, 1967), pp. 60–96.

64. Emanuel Levy, *Small-Town America in Film: The Decline and Fall of Community* (New York: Continuum, 1991). In a certain sense, Levy's analysis has done for Hollywood's rural romance what Arthur J. Vidich and Joseph Bensman did for American sociology's *Gemeinschaft* mystique in their *Small Town in Mass Society: Class, Power and Religion in a Rural Community,* 2d ed. (Princeton, N.J.: Princeton University Press, 1968). See also Arthur J. Vidich and Stanford M. Lyman, "Qualitative Methods: Their History in Sociology and Anthropology," in *Handbook of Qualitative Research,* ed. Norman K. Denzin and Yvonna S. Lincoln (Thousand Oaks, Calif.: Sage Publications, 1994), pp. 23–59, esp. pp. 31–35.

65. Lawrence H. Suid, *Guts and Glory: Great American War Movies* (Reading, Mass.: Addison-Wesley, 1978).

66. Joe Morella, Edward Z. Epstein, and John Griggs, *The Films of World War II* (Secaucus, N.J.: Citadel Press, 1975); Jeanine Basinger, *The World War II Combat Film: Anatomy of a Genre* (New York: Columbia University Press, 1986); Thomas Doherty, *Projections of War: Hollywood, American Culture, and World War II* (New York: Columbia University Press, 1993); Clayton R. Koppes and Gregory D. Black, *Hollywood Goes to War: How Politics, Profits, and Propaganda Shaped World War II Movies* (New York: Free Press, 1987); Roy Hoopes, *When the Stars Went to War: Hollywood and World War II* (New York: Random House, 1994); Michael Renov, *Hollywood's Wartime Woman: Representation and Ideology* (Ann Arbor, Mich.: UMI Research Press, 1988); Antonia Lant, *Blackout: Reinventing Women for Wartime British Cinema* (Princeton, N.J.: Princeton University Press, 1991).

67. Michael Rogin, *Ronald Reagan, the Movie and Other Episodes in Political Demonology* (Berkeley: University of California Press, 1987); and Stephen Vaughn, *Ronald Reagan in Hollywood: Movies and Politics* (New York: Cambridge University Press, 1994).

68. Steve Vineberg, *No Surprises, Please: Movies in the Reagan Decade* (New York: Schirmer Books, Macmillan, 1993).

69. See Edward Wagenknecht, *The Movies in the Age of Innocence* (New York: Ballantine, 1971); Lewis Jacobs, *The Rise of the American Film: A Critical History with an Essay, Experimental Cinema in America, 1921–1947* (New York: Teachers College Press,1968); Kevin Brownlow, *The Parade's Gone By . . .* (New York: Ballantine Books, 1968); Charles Musser, *The Emergence of Cinema: The American Screen to 1907* (New York: Charles Scribner's Sons,1990); Eileen Bowser, *The Transformation of Cinema: 1907–1915* (New York: Charles Scribner's Sons, 1990); Richard Koszarski, *An Evening's Entertainment: The Age of the Silent Feature Picture, 1915–1928* (New York: Charles Scribner's Sons, 1990); and Tino Balio, *Grand Design: Hollywood as a Modern Business Enterprise, 1930–1939* (New York: Charles Scribner's Sons, 1993); Ted Sennett, *Hollywood's Golden Year, 1939: A Fiftieth Anniversary Celebration* (New York: St. Martin's Press, 1989); and Gerald Mast, *A Short History of the Movies,* 5th ed., rev. by Bruce F. Kawin (New York: Macmillan, 1992); Charles Champlin, *The Movies Grow Up, 1940–1980* (Chicago: Swallow Press, 1977, 1981). See also Thomas Schatz, *The Genius of the System: Hollywood Filmmaking in the Studio Era* (New York: Henry Holt-Metro, 1988, 1996); and Norman Ziebold, *The Moguls: Hollywood's Merchants of Myth* (Los Angeles: Selman-James Press, 1969, 1991).

70. Gerald Mast, *A Short History of the Movies,* 4th ed. (New York: Macmillan, 1986), p. 492.

71. See, e.g., Stuart Hall, "Notes on Deconstructing 'the Popular,'" in *Cultural Theory and Popular Culture: A Reader,* ed. John Storey (New York: Harvester, Wheatsheaf, 1994), pp. 455–66.

72. Richard Hofstadter, *The Paranoid Style in American Politics and Other Essays* (New York: Alfred A. Knopf, 1965), pp. 3–141.

73. Biskind, op. cit., pp. 101–245; and Michael Paul Rogin, "Kiss Me Deadly: Communism, Motherhood, and Cold War Movies," in *Invasion of the Body Snatchers: Don Siegel, Director,* ed. Al LaValley (New Brunswick, N.J.: Rutgers University Press, 1989), pp. 201–5.

74. See Nora Sayre, *Running Time: Films of the Cold War* (New York: Dial, 1982); and Lary May, "Movie Star Politics: The Screen Actors Guild, Cultural Conversion, and the Hollywood Red Scare," in *Recasting America: Culture and Politics in the Age of the Cold War,* ed. Lary May (Chicago: University of Chicago Press, 1989), pp. 125–53.

75. Michael Barson, *"Better Dead Than Red!"—A Nostalgic Look at the Golden Years of Russiaphobia, Red-baiting, and Other Commie Madness* (New York: Hyperion, 1992).

76. See two works by Hortense Powdermaker: *Hollywood: The Dream Factory* (Boston: Little, Brown and Co., 1950); and *Stranger and Friend: The Way of an Anthropologist* (New York: W. W. Norton, 1966), pp. 209–31.

77. Geoffrey Hill, *Illuminating Shadows: The Mythic Power of Film* (Boston: Shambhala Publications, 1992), pp. 297–306. Quotation from p. 306.

78. The following draws on Arthur Kroker and Michael A. Weinstein, *Data Trash: The Theory of the Virtual Class* (New York: St. Martin's Press, 1994).

79. Ibid., pp. 156–57.

80. Peter Roffman and Jim Purdy, *The Hollywood Social Problem Film: Madness, Despair, and Politics from the Depression to the Fifties* (Bloomington: Indiana University Press, 1981).

81. Angela McRobbie, *Postmodernism and Popular Culture* (London: Routledge, 1994), pp. 198–219.

82. Denzin, *Symbolic Interaction and Cultural Studies: The Politics of Interpretation,* op. cit., p. 168.

83. Loc. cit.

84. Keyan Tomaselli, *The Cinema of Apartheid: Race and Class in South African Film* (New York: Smyrna Press, 1988), p. 71.

85. Keyan Tomaselli, Alan Williams, Lynette Steenveld, and Ruth Tomaselli, *Myth, Race and Power: South Africans Imaged on Film and TV* (Bellville: South Africa: Anthropos Publishers, 1986), p. 105.

86. Ella Shohat, *Israeli Cinema: East/West and the Politics of Representation* (Austin: University of Texas Press, 1989), p. 272.

87. Ibid., p. 245.

88. Ibid., p. 273.

89. Joseph L. Anderson and Donald Richie, *The Japanese Film: Art and Industry,* expanded ed. (Princeton, N.J.: Princeton University Press, 1982), p. 129.

90. See David Stewart Hull, *Film in the Third Reich: A Study of the German Cinema* (Berkeley: University of California Press, 1969), pp. 10–41.

91. Anderson and Richie, op. cit., p. 129.

92. It is worth noting that Sessue Hayakawa (1890–1973)— whose silent films, especially *The Cheat* (1915), were not popular in Japan—made one Franco-Japanese-German film, *Die Tochter des Samurai* (*The Daughter of the Samurai,* sometimes called *New Earth,* 1942?). According to David Stewart Hull, op. cit., p. 121: "Arnold Fanck was selected as director . . . Fanck's idea of Japan had little in common with reality, but to the amazement of the Japanese advisors and crew, he insisted on filming the story exactly as it had been scripted in Berlin. The result was a movie which rather resembled a mixture of *Madame Butterfly* and shop-worn Nazi clichés of self-sacrifice for the cause. Viewed today, the picture is of interest only for the performance of Sessue Hayakawa and some beautiful scenery. The film was a great success in Berlin but the Japanese found it mystifying and ridiculous." Perhaps, understandably, Hayakawa, op. cit., pp. 189–212, made no mention of this film in his account of his sojourn in France, 1937–1948. As an alien ineligible because of his race for United States citizenship, but also an opponent of Japan's militaristic adventurism in Asia and the Pacific and in self-exile from Hollywood's racism and ill treatment—he had resided in the United States since 1909—Hayakawa lived a truly marginal life. His great acting skills were eventually put to use on screen in *The Bridge on the River Kwai* (1957). For two sensitive analyses of his early career in silent films, see Kevin Brownlow, *Behind the Mask of Innocence,* op. cit., pp. 346–52, and Sklar, op. cit., pp. 85–87, 92, 109. The miscegenationist racism that typified Hayakawa's early career was noticed by Deems Taylor,

Marcelene Peterson and Bryant Hale, *A Pictorial History of the Movies* (New York: Simon and Schuster, 1943), p. 85: "Sessue Hayakawa became the only Oriental actor ever to play romantic leads in American pictures. Because of racial prejudices, however, he always had to relinquish the girl in the final reel." For a feminist reading of his role in *The Cheat,* see Sumiko Higashi, "Ethnicity, Class and Gender in Films: DeMille's *The Cheat,"* in *Unspeakable Images: Ethnicity ad the American Cinema,* ed. Lester D. Friedman (Urbana: University of Illinois Press, 1991), pp. 112–39.

93. Donald Richie, *Japanese Cinema* (Garden City, N.Y.: Doubleday, Anchor, 1971). pp. 56–57.

94. For the debate, see two works by Joan Mellen, *Voices from the Japanese Cinema* (New York: Liveright, 1975), pp. 8, 73, 109–10n, 131, 138, 149, 208, 228; and *The Waves at Genji's Door: Japan through Its Cinema* (New York: Pantheon Books, 1976), pp. 106, 122, 165–73, 219–31, 330, 350, 357, 397, 405, 435; Tadao Sato, *Currents in Japanese Cinema: Essays,* trans. Gregory Barrett (Tokyo: Kodansha, 1982), pp. 46, 91–114, 133, 141–42 162, 214, 233–41, 256–58, 266; Anderson and Richie, op. cit., pp. 372–76 et passim; and Nagisa Oshima, *Cinema, Censorship, and the State: The Writings of Nagisa Oshima, 1956–1978,* trans. Dawn Lawson, ed. Annette Michelson (Cambridge, Mass.: MIT Press, 1992), pp. 21–22 n. 2.

95. Richie, op. cit., p. 57.

96. Ibid., p. 55.

97. Sato, op. cit., p. 102.

98. Ibid., pp. 57–58.

99. Ian Buruma, *The Wages of Guilt: Memories of War in Germany and Japan* (New York: Farrar, Straus, and Giroux, 1994), p. 176.

100. Loc. cit.

101. Oshima, op. cit., pp. 280–81.

102. Prince, op. cit., pp. 67–113.

103. David Bordwell, *Ozu and the Poetics of Cinema* (Princeton, N.J.: Princeton University Press, 1988), pp. 11–15, 129–31, 302–6.

104. Sato, op. cit., pp. 104–15.

105. See Alain Silver, *The Samurai Film* (Woodstock, N.Y.: Overlook Press, 1983).

106. Oshima, op. cit., pp. 8–9.

107. Ibid., esp. pp. 233–88.

108. Ibid., pp. 285–86.

109. Sandra A. Wawrytko, "The Murky Mirror: Women and Sexual Ethics as Reflected in Japanese Cinema," in *Japan in Traditional and Postmodern Perspectives,* ed. Charles Wei-hsun Fu and Steven Heine (Albany: State University of New York Press, 1995), pp. 121–68. Quotation from p. 121.

110. Ibid., pp. 161–62.

111. Ibid., p. 162.

112. Loc. cit.

113. Sato, op. cit., pp. 213–21.

114. Oshima, op. cit., p. 261; Sato, op. cit., pp. 245–46. The screenplay is based on an actual incident that occurred in Japan in 1936.

115. Oshima, op. cit., p. 285. See also Sato, pp. 17–27, 34–37, 201, 244–46.

116. Oshima, op. cit., pp. 247–48.

117. See, e.g., the critique of Kracauer in E. Ann Kaplan's essay entitled "Fritz Lang and German Expressionism: A Reading of *Dr. Mabuse, der Spieler*," in *Passion and Rebellion: The Expressionist Heritage,* ed. Stephen Eric Browner and Douglas Kellner (New York: Columbia University Press, 1983, 1988), pp. 398–408.

118. Siegfried Kracauer, *From Caligari to Hitler: A Psychological History of the German Film* (Princeton, N.J.: Princeton University Press, 1947, 1971), pp. 72–73.

119. See Mike Budd, ed., *The Cabinet of Dr. Caligari: Texts, Contexts, Histories* (New Brunswick, N.J.: Rutgers University Press, 1990); and S. S. Prawer, *Caligari's Children: The Film as Tale of Terror* (New York: Oxford University Press, 1980).

120. For the argument that American economic policy and Hollywood's studios had a profound effect on Weimar's films, see Thomas J. Saunders, *Hollywood in Berlin: American Cinema and Weimar Germany* (Berkeley: University of California Press, 1994), pp. 117–70, 221–50.

121. Kracauer, op. cit., pp. 43–202.

122. Hans Mommsen, *The Rise and Fall of Weimar Democracy,* trans. Elborg Forster and Larry Eugene Jones (Chapel Hill: University of North Carolina Press, 1996), pp. 68, 253–97, 314–15, 402–8, 458, 486, 519–42.

123. Klaus Kremeier, *The UFA Story: A History of Germany's Greatest Film Company, 1918–1945,* trans. Robert and Rita Kimber (New York: Hill and Wang, 1996), pp. 182–83.

124. Kremeier, op. cit., pp. 205–6.

125. Kracauer, op. cit., p. 74.

126. For the director's screenplay, see Lotte H. Eisner, *Murnau* (Berkeley: University of California Press, 1973), pp. 227–72. In the American movie *Batman Returns* (1992), Christopher Walken (b. 1943) essays the role of the principal villain, "Max Shreck," a corrupt businessman who seeks to wreck Gotham City's celebration of Christmas. Walken's "Shreck" could be a Jew. As Paul Moncao observes in *Cinema and Society: France and Germany during the Twenties* (New York: Elsevier Scientific Publishing Co., 1976), p. 134: "The foreigner as well as the 'foreign element,' of the Weimar popular cinema refers to the Jew . . . [The Transylvanian] Count who buys property in Bremen is really a vampire . . . According to anti-Semitic dogma, Jews were not quite what they passed themselves off to be . . . The Jew as an outsider posing as an insider is a stock notion in the pantheon of anti-Jewish sentiments." Walken's "Shreck" uses Yiddish slang—referring to himself as a "schmoe," the evil Penguin (Danny deVito) as a "Mensch," and a pet monkey as a "Schmuck"—and, insofar as this characterization might awaken antisemitic sentiments, this imagery was severely taken to task by two Columbia University graduate students. See Rebecca Roiphe and Daniel Cooper, "Batman and the Jewish Question," *New York Times,* July 2, 1992, p. A13. It should be noted that, while respected historical scholars, e.g., Joshua Trachtenberg (in *The Devil and the Jews: The Medieval Conception of the Jew and Its Relation to Modern Anti-Semitism* [Philadelphia: Jewish Publication Society of America, 1983], pp. 1–75) and R. Po-chia Hsia (in *The Myth of Ritual Murder: Jews and Magic in Reformation*

Germany [New Haven, Conn.: Yale University Press, 1988], pp. 62–64, 133, 213; and *Trent 1475: Stories of a Ritual Murder Trial* [New Haven, Conn.: Yale University Press, 1992]), have documented the demonization of the Jews in medieval European thought, such American analysts of vampire movies as David Pirie (in *The Vampire Cinema* [New York: Crescent Books, 1977], pp. 32–41) and Denis Gifford (in *A Pictorial History of Horror Movies* [London: Hamlyn Publishing Group, 1973], pp. 54–58) have not connected *Nosferatu* to anti-Semitism. Nor does Jan L. Perkowski make any mention of Jews or anti-Semitism in his otherwise comprehensive work, *The Darkling: A Treatise on Slavic Vampirism* (Columbus, Ohio: Slavica Publishers, 1989).

127. Quoted from the distribution flyer for *Dr. Mabuse der Spieler* in Lotte H. Eisner, *Fritz Lang*, trans. Gertrud Mander, ed. David Robinson (New York: Oxford University Press, 1977), p. 57.

128. Ibid., p. 129.

129. Frederick W. Ott, *The Great German Films: From before World War I to the Present* (Secaucus, N.J.: Citadel Press, 1986), p. 58.

130. Ibid., p. 59.

131. Ibid., pp. 58–60.

132. Fritz Schmalenbach, "The Term *Neue Sachlichkeit*," *The Art Bulletin* 22:3 (September 1940): 161, 164–65. Quoted in Kracauer, op. cit., p. 165.

133. Kracauer, op. cit., pp. 178–79; Ott, op. cit., pp. 88–91.

134. Barry Paris, *Louise Brooks* (New York: Doubleday, Anchor, 1989), p. 305.

135. Maria Tatar, *Lustmord: Sexual Murder in Weimar Germany* (Princeton, N.J.: Princeton University Press, 1995), p. 159.

136. Paul Monaco, *Cinema and Society*, op. cit., p. 125.

137. Loc. cit.

138. Loc. cit.

139. Loc. cit.

140. Loc. cit.

141. Loc. cit.

142. Kracauer, op. cit., pp. 88–91.

143. Ibid., pp. 31–33. Ott, op. cit., pp. 52–53.

144. Ott, op. cit., pp. 52–55.

145. Kracauer, op. cit., pp. 112–13.

146. Monaco, *Cinema and Society*, op. cit., pp. 52–53.

147. For analyses of the screenplay, see David Welch, *Propaganda and the German Cinema 1933–1945* (Oxford, U.K.: Clarendon Press, 1983, 1985), pp. 284–92; and Hull, op. cit., pp. 160–74.

148. Welch, op. cit., p. 291.

149. Hull, op. cit., pp. 171–72, 269; Kreimeier, op. cit., pp. 296–97; Sklar, op. cit., p. 274.

150. Veidt is reported to have said, "No matter what roles I play, I can't get Caligari out of my mind." Quoted in Leslie Halliwell, *Halliwell's Filmgoer's Companion*, 8th ed. (New York: Charles Scribner's Sons, 1985), p. 1037. More to the point is Herman G.

Weinberg's lament: "Why is it that the infamous distortion of Feuctwanger's *Jew Süss* by Veit Harlan survives and that honest and powerful filming of it by Lothar Mendes (with Conrad Veidt in the title role) has not survived?" Herman G. Weinberg's "Coffee, Brandy and Cigars (autumn 1965)" *Saint Cinema,* op. cit., p. 244.

151. Kracauer, op. cit., pp. 84–87, 89, 272; Ott, op. cit., pp. 61–62.

152. Monaco, *Cinema and Society,* op. cit., p. 119, 123, 131, 134, 137, 142–48; Kracauer, op. cit., p. 153.

153. Jeff Siegel, *The Casablanca Companion: The Movie and More* (Dallas: Taylor Publishing Co., 1992), p. 57.

154. But Hull, op. cit., p. 161, disagrees: "[Jew Süss] was filmed in England in 1932 by the Jewish director Lothar Mendes and a large cast including Conrad Veidt and Frank Vosper. The film followed [Lion] Feuchtwanger's novel with some fidelity, and Veidt played the title role of Josef Süss Oppenheimer with satanic brilliance. Indeed, with a little editing, the British movie could have been released in Germany as Goebbels' desired project, and he toyed with the idea; he had the film screened many times."

155. Siegel, op. cit., pp. 56–57.

156. Ibid., pp. 15–16, 52–56, 61, 124.

157. Ibid., p. 109.

158. Prawer, op. cit., pp. 61–62.

159. Kremeier, op. cit., pp. 255–302.

160. Hull, op. cit., pp. 42–43; Ott, op. cit., p. 139.

161. *New York Times,* February 17, 1934, p. 3. Quoted in Hull, op. cit., p. 44.

162. Hull, op. cit., p. vii.

163. See Evelyn Ehrlich, *Cinema of Paradox: French Filmmaking under the German Occupation* (New York: Columbia University Press, 1985), pp. 1–12, 189–92.

164. Ibid., pp. 57–70.

165. Ibid., pp. 93–134.

166. Ibid., p. 137.

167. Ibid., pp. 13–38, 135–88. For example, Sessue Hayakawa, op. cit., p. 202, would later recall that *Macao, L'Enfer Du Jeu* (*Macao, The Gambling Hell,* 1939, 1941), the only film in which he co-starred with the Austrian actor, Erich von Stroheim (1885–1957), who, in 1936, like Hayakawa a year later, had abandoned Hollywood for Paris, was recalled by the German authorities who objected to von Stroheim's sensitive portrayal of a Prussian officer in *La Grande Illusion* (*Grand Illusion,* 1937), so that "All of Von's scenes [could be] remade with Pierre Renoir playing the role of Werner Krall. Only after this was done did the Nazis allow Macao to be shown during the Occupation . . . The deletion of Von's scenes from his French pictures was not limited to *Macao.* The Germans also cut him out of another of his films, *Derrière la Facade.* The rest of the twenty-four French films he made prior to the German Occupation of France were either burned, banned, or buried." For the career of Pierre Renoir (1885–1952), see Ehrlich, op. cit., pp. 59, 88, 115, 140, 152, 166, 170. For the life and career of Erich von Stroheim—who returned to Hollywood in 1939, essaying the role of General Rommel

in *Five Graves to Cairo* (1943) and of the faithful butler in *Sunset Boulevard* (1950)—see two works by Herman G. Weinberg, "Erich von Stroheim (April 1958)," *Saint Cinema: Writings on the Film, 1929–1970,* rev. ed. (New York: Dover, 1973), pp. 127–33; and *Stroheim: A Pictorial Record of His Nine Films* (New York: Dover, 1975); Thomas Quinn Curtis, *Von Stroheim* (New York: Farrar, Straus, and Giroux, 1971); Richard Koszarski, *The Man You Loved to Hate: Erich von Stroheim and Hollywood* (Oxford, U.K.: Oxford University Press, 1983).

168. Ehrlich, op. cit., p. 191.

169. Leonard W. Doob, "Goebbels' Principles of Propaganda," *Public Opinion Quarterly* 14 (fall 1950): 419–42. Reprinted in *Propaganda,* ed. Robert Jackall (New York: New York University Press, 1995), pp. 190–216. Quotations from pp. 198, 211, 213.

170. Z. A. B. Zeman, "The State and Propaganda." Reprinted from idem, *Nazi Propaganda,* new ed. (Oxford, U.K.: Oxford University Press, 1973) in Jackall, ed., op. cit., pp. 174–89. Quotation from p. 185.

171. For Riefenstahl's self-serving claim that she did not wish to make *Triumph des Willens,* and that she agreed to do it only when Hitler personally gave her his complete support, promised her absolute artistic freedom on the project, and assured her that Goebbels would not interfere, see Leni Riefenstahl, *Leni Riefenstahl: A Memoir* (New York: St. Martin's Press, 1993), pp. 156–66. For various analyses of the film, see Welch, op. cit., pp. 147–59; Hull, op. cit., pp. 73–76; Kracauer, op. cit., pp. 300–303; Kreimeier, op. cit., pp. 233, 252–54, 268, 306.

172. Riefenstahl, op. cit., pp. 168–208, 434–36; and Richard D. Mandell, *The Nazi Olympics* (Urbana: University of Illinois Press, 1987), pp. 250–74.

173. Welch, op. cit., pp. 292–301; Kreimeier, op. cit., p. 275; Hull, op. cit., pp. 170–74.

174. Welch, op. cit., pp. 242–55; Kreimeier, op. cit., pp. 230, 282; Hull, op. cit., pp. 59, 86.

175. Welch, op. cit., p. 291.

176. Ibid., pp. 10–17, 30–39, 98, 308.

177. Doob, op. cit., p. 214; Kreimeier, op. cit., pp. 312–13.

178. Zeman, op. cit., pp. 185–86.

179. Kreimeier, op. cit., pp. 208–17, 226–27, 312, 322, 328, 367.

180. Lang's claim—viz., that "after the Nazis had come to power, my anti-Nazi film, *The Last Will of Dr. Mabuse,* in which I put Nazi slogans into the mouth of a pathological criminal, was banned of course. I was called to see Goebbels, not, as I had feared, in order to be called to account for the film but to be told by the Reichs-propaganda minister to my surprise, that Hitler had instructed him to offer me the leading post in the German film industry. 'The Führer saw your film *Metropolis* and announced, "That's the man to make national socialist film . . . !"' I left Germany the same evening." (Fritz Lang, "Autobiography," in Eisner, *Fritz Lang,* op. cit., pp. 14–15) —is a matter of much debate. For example, David Stewart Hull, op. cit., p. 39, that "the elaborate thesis that the film was meant as a parable on the Hitler regime, with Nazi stock phrases put in the mouths of gangsters, seems far-fetched, and, if true,

would certainly have gone over the heads of almost all the audience. Considering that the script was by Thea von Harbou (Frau Lang at the time), a writer who left her husband for the Nazis, the legend of the film's 'true meaning' seems to have no foundation in fact." Herman G. Weinberg (*St. Cinema,* op. cit., pp. 84–85) holds a different opinion: *The Last Will of Dr. Mabuse* "was made as an allegory, to show Hitler's processes of terrorism . . . [It] was made by Lang as a warning and a prophecy—out of the Mabuses come the Heydrichs, Himmlers, and Hitlers." As for Goebbel's offer, Robert Sklar (op. cit., p. 226) observes, "Lang claimed that, after banning the film, Goebbels offered him leadership of the German film industry; though often cited in film histories, this seems wholly mythical." See also the comment by Kreimeier, op. cit., p. 214.

181. Kracauer, op. cit., p. 250.

182. See Stanford M. Lyman, *NATO and Germany: A Study in the Sociology of Supranational Relations* (Fayetteville: University of Arkansas Press, 1995), pp. 5–7, 35–37, 170–75, 188.

183. Robert C. Reimer and Carol J. Reimer, *Nazi-retro Film: How German Narrative Cinema Remembers the Past* (New York: Twayne Publishers, 1992), p. 15.

184. Anton Kaes, *From Hitler to Heimat: The Return of History as Film* (Cambridge, Mass.: Harvard University Press, 1989), pp. 12–13.

185. Reimer and Reimer, op. cit., p. 16.

186. Loc. cit.

187. Kaes, op. cit., pp. 11–12.

188. Ibid., pp. 12–13.

189. Ibid., p. 13.

190. Jean-Paul Bier, "The Holocaust, West Germany, and Strategies of Oblivion, 1947–1949," in *Germans and Jews since the Holocaust: The Changing Situation in West Germany,* ed. Anson Rabinbach and Jack Zipes (New York: Holmes and Meier, 1986), pp. 199–200; Kaes, op. cit., pp. 6–7, 37–72, 93, 153, 214 n. 8; and Reimer and Reimer, op. cit., pp. 59–63, 98, 111–28, 164, 194, 195.

191. See Ilan Avisar, *Screening the Holocaust: Cinema's Images of the Unimaginable* (Bloomingdale: Indiana University Press, 1988), and Annette Insdorf, *Indelible Shadows: Film and the Holocaust,* 2d ed. (Cambridge, U.K.: Cambridge University Press, 1989).

192. Reimer and Reimer, op. cit., pp. 8–10, 38, 91–92, 127, 172; Kaes, op. cit., pp. 163–78.

193. Mark Koenigil, *Movies in Society: Sex, Crime and Censorship* (New York: Robert Speller and Sons, Publishers, 1962), p. 79.

194. Reimer and Reimer, op. cit., pp. 15–204.

195. Peter Baldwin, ed., *Reworking the Past: Hitler, the Holocaust, and the Historians' Debate* (Boston: Beacon Press, 1990). See also two essays by Stanford M. Lyman: "History and Sociology: Some Unresolved Epistemological Issues," *International Journal of Politics, Culture and Society* 9:1 (fall 1995): 29–55; and "Some Dilemmas of History and Memory," *International Journal of Politics, Culture and Society* 9:4 (summer 1996): 623–35.

196. Dan Diner, "Between Aporia and Apology: On the Limits of Historicizing National Socialism," in Baldwin, op. cit., pp. 133–45.

197. Hans Mommsen, "Reappraisal and Repression: The Third Reich in West German Historical Consciousness," in Baldwin, op. cit., pp. 173–84.

198. Wolfgang Benz, "Warding Off the Past: A Problem Only for Historians and Moralists?" in Baldwin, op. cit., pp. 196–213.

199. Andrei S. Markovitz, "Negative Symbiosis: Germans and Jews after Auschwitz," in Baldwin, op. cit., pp. 251–61. See also Franco Ferrarotti, *The Temptation to Forget: Racism, Anti-Semitism, Neo-Nazism* (Westport, Conn.: Greenwood Press, 1994).

200. Reimer and Reimer, op. cit., pp. 18–22.

201. Ibid., pp. 60, 62.

202. Kaes, op. cit., p. 17.

203. Reimer and Reimer, op. cit., p. 102.

204. Ibid., pp. 117–22.

205. Ibid., pp. 131–68.

206. Bier, op. cit., pp. 199–200.

207. Reimer and Reimer, op. cit., p. 171.

208. See Judith Mayne, "Fassbinder's *Ali: Fear Eats the Soul* and Spectatorship," in *Close Readings: An Anthology of New Film Criticism,* ed. Peter Lehman (Tallahassee: Florida State University Press, 1990), pp. 353–69.

209. Sklar, op. cit., pp. 455–57.

210. Kaes, op. cit., p. 81.

211. Ibid., p. 93.

212. Reimer and Reimer, op. cit., pp. 173–76.

213. Ibid., pp. 35–38, 152–53, 171.

214. Ibid., pp. 171–73, 203–4.

215. Sklar, op. cit., p. 457.

216. Lyman, *NATO and Germany,* op. cit., p. 10.

217. Dmitry Shlapentokh and Vladimir Shlapentokh, *Soviet Cinematography, 1918–1991: Ideological Conflict and Social Reality* (New York: Aldine de Gruyter, 1993).

218. Sklar, op. cit., p. 150.

219. Shlapentokh and Shlapentokh, op. cit., p. 21.

220. Loc. cit.

221. Richard Pipes, *Russia Under the Bolshevik Regime* (New York: Alfred A. Knopf, 1993), pp. 287, 308.

222. Ibid., p. 285.

223. Shlapentokh and Shlapentokh, op. cit., p. 27; Sklar, op. cit., pp. 151, 163.

224. Shlapentokh and Shlapentokh, op. cit., p. 21.

225. Pipes, op. cit., pp. 308–9. For the Agit trains, see Sklar, op. cit., pp. 150–51.

226. Pipes, op. cit., p. 309.

227. Loc. cit.

228. Richard Schickel, *D. W. Griffith: An American Life* (New York: Simon and Schuster, Touchstone Books, 1984), p. 435.

229. Ibid., p. 335. See also Tom Gunning, *D. W. Griffith and the Origins of American Narrative Film: The Early Years at Biograph* (Urbana: University of Illinois Press, 1991), pp. 10–30, 112–29.

230. Sklar, op. cit., p. 151.

231. For a brief synopsis, see Sklar, op. cit., pp. 152–57.

232. Shlapentokh and Shlapentokh, op. cit., p. 7.

233. Shlapentokh and Shlapentokh, op. cit., p. 11.

234. Ibid., p. 10.

235. Cf. Sklar, op. cit., p. 157 and Pipes, op. cit., p. 309.

236. Shlapentokh and Shlapentokh, op. cit., pp. 52–53.

237. Sklar, op. cit., p. 157.

238. Sergei Mikhailovitch Eisenstein, "'Wie sag ich's meinem Kind?' and My First Film," in *Cinema in Revolution: The Heroic Era of the Soviet Film,* ed. Luda and Jean Schnitzer and Marcel Martin, trans. David Robinson (New York: Hill and Wang, 1973), pp. 43–50. Quotation from p. 47.

239. D. J. Wendon, "*Battleship Potemkin*—Film and Reality," in *Feature Films as History,* ed. K. R. M. Short (Knoxville: University of Tennessee Press, 1981), pp. 37–61.

240. Ibid., p. 37.

241. Judith Mayne, *Kino and the Woman Question: Feminism and Soviet Silent Film* (Columbus: Ohio State University Press, 1989).

242. Ibid., p. 33.

243. Ibid., p. 37.

244. Ibid., p. 56.

245. For Kuleshov's statement on the matter, see Lev Vladimirovitch Kuleshov, *"The Origins of Montage,"* in Luda and Jean Schnitzer and Marcel Martin, eds., op. cit., pp. 65–76.

246. See Dziga Vertov, "Kino-Eye: The Embattled Documentarists," in Luda and Jean Schnitzer and Marcel Martin, eds., op. cit., pp. 77–88.

247. Mayne, op. cit., p. 33.

248. Ibid., pp. 191–92.

249. Shlapentokh and Shlapentokh, op. cit., pp. 91–98, 117–18, 160–62, 166–69.

250. Ibid., pp. 41–42.

251. Ibid., pp. 87–88, 145, 188–94.

252. Ibid., pp. 223–24.

253. Ibid., p. 31.

254. Ibid., pp. 75–128.

255. Ibid., pp. 181, 259.

256. Ibid., pp. 181–82.

257. Ibid., p. 185.

258. Ibid., pp. 185–96.

259. Ibid., pp. 201–7.

260. Ibid., pp. 214–17.

261. Ibid., pp. 218–24.

262. Ibid., pp. 224–32.

263. Sklar, op. cit., p. 150.

264. Shlapentokh and Shlapentokh, op. cit., p. 242.

265. Ibid., p. 226.

266. Perkowski, op. cit., p. 14.

267. Loc. cit. See also Paul Barber, *Vampires, Burial, and Death: Folklore and Reality* (New Haven, Conn.: Yale University Press, 1988). For Vlad Tepes as the model for Bram Stoker's Dracula, see Raymond T. McNally and Radu R. Florescu, *In Search of Dracula: A True History of Dracula and Vampire Legends* (Greenwich, Conn.: New York Graphic Society, 1972); and Radu R. Florescu and Raymond T. McNally, *Dracula: Prince of Many Faces* (Boston: Little, Brown and Co., 1989); and *The Annotated Dracula: Dracula by Bram Stoker,* intro., notes, biblio. by Leonard Wolf (New York: Clarkson N. Potter, 1975). For the most recent biography of Bram Stoker, see Barbara Belford, *Bram Stoker: A Biography of the Author of Dracula* (New York: Alfred A. Knopf, 1996).

There is, perhaps, another irony here. The vampire appears at the onset and after the downfall of communism. Bela Lugosi (Bela Ferenc Dezsö Blasko, 1882–1956), the preeminent portrayer of the vampire, Dracula, had established the Free Organization of Theater Employees in Hungary in 1918 and lent his support to the short-lived Bela Kun regime. "The definite aim of my organizing activity," he wrote, "was the raising of the moral, economic, and cultural level of the actor's society." Quoted from Bela Lugosi, "History of the Formation of Our Trade Union," *Színészek Lapja,* May 1, 1919, in Arthur Lennig, *The Count: The Life and Films of Bela "Dracula" Lugosi* (New York: G. P. Putnam's Sons, 1974), p. 43. See also the excerpt from Bela Lugosi, "Love the Actor," *Színészek Lapja,* May 15, 1919, in Lennig, op. cit., p. 45; and in Robert Cremer, *Lugosi: The Man behind the Cape* (Chicago: Henry Regnery, 1976), p. 67.

268. See Fred Block, *The Vampire State and Other Myths and Fallacies about the U.S. Economy* (New York: New Press, 1996).

269. Richard J. Blackburn, *The Vampire of Reason: An Essay in the Philosophy of History* (London: Verso, 1990), pp. 13–34, 75–214; and Noël Carroll, op. cit., pp. 195–214; and Block, op. cit.

270. See three works by Stanford M. Lyman: *The Seven Deadly Sins: Society and Evil,* rev. ed. (Dix Hills, N.Y.: General Hall, 1989), pp. 239–68; *Militarism, Imperialism, and Racial Accommodation: An Analysis and Interpretation of the Early Writings of Robert E. Park* (Fayetteville: University of Arkansas Press, 1992), pp. 41–135; *Color, Culture, Civilization: Race and Minority Issues in American Society* (Urbana: University of Illinois Press, 1994), pp. 85–102; and Block, op. cit., pp. 1–94.

271. Cf. Mary Beth Inverso, *The Gothic Impulse in Contemporary Drama* (Ann Arbor: UMI Research Press, 1990).

272. Ken Gelder, *Reading the Vampire* (London: Routledge, 1994), p. 141.

273. Cf. George Herbert Mead, *Selected Writings,* ed. Andrew J. Reck (Indianapolis: Bobbs-Merrill, 1964), pp. 82–93, 114–49, 355–70.

274. Gelder, loc. cit.

275. Manuela Dunn Mascetti, *Vampire: The Complete Guide to the World of the Undead* (New York: Viking Studio Books, 1992), p. 11.

276. Shlapentokh and Shlapentokh, op. cit., p. 242. By the same token, Barbara Belford, author of the latest biography of Bram Stoker, cited supra, "ignores . . . the once-fashionable Marxist equation of Count Dracula with the bloodsucking capitalist who feeds off his workers . . . [preferring, instead, to assert] that all works of the occult stem from primordial human fears of sex, incest, disease, death, and the unknown." Margot Peters, "The Boss from Hell: A Life of Bram Stoker, Who Modeled Dracula Largely on His Employer, Henry Irving," *New York Times Book Review,* Sec. 7 (April 7, 1996), p. 20.

277. Ibid., p. 244.

278. Berman, op. cit., p. 197.

279. Daniel Bell, *The End of Ideology: On the Exhaustion of Political Ideas in the Fifties—with a new Afterword* (Cambridge, Mass.: Harvard University Press, 1988). See also Howard Brick, *Daniel Bell and the Decline of Intellectual Radicalism: Social Theory and Political Reconciliation in the 1940s* (Madison: University of Wisconsin Press, 1986).

280. See three works by Francis Fukuyama: "The End of History?" *National Interest* 16 (summer 1989): 3–18; *The End of History and the Last Man* (New York: Free Press, 1992); and "Reflections on the End of History Five Years Later," in *After History? Francis Fukuyama and His Critics,* ed. Timothy Burns (London: Littlefield Adams, Rowman and Littlefield, 1994), pp. 239–58.

281. Fukuyama, "The End of History," op. cit., p. 3.

282. Fukuyama, "Reflections . . . ," op. cit., p. 257.

283. Weber, "Science as a Vocation," in Gerth and Mills, op. cit., p. 147.

284. See Lyman, *NATO and Germany,* op. cit., pp. 3–11.

285. Fukuyama, "Reflections . . . ," op. cit., p. 243.

286. Francis Fukuyama, *Trust: The Social Virtues and the Creation of Prosperity* (New York: Free Press, 1995), p. 353.

287. Ibid., p. 26.

288. Loc. cit.

289. Ferdinand Tönnies, *Community and Society (Gemeinschaft und Gesellschaft),* trans. and ed. Charles P. Loomis (East Lansing: Michigan State University Press, 1957), pp. 31–260.

290. Fukuyama, *Trust* . . . , op. cit., p. 356.

291. Fukuyama, *Reflections* . . . , op. cit., p. 242. Emphasis in original.

292. Ibid., p. 257.

293. Leo Lowenthal, "Against Postmodernism: Interview with Emilio Galli Zugaro," in *An Unmastered Past: The Autobiographical Reflections of Leo Lowenthal,* ed. Martin Jay (Berkeley: University of California Press, 1987), pp. 263, 264, 265.

294. See Ernest Lee Tuveson, *Redeemer Nation: The Idea of America's Millennial Role* (Chicago: University of Chicago Press, 1968); and Mona Harrington, *The Dream of Deliverance in American Politics* (New York: Alfred A. Knopf, 1986).

295. See Stanley G. Payne, *A History of Fascism, 1914–1945* (Madison: University of Wisconsin Press, 1995).

296. J. P. Mayer, *Sociology of Film,* op. cit., p. 34.

297. Loc. cit.

298. Ibid., p. 309.

299. Immanuel Wallerstein, *After Liberalism* (New York: New Press, 1995), p. 1. Emphasis in original.

300. Walter Laquer, "Postmodern Terrorism," *Foreign Affairs* 75:5 (September–October 1996): 24–36.

301. Joseph Zulaika and William A. Douglass, *Terror and Taboo: The Follies, Fables, and Faces of Terrorism* (New York: Routledge, 1996), p. 3.

302. Laquer, "Postmodern Terrorism," op. cit., p. 32 n. 2.

303. Weber, "Politics as a Vocation," in Gerth and Mills, op. cit., p. 128.

304. ". . . *charisma:* it is a gift of grace (*Gnadengabe*) for a people or a nation to have a great (charismatic) political leader." J. P. Mayer, *Max Weber and German Politics* (London: Faber and Faber, Ltd., 1944), p. 20.

305. See Ellen Jaffe McClain, *Embracing the Stranger: Intermarriage and the Future of the American Jewish Community* (New York: Basic Books, 1995), pp. 32–33.

306. Louis Wirth, *The Ghetto* (Chicago: University of Chicago Press, Phoenix Books, 1956 [1928]), pp. 195–281.

307. Jacqueline P. Wiseman, *Stations of the Lost: The Treatment of Skid Row Alcoholics* (Englewood Cliffs, N.J.: Prentice-Hall, 1970).

308. Cf. the remark by Julia Kristeva (*Tales of Love,* trans. Leon S. Roudiez [New York: Columbia University Press, 1987], pp. 382–83): "Today Narcissus is an exile, deprived of his psychic space, an extraterrestrial with a prehistory bearing, wanting for love. An uneasy child, all scratched up, somewhat disgusting, without a precise body or image, having lost his specificity, an alien in a world of desire and power, he longs only to reinvent love. The ET's are more and more numerous. We are all ET's."

309. The inside joke of his remark references Steven Spielberg's *E.T.: The Extra-Terrestrial* (1982), in which American children outwit adults and help a being from another planet return home. By 1996, the cute extraterrestrial with whom the children had played had—it might be inferred—grown to become one of the earth-threatening monsters of *Independence Day.*

310. Jean Franco, "The Nation as an Imagined Community," in *The New Historicism,* ed. H. Aram Veeser (New York: Routledge, 1989), p. 212.

Chapter Eight. Community: A Theoretical Perspective on Its Dilemmas, Contradictions, and Possible Future

1. Timothy Egan, "Many Seek Security in Private Communities," *New York Times,* CXLIV:50, 173 (September 3, 1995), pp. 1, 10.

2 . Edward Tivnan, *The Moral Imagination: Confronting the Ethical Issues of Our Day* (New York: Simon and Schuster, 1995), p. 220.

3. Loc. cit.

4. Egan, op. cit., p. 1.

5. Loc. cit.

6. Ibid., p. 10.

7. For the concept of territoriality, see Stanford M. Lyman and Marvin B. Scott, *A Sociology of the Absurd,* 2d ed. (Dix Hills, N.Y.: General Hall, 1989), pp. 22–34.

8. Quoted in Egan, op. cit., p. 10.

9. Cf. two essays by Stanford M. Lyman, "Territoriality as a Global Concept," *Revija za Sociologiju,* XXV:3–4 (Srpanj-Prosinac, 1994): 139–50; and "Interstate Relations and the Sociological Imagination Revisited: From Social Distance to Territoriality," *Sociological Inquiry* 65:2 (spring 1995): 125–42.

10. See Charles Lemert, *Sociology after the Crisis* (Boulder, Colo.: Westview Press, 1995), pp. 38–39, 62–69, 103–11, 168–95, 206–11.

11. See Richard Thompson Ford, "The Boundaries of Race: Political Geography in Legal Analysis," *Harvard Law Review* 107:8 (June 1994): 1841–1922. For the role of commercial media in depicting African Americans in stereotypes that would instantiate their subcultural differences and social distance from white, middle-class Americans, see William M. O'Barr, *Culture and the Ad: Exploring Otherness in the World of Advertising* (Boulder, Colo.: Westview Press, 1994), pp. 107–56.

12. Quoted in Egan, op. cit., p. 10.

13. Loc. cit.

14. William Prosser, "Trespassing Children," *California Law Review* 47:3 (August 1959): 427–69. Quotation from p. 427.

15. On Toennies (also Tönnies), see Werner J. Cahnman and Rudolf Heberle, eds., *Ferdinand Tönnies on Sociology: Pure, Applied, and Empirical* (Chicago: University of Chicago Press, 1971); Werner J. Cahnman, ed., *Ferdinand Tönnies: A New Evaluation—Essays and Documents* (Leiden, The Netherlands: E. J. Brill, 1973); Werner J. Cahnman, *Weber and Toennies: Comparative Sociology in Historical Perspective* (New Brunswick, N.J.: Transaction Publishers, 1995).

16. Ferdinand Tönnies, *Community and Society: (Gemeinschaft und Gesellschaft),* trans. and ed. Charles P. Loomis (East Lansing: Michigan State University Press, 1957).

17. Ferdinand Toennies, "The Concept of Gemeinschaft," in Cahnman and Heberle, op. cit., pp. 62–72. Quotation from p. 65.

18. Loc. cit.

19. Tönnies, *Community and Society,* op. cit., p. 33.

20. Quoted from Johann Caspar Bluntschli, *Staatsworterbuch IV* in Tönnies, *Community and Society,* op. cit., pp. 34–35.

21. Ibid., pp. 33–34.

22. Ibid., p. 34.

23. Ferdinand Toennies, "Social Values: Economic Values," in Cahnman and Heberle, eds., op. cit., pp. 157–69. Quotation from p. 165.

24. Loc. cit.

25. Ferdinand Tönnies, "The Revision of the Medieval World View," in idem, *On*

Social Ideas and Ideologies, ed. and trans. E. G. Jacoby (New York: Harper and Row, 1974), pp. 3–36. Quotation from p. 12.

26. Ibid., p. 13.

27. Ibid., pp. 13–14.

28. Ibid., pp. 17–24.

29. Tönnies, *Community and Society,* op. cit., p. 34.

30. Loc. cit.

31. Ibid., pp. 162–63.

32. Ibid., p. 165. Emphasis supplied.

33. Max Weber, "Politics as a Vocation," in *From Max Weber: Essays in Sociology,* trans. and ed. H. H. Gerth and C. Wright Mills (New York: Oxford University Press, 1946), pp. 77–128.

34. Tönnies, *Community and Society,* op. cit., p. 165.

35. Ibid., p. 165.

36. Ibid., pp. 165–66.

37. Ibid., p. 166.

38. Rudolf Heberle, "Introduction," in Ferdinand Tönnies, *Custom: An Essay on Social Codes,* trans. A. Farrell Borenstein (Chicago: Henry Regnery, Gateway, 1971) [1909]), pp. 26–27.

39. Ibid., p. 26.

40. Tönnies, *Community and Society,* op. cit., p. 167.

41. Loc. cit.

42. Loc. cit.

43. Ibid., p. 168.

44. Ibid., p. 166.

45. Loc. cit.

46. Loc. cit.

47. See Russell Kirk, *The Conservative Mind: From Burke to Eliot,* 7th ed., rev. (Washington, D.C.: Regnery Publishing, 1995), pp. 482–88.

48. Ferdinand Toennies, "The Individual and the World in the Modern Age," in Cahnman and Heberle, op. cit., pp. 288–317, esp. pp. 306–8.

49. See Arthur J. Vidich and Stanford M. Lyman, *American Sociology: Worldly Rejections of Religion and Their Directions* (New Haven, Conn.: Yale University Press, 1985).

50. Ferdinand Toennies, "The Active Forces of Social Development in the Modern Age," in Cahnman and Heberle, op. cit., pp. 318–32. Quotation from p. 332.

51. Alan Ryan, *John Dewey and the High Tide of American Liberalism* (New York: W. W. Norton, 1995), p. 21.

52. John Dewey, *The Public and Its Problems* (New York: Henry Holt and Co., 1927), pp. 143–84.

53. Robert Redfield, *The Little Community and Peasant Society and Culture* (Chicago: University of Chicago Press, 1960).

54. Alan Ryan, op. cit., pp. 35–60, 154–242, 284–327.

55. Dewey, *The Public and Its Problems,* op. cit., pp. 152–54, 176–79, 211–19. See also John Dewey, *German Philosophy and Politics* (New York: G. P. Putnam's Sons, 1942), pp. 45–48.

56. Jürgen Habermas, *The Theory of Communicative Action,* Vol. 1: *Reason and the Rationalization of Society;* Vol. 2: *Lifeworld and System: A Critique of Functionalist Reason,* trans. Thomas McCarthy (Boston: Beacon Press, 1984, 1987).

57. John Dewey, "Science and Social Philosophy," *Lectures in China, 1919–1920,* ed. and trans. Robert W. Clopton and Tsuin-chen Ou (Honolulu: University Press of Hawaii, 1973), pp. 54–63. Quotation from p. 54.

58. Dewey, *The Public and Its Problems,* op. cit., p. 148.

59. John Dewey, *The Child and the Curriculum and the School and Society* (Chicago: University of Chicago Press, 1971).

60. John Dewey, "Criteria for Judging Systems of Thought," *Lectures in China, 1919–1920,* op. cit., pp. 82–89. Quotation from p. 89.

61. John Dewey, "Political Liberalism," *Lectures in China, 1919–1920,* op. cit., pp. 141–46.

62. John Dewey, "Discipline for Associated Living," *Lectures in China, 1919–1920,* op. cit., pp. 217–22.

63. John Dewey, "Moral Education: The Social Aspects," *Lectures in China, 1919–1920,* op. cit., pp. 294–302, esp. pp. 296–98.

64. John Dewey, "Creative Dramatics and Work," *Lectures in China, 1919–1920,* op. cit., 203–9.

65. John Dewey, "Nationalism and Internationalism," *Lectures in China, 1919–1920,* op. cit., pp. 156–63. Quotation from p. 163.

66. Barry Keenan, *The Dewey Experiment in China: Educational Reform and Political Power in the Early Republic* (Cambridge, Mass.: Harvard University Press, 1977), p. 161.

67. Walter Lippmann, *The Phantom Public* (New York: Harcourt, Brace and Co., 1925). Dewey's favorable review of this book appeared as "Practical Democracy," in *New Republic* 2 (December 1925): 52–54.

68. George Dykhuizen, *The Life and Mind of John Dewey,* ed. Jo Ann Boydston (Carbondale: Southern Illinois University Press, 1973), p. 72.

69. Dewey, *The Public and Its Problems,* op. cit., p. 115.

70. Loc. cit.

71. Ibid., pp. 115–16.

72. Ibid., p. 126.

73. Ibid., p. 131.

74. Ibid., p. 135.

75. Ibid., p. 141.

76. Ibid., p. 142.

77. Loc. cit.

78. Loc. cit.

79. Ibid., p. 140.

80. John Dewey, "Moral Education: The Social Aspects," *Lectures in China,* op. cit., p. 308.

81. Quoted in Ryan, op. cit., p. 320.

82. John Dewey, "The Lost Individual," in *The Philosophy of John Dewey,* ed. John J. McDermott (Chicago: University of Chicago Press, 1981), pp. 598–608. Quotation on p. 601.

83. Quoted in Ryan, op. cit., p. 320.

84. Dewey, "The Lost Individual," op. cit., p. 607.

85. Kirk, op. cit., p. 419.

86. Loc. cit.

87. Michael A. Weinstein, *The Wilderness and the City: America's Classical Philosophy as a Moral Quest* (Amherst: University of Massachusetts Press, 1982), p. 155.

88. Robert A. Nisbet, *The Quest for Community: A Study in the Ethics of Order and Freedom* (New York: Oxford University Press, 1953), p. 73.

89. Jean-Jacques Rousseau, "Discourse on the Origin and the Foundation of Inequality among Mankind," in idem, *The Social Contract and Discourse on the Origin of Inequality,* ed. Lester G. Crocker (New York: Washington Square Press, 1967), pp. 151–258, esp. pp. 178–211.

90. Ibid., p. 179.

91. Ibid., p. 182.

92. Loc. cit.

93. Ibid., pp. 216–18.

94. Ibid., p. 211.

95. Ibid., p. 212.

96. Ibid., p. 183.

97. For a thoughtful and sympathetic analysis of Rousseau on these issues, see Alessandro Ferrara, *Modernity and Authenticity: A Study of the Social and Ethical Thought of Jean-Jacques Rousseau* (Albany: State University of New York Press, 1993).

98. The following draws on Arthur J. Vidich and Stanford M. Lyman, "Qualitative Methods: Their History in Sociology and Anthropology," in Norman K. Denzin and Yvonna S. Lincoln, eds., *Handbook of Qualitative Research* (Thousand Oaks, Calif.: Sage Publications, 1994), pp. 23–59, esp. 34–35.

99. See, e.g., the following works by Robert Redfield: *Tepoztlan-a Mexican Village: A Study of Folk Life* (Chicago: University of Chicago Press, 1930); *The Folk Culture of Yucatan* (Chicago: University of Chicago Press, 1941); *The Little Community and Peasant Society and Culture,* op. cit.; and the 21 essays collected under the title, "The Folk Society and Civilization," in Margaret Park Redfield, ed., *The Papers of Robert Redfield,* Vol. 1: *Human Nature and the Study of Society* (Chicago: University of Chicago Press, 1962), pp. 143–414.

100. Quoted from an essay by Margaret Park Redfield, "The American Family: Consensus and Freedom," in *The American Journal of Sociology* of November 1946, in Nisbet, op. cit., p. 287 n. 4.

101. Robert Redfield, "Talk with a Stranger," in Margaret Park Redfield, ed., op. cit.,

Vol. 2: *The Social Uses of Social Science* (Chicago: University of Chicago Press, 1963), pp. 270–84.

102. Stow Persons, *Ethnic Studies at Chicago, 1905–1945* (Urbana: University of Illinois Press, 1987).

103. Louis Wirth, "Urbanism as a Way of Life," *American Journal of Sociology* 44 (July 1938): 1–24.

104. The principal works of Charles Louis de Secondat, Baron de La Breda et de Montesquieu, are *The Spirit of the Laws,* trans. Thomas Nugent (New York: Hafner Press, 1949); *The Greatness of the Romans and Their Decline,* trans. David Lowenthal (Ithaca, N.Y.: Cornell University Press, 1968); *The Persian Letters,* ed. and trans. J. Robert Loy (New York: World Publishing Co., Meridian, 1961). For commentaries, see Albert Sorel, *Montesquieu,* trans. Melville B. Anderson and Edward Playfair Anderson (Port Washington, N.Y.: Kennikat Press, 1969) [1888]); Thomas L. Pangle, *Montesquieu's Philosophy of Liberalism: A Commentary on the Spirit of the Laws* (Chicago: University of Chicago Press, 1973); Mark Hulliung, *Montesquieu and the Old Regime* (Berkeley: University of California Press, 1976); and Melvin Richter, *The Political Theory of Montesquieu* (Cambridge, U.K.: Cambridge University Press, 1977). See also the many commentaries on Montesquieu in Christopher Fox, Roy Porter, and Robert Wolker, eds., *Inventing Human Science: Eighteenth-Century Domains* (Berkeley: University of California Press, 1995).

105. Hulliung, op. cit., p. 217.

106. Ibid., p. 220.

107. Loc. cit.

108. Robert E. Park, "Human Migration and the Marginal Man," in *Personality and the Social Group,* ed. Ernest W. Burgess (Chicago: University of Chicago Press, 1929; reprint, Freeport, N.Y.: Books for Libraries Press, 1969), pp. 64–77.

109. Everett Cherrington Hughes, "Preface," to Robert Ezra Park, *Human Communities: The Collected Papers of Robert Ezra Park,* Vol. 2, ed. Everett Cherrington Hughes, Charles S. Johnson, Jitsuichi Masuoka, Robert Redfield, and Louis Wirth (Glencoe, Ill.: Free Press, 1952), pp. 5–7. Quotation from p. 6.

110. Robert E. Park, "Culture and Civilization," in idem, *Race and Culture: The Collected Papers of Robert Ezra Park,* Vol. 1, ed. Everett Cherrington Hughes, Charles S. Johnson, Jitsuichi Masuoka, Robert Redfield, and Louis Wirth (Glencoe, Ill.: Free Press, 1950), pp. 15–23. Quotation from pp. 20–21.

111. Robert E. Park, "The City: Suggestions for the Investigation of Human Behavior in the Urban Environment," in *The City,* ed. Robert E. Park, Ernest W. Burgess, and Roderick D. McKenzie (Chicago: University of Chicago Press, 1967 [1925]), pp. 1–46. Quotation from pp. 45–46.

112. See, e.g., Ruth Shonle Cavan, *Suicide* (New York: Russell and Russell, 1965 [1928]); and Robert E. L. Faris and H. Warren Dunham, *Mental Disorders in Urban Areas: An Ecological Study of Schizophrenia and Other Psychoses* (Chicago: University of Chicago Press, 1965 [1939]).

113. See, e.g., Norman S. Hayner, "Hotel Life and Personality," in Burgess, ed., op.

cit., pp. 108–20; and Paul C. P. Siu, *The Chinese Laundryman: A Study of Social Isolation,* ed. John Kuo Wei Tchen (New York: New York University Press, 1987).

114. Bingham Dai, *Opium Addiction in Chicago* (Montclair, N.J.: Patterson Smith, 1970 [1937]).

115. Frederic M. Thrasher, *The Gang: A Study of 1,313 Gangs in Chicago,* abr. ed. (Chicago: University of Chicago Press, 1963 [1927]); and Clifford R. Shaw, "Correlation of Rate of Juvenile Delinquency with Certain Indices of Community Organization and Disorganization," in Burgess, ed., op. cit., pp. 206–11.

116. See Ernest W. Burgess and Donald J. Bogue, eds., *Contributions to Urban Sociology* (Chicago: University of Chicago Press, 1964).

117. See Fred Davis, *Yearning for Yesterday: A Sociology of Nostalgia* (New York: Free Press, 1979).

118. Talcott Parsons, "Note on *Gemeinschaft* and *Gesellschaft,*" *The Structure of Social Action: A Study in Social Theory with Special Reference to a Group of Recent European Writers* (New York: McGraw-Hill Book Co., 1937; reprint, Glencoe, Ill.: Free Press, 1949), pp. 686–94. Quotation from pp. 687–88.

119. Both essays are found in *The Sociology of Georg Simmel,* trans. and ed. Kurt H. Wolff (Glencoe, Ill.: Free Press, 1950), pp. 402–26.

120. Louis Wirth, "Urbanism as a Way of Life," reprinted in *Louis Wirth on Cities and Social Life: Selected Papers,* ed. Albert J. Reiss Jr. (Chicago: University of Chicago Press, 1964), pp. 60–83. Quotation from p. 71.

121. Loc. cit.

122. Ibid., p. 82.

123. Thomas C. Wilson, "Urbanism and Kinship Bonds: A Test of Four Generalizations," *Social Forces* 71:3 (March 1993): 703–12. Quotation from pp. 710–11.

124. Thomas C. Wilson, "Urbanism and Racial Attitudes: A Test of Some Urban Theories," *Urban Affairs Quarterly* 20:2 (December 1984): 201–9. Quotation from p. 205.

125. Thomas C. Wilson, "Urbanism, Misanthropy and Subcultural Processes," *Social Science Journal* 22:3 (July 1985): 89–101. Quotation from p. 97.

126. Thomas C. Wilson, "White Response to Neighborhood Racial Change," *Sociological Focus* 16:4 (October 1983): 305–18. Quotation from pp. 315–16.

127. Thomas C. Wilson, "The Impact of Cohort Prejudice toward Four Minority Groups." Paper presented at the 23d conference of The National Association of Ethnic Studies, Boulder, Colorado, March 8–12, 1995. In a related paper, entitled "Compliments Will Get You Nowhere: Benign Stereotypes, Prejudice and Anti-Semitism," presented August 23, 1995, to the 90th annual meeting of the American Sociological Association, at Washington, D.C., Wilson noted that "ostensibly benign Jewish stereotypes are not generally pro-Semitic, but are likely instead to veil underlying anti-Semitism."

128. Wilson, "The Impact of Cohort Prejudice . . . ," op. cit.

129. Arthur J. Vidich and Joseph Bensman, *Small Town in Mass Society: Class, Power and Religion in a Rural Community,* 2d ed., rev. (Princeton, N.J.: Princeton University Press, 1968).

130. Ibid., p. xi.

131. Roland L. Warren, *The Community in America,* 2d ed. (Chicago: Rand, McNally, 1972), pp. 53–94. Quotation from p. 53.

132. Peter Schrag, *The Decline of the WASP* (New York: Simon and Schuster, 1970).

133. Michael Novak, *The Rise of the Unmeltable Ethnics: Politics and Culture in the Seventies* (New York: Macmillan, 1972).

134. Alejandro Portes and Alex Stepick, *City on the Edge: The Transformation of Miami* (Berkeley: University of California Press, 1993).

135. Ibid., p. 221.

136. Joseph Bensman and Arthur J. Vidich, eds., *Metropolitan Communities: New Forms of Urban Sub-Communities* (New York: New Viewpoints, Franklin Watts, 1975), p. 62.

137. Loc. cit.

138. "In North America . . . the time will come when the population will have become dense. The struggle for existence will have to be more carefully planned. Then the people of America will be forced to stop and reflect . . . When that situation comes about, the memory of racial extraction may at last be reawakened. The different languages may become the rallying centers for the different interests. Thereupon for the first time will America confront decisively the problem of its national unity." Gustav Ratzenhofer, *Wesen und Zweck der Politik,* translated into English and quoted by Albion W. Small, *General Sociology: An Exposition of the Main Developments in Sociological Theory from Spencer to Ratzenhofer* (Chicago: University of Chicago Press, 1905; reprint, New York: Arno Press, 1974), p. 256.

139. Loc. cit. See also the discussion in Stanford M. Lyman, *Color, Culture, Civilization: Race and Minority Issues in American Society* (Urbana: University of Illinois Press, 1994), pp. 105–47, 326–84.

140. Michael W. Hughey and Arthur J. Vidich, "Ethnicity and Community in America," in idem, eds., *The Ethnic Quest for Community: Searching for Roots in the Lonely Crowd,* Research in Community Sociology, vol. 3 (Greenwich, Conn.: JAI Press, 1993), pp. 3–16. Quotation from pp. 7–8.

141. Ibid., p. 8.

142. See Ernest Gellner, *Conditions of Liberty: Civil Society and Its Rivals* (New York: Allen Lane, Penguin Press, 1994).

143. See Stanford M. Lyman and Marvin B. Scott, *A Sociology of the Absurd,* rev. ed. (Dix Hills, N.Y.: General Hall, 1989).

144. Ernst Bloch, *Natural Law and Human Dignity,* trans. Dennis J. Schmidt (Cambridge, Mass.: MIT Press, 1986; originally published under the title *Naturrecht und menschliche Würde,* Frankfurt, FRG: Suhrkamp Verlag, 1961), p. 279.

145. Ibid., pp. 279–80.

146. Max Weber, "Politics as a Vocation," in Hans H. Gerth and C. Wright Mills, trans. and eds., op. cit., pp. 77–128.

147. Friedrich Engels, *Herr Eugen Dühring's Revolution in Science (Anti-Dühring),* trans. Emil Burns (New York: International Publishers, 1939), p. 309. Quoted in Frank Manuel, *A Requiem for Karl Marx* (Cambridge, Mass.: Harvard University Press, 1995), p. 179.

148. Jean B. Quandt, *From the Small Town to the Great Community: The Social Thought of Progressive Intellectuals* (New Brunswick, N.J.: Rutgers University Press, 1970), p. 157.

149. See, e.g., Larry Diamond and Marc F. Plattner, eds., *The Global Resurgence of Democracy* (Baltimore: Johns Hopkins University Press, 1993).

150. Richard Edward DeLeon, *Left Coast City: Progressive Politics in San Francisco, 1975–1991* (Lawrence: University Press of Kansas, 1992), p. 174.

151. Witold Rybczynski, *City Life: Urban Expectations in a New World* (New York: Scribner, 1995), pp. 231–32.

152. Wayne S. Wooden, *Return to Paradise: Continuity and Change in Hawaii* (Lanham, Md.: University Press of America, 1995), pp. v, 10, 157–58.

153. See Joseph R. Gusfield, *Community: A Critical Response* (New York: Harper Colophon, 1975), pp. 83–106; Larry Lyon, *The Community in Urban Society* (Chicago: Dorsey Press, 1987), pp. 95–142, 240–51; Robert Booth Fowler, *The Dance with Community: The Contemporary Debate in American Political Thought* (Lawrence: University Press of Kansas, 1991).

154. Wataru Ebihara, comp. and ed., *An Asian American Internet Guide* (Los Angeles: Amerasia Journal and APNet, 1995), p. 7.

155. Quoted in Lance deHaven Smith, *Philosophical Critiques of Policy Analysis: Lindblom, Habermas, and the Great Society* (Gainesville: University of Florida Press, 1988), p. 95.

156. William Gibson, *Neuromancer* (New York: Ace, 1984). Quoted in Allucquère Rosanne Stone, *The War of Desire and Technology at the Close of the Mechanical Age* (Cambridge, Mass.: MIT Press, 1995), p. 33.

157. Stone, op. cit., p. 37.

158. Ibid., p. 167.

159. Ibid., p. 182.

160. Doreen Massey, "Double Articulation: *A Place in the World*," in Angelika Bammer, ed., *Displacements: Cultural Identities in Question* (Bloomington: Indiana University Press, 1994), pp. 110–21. Quotation from p. 120.

161. See William K. Rawlins, *Friendship Matters: Communication, Dialectic, and the Life Course* (New York: Aldine deGruyter, 1992), for a thoroughgoing analysis of the issues entailed-issues that necessarily go beyond the scope of this paper.

162. See Gerald D. Suttles, *The Social Construction of Communities* (Chicago: University of Chicago Press, 1972), pp. 3–110, 233–68.

163. Donald L. Parman, *Indians and the American West in the Twentieth Century* (Bloomington: Indiana University Press, 1994), p. 184. For an angry but informed critique of how Native American culture differs from and has been subverted by Occidental scientific, rational, and technological values, see Vine Deloria Jr., *Red Earth, White Lies: Native Americans and the Myth of Scientific Fact* (New York: Scribner, 1995).

164. Sam Bass Warner Jr., "Eco-Urbanism and Past Choices for Urban Living," in *Urban Policy in Twentieth-Century America*, ed. Arnold R. Hirsch and Raymond A. Mohl (New Brunswick, N.J.: Rutgers University Press, 1993), pp. 213–28. Quotation from p. 226.

165. Lance deHaven-Smith, *Environmental Concern in Florida and the Nation* (Gainesville: University of Florida Press, 1991), p. 98.

166. Ibid., pp. 15–22, 49–81, 93–100.

167. Ibid., p. 99.

168. For the racial situation in Florida's largest city, see Raymond A. Mohl, "Race and Space in the Modern City: Interstate-95 and the Black Community in Miami," in Hirsch and Mohl, eds., op. cit., pp. 100–158. For the national situation, see in the same volume (pp. 65–99), the essay by Arnold R. Hirsch, "With or without Jim Crow: Black Residential Segregation in the United States."

169. See Jim Schwab, *Deeper Shades of Green: The Rise of Blue-Collar and Minority Environmentalism in America* (San Francisco: Sierra Club Books, 1994).

170. Douglas S. Massey and Nancy A. Denton, *American Apartheid: Segregation and the Making of the Underclass* (Cambridge, Mass.: Harvard University Press, 1993), p. 236.

171. Amitai Etzioni, *The Spirit of Community: The Reinvention of American Society* (New York: Touchstone, Simon and Schuster, 1994). The "Responsive Communitarian Platform" will be found on pp. 251–67.

172. Ibid., p. 248.

173. For varying histories of that era, see: Joseph C. Goulden, *The Best Years: 1945–1950* (New York: Atheneum, 1976); Douglas T. Miller, *The Fifties: The Way We Really Were* (Garden City, N.Y.: Doubleday, 1977); William L. O'Neill, *American High: The Years of Confidence, 1945–1960* (New York: Free Press, 1986); David Halberstam, *The Fifties* (New York: Villard Books, 1993). For depictions of the ideological differences of the same era, see Richard H. Pells, *The Liberal Mind in a Conservative Age: American Intellectuals in the 1940s and 1950s* (New York: Harper and Row, 1985); and Peter Clecak, *Radical Paradoxes: Dilemmas of the American Left, 1945–1970* (New York: Harper and Row, 1973.) For personal evidence that the repression of the fifties was more severe than Etzioni's rhetoric implies, see Bud Schultz and Ruth Schultz, eds., *It Did Happen Here: Recollections of Political Repression in America* (Berkeley: University of California Press, 1989).

174. Stephanie Coontz, *The Way We Never Were: American Families and the Nostalgia Trap* (New York: Basic Books, 1992).

175. Etzioni, op. cit., p. 248.

176. Ibid., p. 249.

177. Ibid., p. 249.

178. Loc. cit.

179. Quoted in ibid., p. 249.

180. See Stanford M. Lyman, "Social Theory and Social Movements: Sociology as Sociodicy," in idem, ed., *Social Movements: Critiques, Concepts, Case-Studies* (New York: New York University Press, 1995), pp. 397–435.

181. Etzioni, op. cit., p. 122.

182. See Stephen Innes, *Creating the Commonwealth: The Economic Culture of Puritan New England* (New York: W. W. Norton, 1995), pp. 107–59.

183. Homi K. Bhabha, "Frontlines/Borderposts," in Bammer, op. cit., pp. 269–72. Quotation from p. 270.

184. Bhabha, op. cit., p. 270.

185. Yi-Fu Tuan, *Passing Strange and Wonderful: Aesthetics, Nature, and Culture* (New York: Kodansha International, 1995), p. 209.

186. Loc. cit.

187. See George E. Marcus, "The Redesign of Ethnography after the Critique of Its Rhetoric," in Robert F. Goodman and Walter R. Fisher, eds., *Rethinking Knowledge: Reflections across the Disciplines* (Albany: State University of New York Press, 1995), pp. 103–21.

188. See Thomas Bridges, *The Culture of Citizenship: Inventing Postmodern Civic Culture* (Albany: State University of New York Press, 1994); and Don E. Eberly, ed., *Building a Community of Citizens: Civil Society in the 21st Century* (Lanham, Md.: University Press of America, 1994).

Index